James T.

Steroid Biochemistry
and Pharmacology

Steroid Biochemistry and Pharmacology

M. H. BRIGGS

Schering Chemicals Ltd.
Burgess Hill, Sussex
England

J. BROTHERTON

Biochemistry Department
University of Surrey
Guildford, England

1970

ACADEMIC PRESS LONDON AND NEW YORK

ACADEMIC PRESS INC. (LONDON) LTD.
Berkeley Square House
Berkeley Square
London W1X 6BA

U.S. Edition published by
ACADEMIC PRESS INC.
111 Fifth Avenue,
New York, New York 10003

SBN: 12-134650-1
Library of Congress Catalog Card Number: 75-109036

Printed in Great Britain by
Spottiswoode, Ballantyne and Co. Ltd
London and Colchester

PREFACE

During 1968 and 1969 one of us (MHB) gave courses of lectures on steroid biochemistry at the Universities of Surrey and Sussex. It became clear that there existed no book on the subject that could be recommended to advanced students as providing an adequate introduction to the subject and, at the same time, providing background information and indications for further reading. The coverage of steroid biochemistry by general textbooks is too slight, and while advanced texts are available on steroid endocrinology, metabolism and pharmacology, there is no book that surveys the whole field.

We offer this book to fill the gap. It is aimed at graduates in biochemistry, medicine or pharmacology either taking post-graduate courses, or beginning research involving steroids.

It is our experience that many students, especially of medicine or of biological sciences, approach the study of steroids with considerable trepidation. This appears to be due mainly to their difficulties in distinguishing one steroid structure from another. Yet surely it is this chemical similarity, associated with vastly different physiological effects, that is the fascination of steroid biochemistry? The difference between masculinity and femininity is only four H and one C atoms (testosterone and estradiol).

Our first chapter consequently sets out the rules for the recognition and naming of steroids. We do not pretend that this is easy, but it is essential to master the various rules before proceeding.

Throughout the book we have attempted not to present steroid biochemistry in isolation. Wherever possible we have dealt with the biological and physiological backgrounds to the metabolism and actions of particular steroids.

As far more is known of steroid biochemistry in the human than for any other species, we have emphasized this in most chapters. We have consequently presented a good deal of material on human abnormalities involving steroids, and wherever relevant we have discussed steroid pharmaceuticals used in medicine. We have also briefly mentioned non-steroid pharmaceuticals that have profound effects on steroid biochemistry.

We have included a chapter on plant steroids in which we have largely dealt with substances of medicinal interest. The final chapter deals briefly with the production of steroid pharmaceuticals on an industrial scale.

For the sake of ease of reading we have not included literature references in the text. A selected bibliography is, however, provided at the end of the book.

While we have adopted our native English spelling throughout the book, we have bowed to the I.U.P.A.C. rule and used the spelling "estrogen" rather than "oestrogen". We have also used the term "progestogen" rather than "progestin" or "gestogen".

We would like to thank Miss Virginia C. Baines, B.Sc., for extensive proof reading.

May, 1970   MICHAEL H. BRIGGS
                                               JANET BROTHERTON

FOREWORD

Steroids represent a class of chemical compounds to be found in the whole animal and plant kingdoms. For a very long time, their structure has fascinated chemists and stimulated them into continuous endeavours towards total syntheses. The very reasons for this were the various biological activities found in this class of compounds which one has learned to augment or to differentiate by synthetic changes.

The importance of sexual and adrenal cortex hormones, and the interest in them, is so great that one might incline to forget other non-steroidal hormones. The catch-word "the pill" needs no further explanation!

The corticoids should not be overlooked in the series of available drugs. The cardio-active steroids still await an amelioration of their therapeutic index. The discovery of a steroidal insect hormone has led to an interesting speculation on mechanisms of hormonal action, thus reminding us of the present lack of knowledge in this field. On the other hand, the multiple and various metabolic pathways are much better known and understood. The extent to which fundamental knowledge and practical applications may still be discovered in the steroidal area can scarcely be estimated. Inevitably, pharmacologists, endocrinologists, physicians active in clinical chemistry, and biochemists sooner or later get into at least some contact with the steroids.

This textbook should stimulate advanced students of science and medicine, or scientists without experience in this field, to become theoretically and practically interested in it; it gives a first, necessarily incomplete, but condensed survey and provides a key to the recent relevant literature and special review articles.

May, 1970
H. GIBIAN
Main Research Laboratories
Schering A.G.
Berlin

CONTENTS

Chapter 1

Nomenclature of the Steroids

Chapter 2

Neuroendocrinology and Sites of Steroid Biosynthesis

Chapter 3

Pathways of Biosynthesis and Metabolism of Steroids

Chapter 4

Target Organ Effects—A. Estrogens and Progestogens

Chapter 5

Target Organ Effects—B. Androgens and Anabolics

Chapter 6

Target Organ Effects—C. Corticoids

Chapter 7

Effects of Non-Hormonal Steroids

Chapter 8

Clinical Aspects of the Pituitary-Adrenal Axis

Chapter 9

Clinical Aspects of the Pituitary-Gonad Axis

Chapter 10

Plant Steroids

Chapter 11

Industrial Production of the Steroids

Appendix I

Index of Trivial and Systematic Names of Steroids

Appendix II

Some Recent Work

1

NOMENCLATURE OF THE STEROIDS

I. DEFINITION

Steroids are a class of organic compounds biologically derived from six isopentenyl pyrophosphate units and containing the perhydrocyclopentanephenanthrene nucleus, i.e. three six-membered rings (A, B and C) and one five-membered ring (D). The carbon atoms are numbered as shown in Fig. 1.1

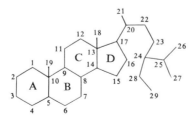

Fig. 1.1. Stigmastane showing the numbering of the carbon skeleton and of the rings.

for stigmastane (24-ethylcholestane), a fully saturated molecule with twenty-nine carbon atoms. If one or more of the side chain carbon atoms is absent, the numbering of the remainder is unaltered. Every ring junction may be either *cis* or *trans*, which gives six centres of asymmetry (C-5, 8, 9, 10, 13 and 14) and therefore sixty-four steroisomeric forms are theoretically possible. With the introduction of a side chain at C-17, a seventh asymmetric centre is produced with 128 theoretical isomers and so on.

II. CONFORMATION AND CONFIGURATION

The six carbon atoms of the cyclohexane ring can exist in either the chair, boat, or twist conformation (Fig. 1.2).

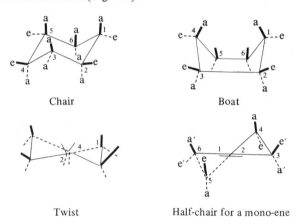

Chair   Boat

Twist   Half-chair for a mono-ene

Fig. 1.2. Conformations of cyclohexane.

Conformation has been defined as denoting different possible spatial arrangements of the atoms in a single organic configuration. The chair form is less strained and therefore preferred. The two hydrogen atoms attached to each carbon atom then take up their positions either in the general plane of the ring, being called equatorial (e), or perpendicular to the plane of the ring, being called axial (a). By convention, the axial atoms are depicted with a solid line if they are projected above the plane of the ring (β-configuration) and with a dotted line if they are projected below the plane of the ring (α-configuration). When the configuration is not known, a wavy line is used with the prefix ξ in the nomenclature. In the chair form each axial hydrogen atom is 2.5 Å from the other two axial hydrogen atoms on the same side of the ring and non-bonded interactions between hydrogen atoms at C-1 and C-2, C-1 and C-3, and C-1 and C-4 are least. A twist form may be regarded as an intermediate boat form which permits the relief of strong 1:4 interactions present in the complete boat form and is a likely form for some steroid ring systems.

In all naturally-occurring steroids, the junction between rings C and B is *trans* and they are both locked in the chair conformation. In the sterols and bile acids, the junction between rings C and D is also *trans,* but in the plant glycosides this

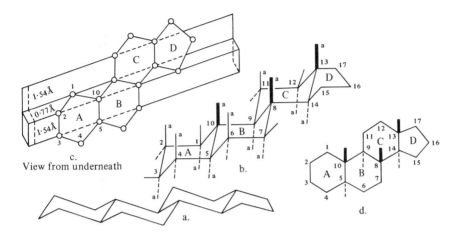

Fig. 1.3. 5α (Allo) series, rings A/B *trans* (from Shoppee, 1964).

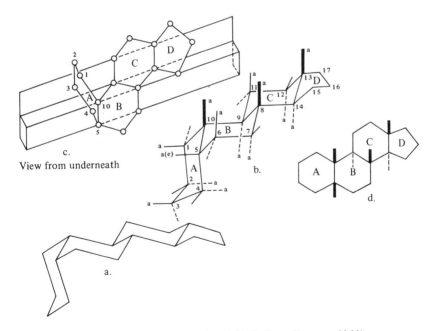

Fig. 1.4. 5β (Normal) series, rings A/B *cis* (from Shoppee, 1964).

junction is *cis*. The junction between rings A and B can be either *trans,* giving the
5α or "allo" series of compounds, or *cis,* giving the 5β or "normal" series of
compounds. Ring A is free to form either the chair or boat conformation but
will form the chair under most circumstances. Most of the biologically-active
steroids have a *trans* junction between rings A and B and belong to the 5α or
"allo" series. This makes the 4-rings almost completely planar as shown in Fig.
1.3, which represents four different ways of showing the same molecule. Figure
1.3a shows a sideways view of the four rings without the hydrogen bonds, Fig.
1.3b shows the same view with the position of the hydrogen bonds, Fig. 1.3c
shows a three-dimensional picture of the carbon skeleton, and Fig. 1.3d shows
the conventional drawing of the basic structure. Note the heavy line at C-10
denoting a H-atom above the ring and the dotted line at C-5 denoting a H-atom
below the ring, i.e. two *trans* H-atoms. The H-atoms at C-8 and C-9, C-13 and
C-14 are also *trans.* Figure 1.4 shows the same four drawings for the normal
series. Note the two heavy lines denoting *cis* H-atoms above the ring at C-5 and
C-10. Until recently, to distinguish between methyl groups and H-atoms
projecting above and below the place of the ring, the hydrogen atoms have been
written into the conventional drawing, i.e. Fig. 1.5a *not* Fig. 1.5b to represent
Fig. 1.5c, but the latest IUPAC rules recommend Fig. 1.5b. It is also common to
insert the configuration of the hydrogen atom at C-5, the configurations of the
remainder being assumed. When configuration of the four rings is known, the
position of the axial and equatorial bonds is as shown in Table 1.1. The

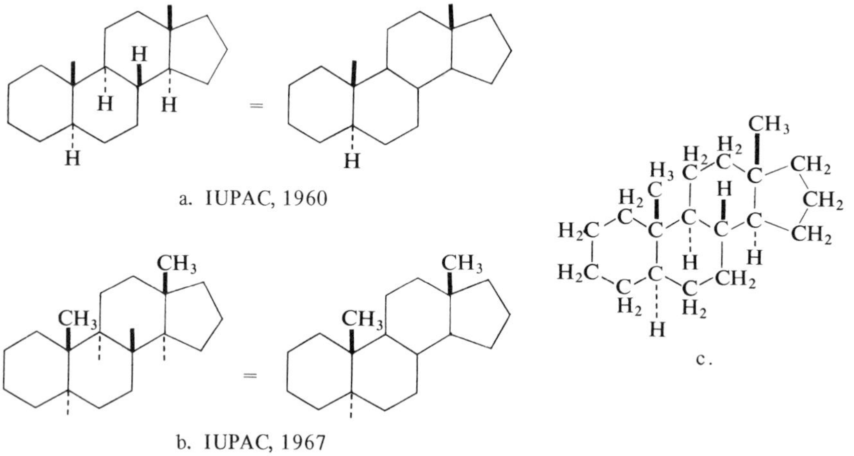

a. IUPAC, 1960

b. IUPAC, 1967

c.

Fig. 1.5. Five ways of drawing 5α-androstane.

Table 1.1. *Configuration and conformation of nuclear substituents*

| Ring | Carbon atom number | 5α ("allo") Ring fusion (rings A and B *trans*) | | 5β ("normal") Ring fusion (rings A and B *cis*) | |
		α-Configuration (axial bonds below ring)	β-Configuration (axial bonds above ring)	α-Configuration (axial bonds below ring)	β-Configuration (axial bonds above ring)
A	1	Axial	Equatorial	Equatorial	Axial
	2	Equatorial	Axial	Axial	Equatorial
	3	Axial	Equatorial	Equatorial	Axial
	4	Equatorial	Axial	Axial	Equatorial
	5	Axial to both rings A and B	—	—	Axial to ring A Equatorial to ring B
	10	—	Axial to both rings A and B	—	Equatorial to ring A Axial to ring B
B and C	6	Equatorial	Axial		
	7	Axial	Equatorial		
	8	—	Axial		
	9	Axial	—		
	11	Equatorial	Axial		
	12	Axial	Equatorial		
	13	—	Axial		
	14	Axial	—		
D	15	Quasi-equatorial to ring C	Quasi-axial to ring C		
	16	Free	Free		
	17	Quasi-axial to ring C	Quasi-equatorial to ring C		

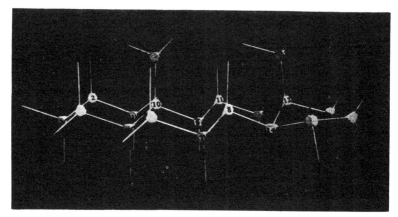

5α-Androstane

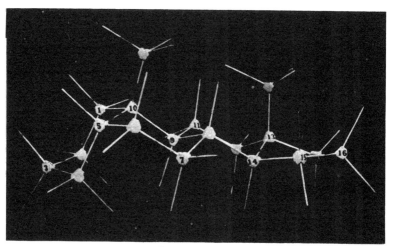

5β-Androstanes

Fig. 1.6. Wire models of 5α- and 5β-androstane.
(Reproduced from Fieser/Fieser:STEROIDS copyright © 1959 by Reinhold Publishing Corporation, with permission of Litton Educational Publishing, Inc.)

configuration of substituents on C-atoms 6-17 is the same for the 5α and 5β series. Unless stated to the contrary, atoms or groups attached at ring junctions are orientated 8β, 9α, 10β, 13β, 14α and a carbon chain attached to C-17 is assumed to be β-orientated. Photographs of wire models of 5α- and 5β-andro-stanes are shown in Fig. 1.6.

III. PARENT HYDROCARBONS

A. SATURATED

The natural steroids are named after the following saturated hydrocarbons: gonane, (C-17) (a theoretical parent compound), estrane (C-18), androstane (C-19), pregnane (C-21), cholane (C-24), and cholestane (C-27) as shown in Fig. 1.7. The Anglo-Saxon diphthong for oestrane and its derivatives is no longer used. Other more rarely used parent compounds are:

ergostane	(24-methylcholestane)
stigmastane	(24-ethylcholestane)
lanostane	(4,4,14-trimethylcholestane).

B. UNSATURATED

Names for the partly unsaturated or aromatic steroids are derived from the saturated compounds by means of the systematic terminations "—ene" and "yne" as shown in Fig. 1.8. The first name is that recommended by the International Union of Pure and Applied Chemistry (IUPAC), the second name the most commonly used alternative, and the third name uses Δ to indicate unsaturation which is a system becoming obsolete. Unsaturation is shown by sequential numbering, except where this is not possible, in which case the exact position of the double bond is shown by the use of bracketed numbers. The IUPAC system for expressing unsaturation by placing the location of the unsaturation in the middle of the name of the parent hydrocarbon, e.g. pregn-4-ene instead of 4-pregnene (or Δ^4-pregnene), is unpopular as it makes the complete molecule unpronounceable.

The insertion of a double bond in one of the six-membered rings causes the ring to assume the half-chair conformation (Fig. 1.2d). The four carbon atoms associated with the olefinic system C-6, C-1, C-2, C-3 lie in a plane, with C-4 above this plane and C-5 below. The bonds extending to hydrogen at C-4 and C-5 have the character of the normal axial or equatorial bonds but those at C-3 and C-6 are only approximately axial (a′) or equatorial (e′). The half-chair conformation is slightly less stable than the chair form.

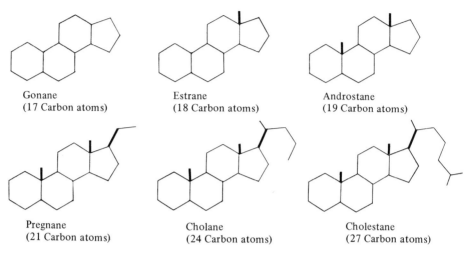

Gonane
(17 Carbon atoms)

Estrane
(18 Carbon atoms)

Androstane
(19 Carbon atoms)

Pregnane
(21 Carbon atoms)

Cholane
(24 Carbon atoms)

Cholestane
(27 Carbon atoms)

Fig. 1.7. Some saturated parent hydrocarbons.

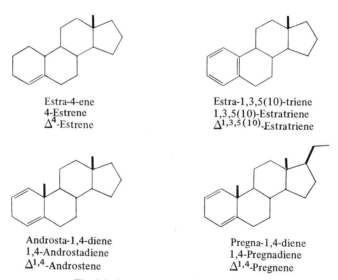

Estra-4-ene
4-Estrene
Δ^4-Estrene

Estra-1,3,5(10)-triene
1,3,5(10)-Estratriene
$\Delta^{1,3,5(10)}$-Estratriene

Androsta-1,4-diene
1,4-Androstadiene
$\Delta^{1,4}$-Androstene

Pregna-1,4-diene
1,4-Pregnadiene
$\Delta^{1,4}$-Pregnene

Fig. 1.8. Some unsaturated parent hydrocarbons.

IV. SUBSTITUENTS

According to the IUPAC rules, substituents are attached to the name of the parent hydrocarbon either as suffixes or as prefixes. Only one suffix is permitted, with the order of priority given by the IUPAC. Once the suffix position has been filled, all other substituents are attached as prefixes. Some substituents, e.g. the halogens, are *always* prefixes. In decreasing preference the order of suffixes for steroids is 'onium salt, acid, lactone, ester, aldehyde, ketone, alcohol, amine, and ether. Examples are given in Table 1.2. This mixed system of prefixes and suffixes is used very little as the parent hydrocarbon has to be elicited from the middle of a chemical name and it widely separates in a

Table 1.2. *IUPAC prefixes and suffixes*

	Prefix	Suffix
1. Carboxylic acids		
(a) No change in number of carbon atoms	Carboxy-	-oic acid or -ic acid
(b) Addition of a carbon atom		-carboxylic acid
2. Esters of carboxylic acids		
(a) No change in number of carbon atoms	Methoxy-carbonyl-	methyl . . . oate or methyl . . . ate
(b) Addition of a carbon atom		methyl . . . carboxylate
3. Lactones of carboxylic acids		
(a) Other than cardanolides and bufanolides		
(i) No change in number of carbon atoms		-lactone
(ii) Addition of a carbon atom		-carbolactone
(b) Cardanolides and bufanolides		-olide
4. Esters of steroid alcohols		
(a) Monohydric alcohols	Acetoxy-, etc.	-yl acetate
(b) Polyols	Acetoxy-, etc.	-diol diacetate
5. Aldehydes (no change in number of carbon atoms)	Oxo-	-al
6. Ketones (no change in number of carbon atoms)	Oxo-	-one
7. Alcohols (no change in number of carbon atoms)	Hydroxy-	-ol
8. Amines	Amino-	-amine
9. Ethers	Methoxy-	methyl ether
10. Hydrocarbons	Methyl-, etc.	
11. Halogens	Chloro-, etc.	
12. Epoxy groups	Epoxy-	epoxide

catalogue or index similar compounds with slightly differing substituents. All the major chemical companies use in their catalogues a slightly different system whereby the parent hydrocarbon is placed first in the name, followed by all the substituents as suffixes. Some examples of both systems are shown in Fig. 1.9. Considering the three alternative correct chemical names for cortisone (Fig. 1.9) (if the Δ system for indicating unsaturation is rejected), the second system has the merit of being pronounceable and giving the quickest picture of the molecule, i.e. 4-pregnen-17α, 21-diol-3, 11, 20-trione.

Details of the IUPAC system of prefixes and suffixes are as follows:

A. CARBOXYLIC ACIDS, THEIR ESTERS AND LACTONES

1. Carboxylic acids

When there is a change from $-CH_3$ to $-COOH$, the suffix is "-oic acid" or "-ic acid", e.g. 5β-cholan-24-oic acid = 5β-cholanic acid. When there is an addition of a carboxylic acid group, i.e. the change is from $>CH$ to $>C\text{-}COOH$, the suffix is "-carboxylic acid", e.g. 5β-androstane-17β-carboxylic acid = 5β, 17 (αH)-etianic acid. (The etianic acids are trivial names for the androstane-17-carboxylic acids, when the orientation of the hydrogen atoms at C-5 and C-17 must be stated in all cases as 5α or 5β, and 17 (αH) or 17(βH), respectively.) Loss of the final "e" from androstane, etc. is variable.

2. Esters of carboxylic acids

Esters of both kinds of carboxylic acids are described as such, e.g.

5β-cholan-24-oic acid methyl ester = 5β-cholanic acid methyl ester,
5β-cholan-24-oic acid sodium salt = 5β-cholanic acid sodium salt.

Alternatively (and more strictly IUPAC) they may be described by placing the ester before the name and using the suffix "-oate" or "-ate", e.g.

methyl 5β-cholan-24-oate = methyl 5β-cholanate,
sodium 5β-cholan-24-oate = sodium 5β-cholanate,
methyl 5β-androstane-17β-carboxylate = methyl 5β, 17 (αH)-etianate.

The prefixes "carboxy-" for a carboxylic acid and "methoxycarbonyl-" (not "carbomethoxy-") for its methyl ester are rarely used, as there is not usually present a suffix which takes precedence over that indicating a carboxylic acid.

3. Lactones of carboxylic acids (other than cardanolides and bufanolides)

For their lactones, the ending "-ic acid" or "carboxylic acid" is changed to "-lactone" or "-carbolactone", respectively, preceded by the locant of the acid

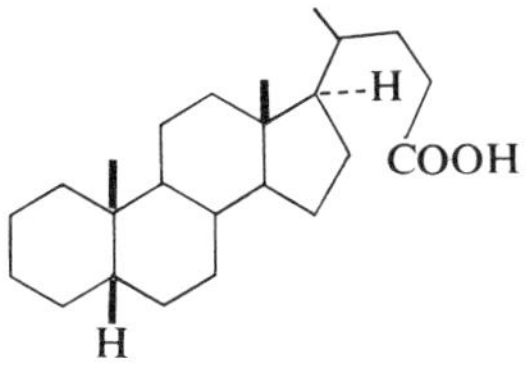

5β-Cholan-24-oic acid
5β-Cholanic acid

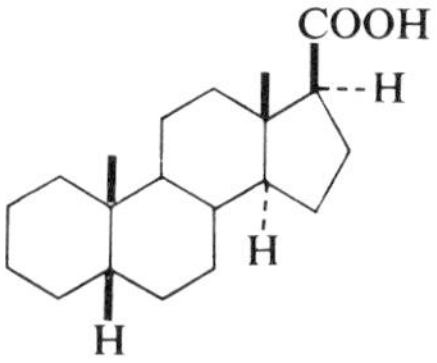

5β-Androstane-17β-carboxylic acid
5β, 17(αH)-Etianic acid

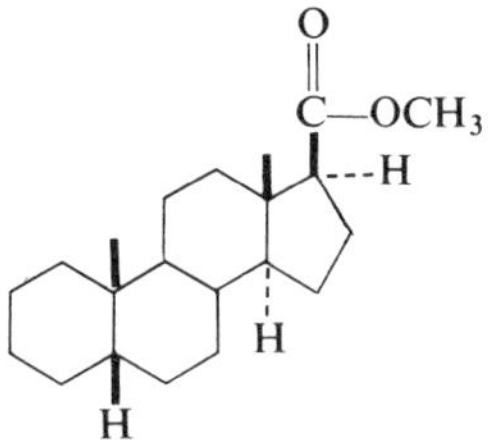

5β-Androstane-17β-carboxylic acid methyl ester
Methyl 5β-androstane-17β-carboxylate
5β,17(αH)-Etianic acid methyl ester
Methyl 5β,17(αH)-etianate

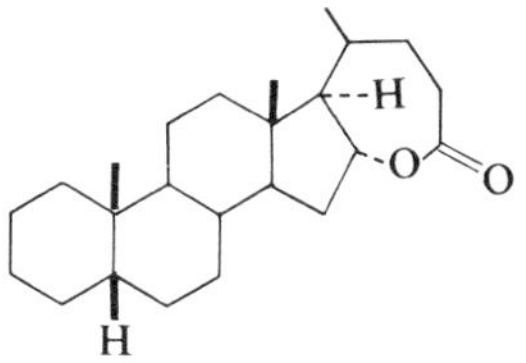

5β-Cholano-24,17α-lactone

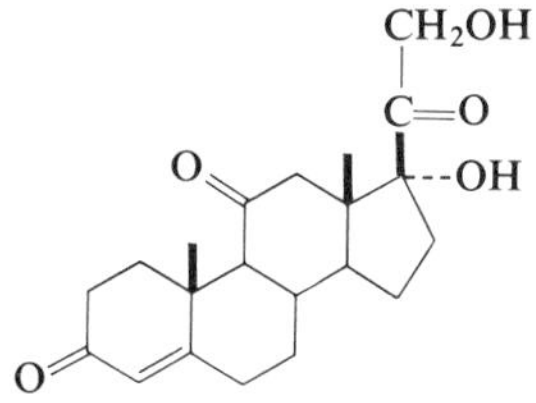

Cortisone
17α,21-Dihydroxy-4-pregnene-3,11,20-
   trione
4-Pregnene-17α,21-diol-3,11,20-trione

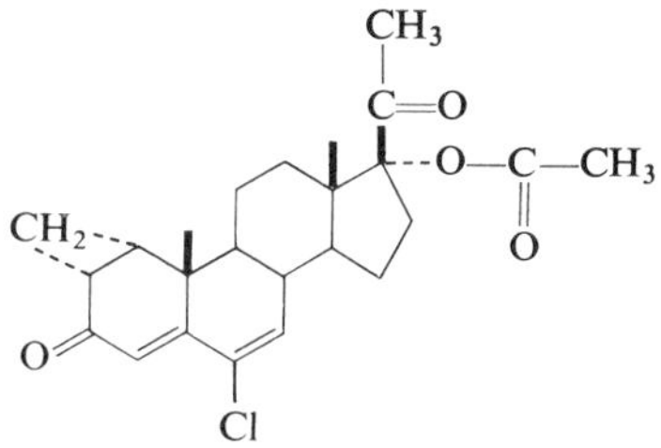

Cyproterone acetate
17α-Acetoxy-6-chloro-1α,2α-methylene-4,6-
   pregnadiene-3,20-dione
6-Chloro-1α,2α-methylene-4,6-pregnadien-
   17α-ol-3,20-dione 17-acetate

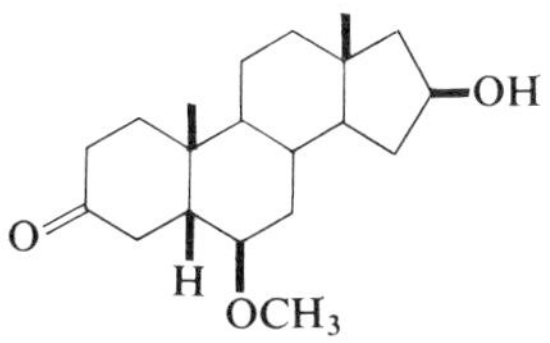

6β,16β-Dihydroxy-5β-androstan-3-one
   6-methyl ether
16β-Hydroxy-6β-methoxy-5β-androstan-
   3-one
5β-Androstan-6β,16β-diol-3-one 6-methyl
   ether

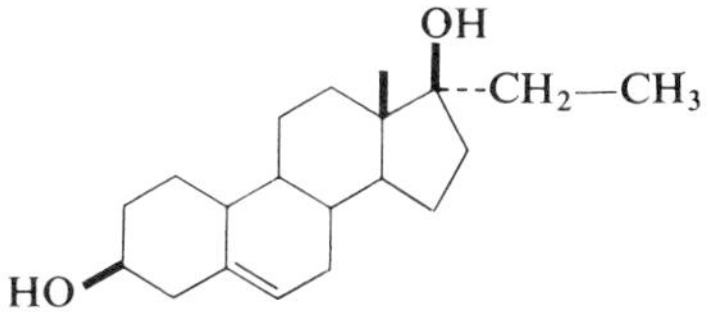

17α-Ethyl-5-estrene-3β,17β-diol

17α-Ethyl-19-nor-5-androstene-3β,17β-diol

19-Nor-17α-pregn-4-ene-3β,17β-diol
19-Nor-(17α),4-pregnen-3β,17-diol

Fig. 1.9. Some examples of nomenclature of substituents.

group and then the locant of the hydroxyl group, and the prefix "hydroxy" is omitted from the lactonized hydroxyl group, e.g.

5β-cholane-24, 17α-lactone
(20R)-5β-pregnane-20, 18-carbolactone.

4. Cardanolides and bufanolides

For the cardanolides and bufanolides, the "-olide" ending denotes the lactone grouping and substituents must be named as prefixes.

B. ESTERS OF STEROID ALCOHOLS

1. Monohydric alcohols

The alcohols themselves take precedence after their esters and after aldehydes and ketones. For esters of the monohydric steroid alcohols, the steroid hydrocarbon radical name is followed by that of the acyloxy group in its anionic form. The steroid radical name is formed by replacing the terminal "e" of the hydrocarbon name by "yl" and inserting before this the locant and Greek letter, with hyphens, to designate the position and configuration, e.g.

5β-cholestan-3β-yl acetate.

2. Polyols

For esters of polyols the name of the polyol is followed by that of the acyloxy group(s) in its anionic form, with locants when necessary, e.g.

5β-cholestane-3α, 12α-diol 3-acetate 12-benzoate.

Many such esters are in common use, e.g. sodium hemisuccinate, cyclopentyl-propionate (cyprionate), sodium sulphate, trimethylacetate (pivalate), glucuro-nide (glucuronoside), caproate, enanthate, etc. When an acid, acid ester, lactone or spirostan group is also present, the ester group is designated by an acyloxy prefix, e.g.

Prefix	Suffix
acetoxy-	acetate
formyloxy- (not formoxy-)	formate
benzoyloxy-	benzoate
propionyloxy-	propionate
3β-carboxypropionyloxy-	succinate
isopropylidenedioxy-	acetonide
cyclopentylpropionyloxy-	cypionate

C. ALDEHYDES, KETONES AND ALCOHOLS

1. Aldehydes

When there is a change from $-CH_3$ to $-CHO$, the suffix is "-al". When there is a change from $-COOH$ to $-CHO$, the suffix is "-aldehyde" and the name is derived from that of the acid. The prefix "oxo-" denotes a change of $-CH_3$ or CH_2 to $-CHO$ or $C=O$, respectively, e.g.

$$11\beta, 21\text{-dihydroxy-20-oxopregn-4-en-18-al}$$
$$5\beta\text{-cholan-24-aldehyde.}$$

When additional carbon atoms are introduced as $-CHO$ groups, other methods of nomenclature are used.

2. Ketones

The suffix is "-one" and the prefix "oxo-", e.g.

$$5\beta\text{-androstane-3-one}$$
$$5\text{-pregnene-3, 20-dione}$$
$$11\text{-oxo-5}\alpha\text{-cholan-24-oic acid.}$$

3. Alcohols

The suffix is "-ol" and the prefix "hydroxy-", e.g.

$$5\beta\text{-cholestane-3, 11-diol}$$
$$3\alpha\text{-hydroxy-5}\alpha\text{-androstan-17-one.}$$

D. AMINES

The suffix is "-amine" and the prefix "amino-", e.g.

$$5\beta\text{-androstane-3}\beta\text{-ylamine or } 5\beta\text{-androstane-3}\beta\text{-amine}$$
$$3\beta\text{-(dimethylamino)-5}\alpha\text{-pregnan-20}\alpha\text{-ol.}$$

E. ETHERS

1. Prefix

Ethers are named as alkoxy derivatives, e.g. 17β-methoxy-5β-androstane-3-one.

2. Suffix for monohydric alcohols

The name of the steroid hydrocarbon radical is stated, followed by the name of the alkyl (or aryl, etc.) radical and lastly by "ether", the three parts as separate words, e.g.

$$5\beta\text{-androstan-3}\beta\text{-yl methyl ether}$$
$$6\beta, 16\beta\text{-dihydroxy-5}\beta\text{-androstan-3-one 6-methyl ether.}$$

3. Suffix for polyols

The same system is used as for the monohydric alcohols but with the name of the steroid hydrocarbon radical replaced by the name of the polyol. For partially etherified polyols locant(s) precede the names of the alkyl (or aryl, etc.) group(s), e.g.

5α-pregnane-3β, 17α, 20α-triol 3,17-dimethyl ether.

F. HYDROCARBON AND HALOGEN ADDITIONS

These are always added as prefixes, as they do not have any suffix forms, e.g. methyl, $-CH_3$, ethyl, $-CH_2$ $-CH_3$, vinyl, $-CH=CH_2$, ethinyl (1-propynyl) $-C\equiv CH$, methylene, CH_2. Halogens also can only act as prefixes, e.g. chloro-. Cholesteryl chloride is 3β-chloro-5-cholestene while cholesteryl palmitate is 5-cholesten-3β-yl palmitate.

G. ADDITIONAL RINGS WITHIN OR ON THE STEROID NUCLEUS

A number of these are known. Prefixes are epoxy-, epidoxy-, methylenedioxy-. Suffixes are epoxide, ethylene ketal, etc.

V. THE SIDE CHAIN

The nomenclature of the side chain at C-17 presents a special problem as its carbon atoms are not in the same plane as the ring system and the limits of the β and α symbols for above and below the ring are exceeded. The true positions of these carbon atoms is shown three-dimensionally in Fig. 1.10a and can be visualized as arranged in a plane curving around to the rear.

Two systems of nomenclature for the substituents are in common use—that of Fieser and Fieser and that of Ingold. Figure 1.10 shows the system of Fieser and Fieser where C-20 is viewed from the front. The other carbon atoms are viewed as the eye passes along the chain, looking to the right and left at the substituents at each junction. Those substituents on the left are arbitrarily labelled as β and those on the right as α. When reaching C-23 the viewer has turned upside down but the methyl group is to the left (β) and the hydrogen to the right (α). The example is thus a 20β,24β-dimethyl-22α, 25-diol and is drawn in the Fischer convention as in Fig. 1.10b. This system has the advantage of simplicity and retains the α and β nomenclature although with a different meaning for side chain substituents to ring substituents.

The Ingold system is related to a much more basic system of correctly describing the three-dimensional position of each substituent on any carbon atom in all molecules. The symbols R for right (Latin—*rectus*) and S for left (Latin and many other languages—*sinister*) are used. A right-handed sequence is defined as in Fig. 1.11a when the sequence of substituents above the central carbon atom X of a → b → c traces a right-handed turn when viewed from an

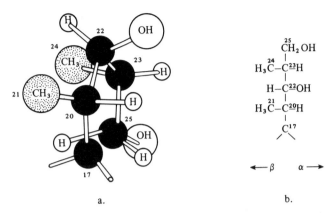

a.   b.

Fig. 1.10. Nomenclature of the side chain at C-17 in the Fieser and Fieser system.

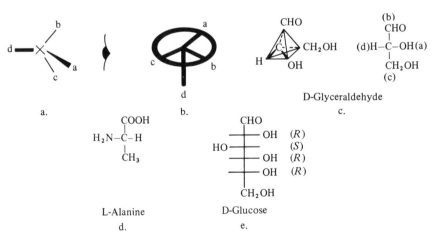

a.   b.   c.

L-Alanine   D-Glucose

d.   e.

Fig. 1.11. The Ingold system or Sequence Rule procedure for nomenclature of substituents in the C-17 side chain.

external point on the side remote from d. This can be visualized as in Fig. 1.11b as the steering-wheel of a car and expressed in Fig. 1.11c in the Fischer convention when it is seen that D-glyceraldehyde appears as *R*-glyceraldehyde as the sequence of the substituents is OH, CHO, CH$_2$OH, H. Similarly L-alanine becomes *S*-alanine (Fig. 1.11d) and the configuration of D-glucose is shown in Fig. 1.11e. The Sequence Rule symbols *R* and *S* are used only in the side chain,

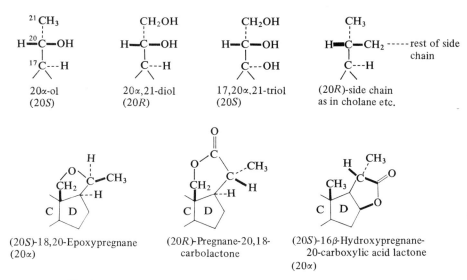

Fig. 1.12. Examples of Sequence Rule nomenclature for the C-20 position.

and *β* being retained for the ring constituents although it is possible and universally correct to use the *R* and *S* symbols for these also. The system needs considerable experience in determining whether a substituent is *R* or *S*, but is needed for a complete description of the structure of the steroidal saponins which are derivatives of stigmastane. For 20-hydroxy, 20-alloxy, 20-amino and 20-halogeno-derivatives of pregnane without a substituent on C-17 or C-21, 20*α* is equivalent to (20*S*)- and 20*β* to (20*R*)-. These equivalencies are sometimes reversed when additional substituents are present (Fig. 1.12). The names cholane, cholestane, ergostane and stigmastane imply the configuration 20*R*, except for some derivatives containing additional substituents. Ergostane implies the 24*S*-configuration and stigmastane the 24*R*-configuration. If one of the two methyl groups attached to C-25 is substituted it is assigned the lower number (26); if both are substituted, that carrying the substituent cited first in the alphabetical order or order of complexity is assigned the lower number.

VI. TRIVIAL NAMES

Many important biological steroids have trivial names, e.g. cortisone, estrone, androsterone, cholesterol, and this gives rise to yet another system of nomenclature depending on the modification of the trivial names. Table 1.3 gives the chemical names equivalent to the trivial names of some of the natural steroids. A comprehensive index of trivial names with their systematic names is given in Appendix I (p. 338). Table 1.4 shows some of the modified or secondary trivial names. The prefixes hydro, dihydro, tetrahydro, dehydro, anhydro, hydroxy, dihydroxy, tetrahydroxy, de(s)oxy, dide(s)oxy, etc. refer to the addition or deletion of hydrogen and oxygen atoms from the parent (trivial) molecule. When no carbon number indicating the exact position of this change is given, a specific position is always understood, e.g. hydrocortisone always refers to the β-isomer produced by the addition of 2H to the keto group at C-11.

The prefix "allo" refers to the 5α or "allo" series when 2H are added across the C-4—C-5 double bond so that rings A and B assume the *trans* configuration as defined above. When there is no prefix, the 5β or "normal" series of rings A and B in the *cis* configuration is assumed. The prefex "epi" refers to the inversion of one of the substituents from below the ring to above or vice versa. Additional substituents are added as prefixes, e.g. 11β-hydroxyprogesterone. This system is very convenient for biochemists when discussing reaction mechanisms but can become very confusing.

VII. RING CONTRACTIONS, ADDITIONS AND CLEAVAGES

Referring back to the numbering of the carbon atoms in Fig. 1.1, it has already been stated that if one or more of the side chain carbon atoms is missing the numbering of the remainder is unaltered. This produces another series of parent hydrocarbons, e.g. 18-nor-pregnane and 21-nor-pregnane shown in Fig. 1.13, the deletions being shown by the prefix "nor" and the appropriate missing carbon atom indicated. In cases of doubt the number attached to "nor" is the highest permissible. The same system applies to ring contraction which is indicated by "nor" preceded by a capital letter indicating the ring affected (see Fig. 1.14). The highest number(s) of the contracted ring, exclusive of ring junction, is deleted. When a compound possesses extra ring carbon atoms, these are numbered in sequence, but given an *a* (or *b* or *c,* etc.) to the highest number in the ring enlarged, exclusive of ring junctions. This letter and number are assigned to the last peripheral carbon atom in the ordering of numbering of the ring affected. The prefix "homo" is used preceded by a capital letter indicating the ring affected as shown in Fig. 1.15. Ring fission, with the addition of a hydrogen atom at each terminal group thus created, is indicated by the prefix "seco", the original steroid numbering being retained, e.g. cholecalciferol (Fig. 1.16).

Table 1.3. *Some primary trivial names of natural steroids*

Trivial names	Systematic names
Derivatives of androstane	
Adrenosterone	4-Androsten-3,11,17-trione
Androstanediol	5α-Androstan-3β,17β-diol
Androstanedione	5α-Androstan-3,17-dione
Androstanolone	5α-Androstan-17β-ol-3-one
Androstenediol	5-Androsten-3β,17β-diol
Androstenedione	4-Androsten-3,17-dione
Androsterone	5α-Androstan-3α-ol-17-one
Etiocholane	5β-Androstane
Testosterone	4-Androsten-17β-ol-3-one
Derivatives of estrane	
(17α)-Estradiol	1,3,5(10)-Estratrien-3,17α-diol
Estriol	1,3,5(10)-Estratrien-3,16α,17β-triol
Estrone	1,3,5(10)-Estratrien-3-ol-17-one
Estrenol	4-Estren-17β-ol
Derivatives of pregnane	
Aldosterone	4-Pregnen-18-al-11β,21-diol-3,20-dione
Cortexolone	4-Pregnen-17α,21-diol-3,20-dione
Cortexone	4-Pregnen-21-ol-3,20-dione
Corticosterone	4-Pregnen-11β,21-diol-3,20-dione
Cortisol	4-Pregnen-11β,17α,21-triol-3,20-dione
Cortisone	4-Pregnen-17α,21-diol-3,11,20-trione
Pregnenolone	5-Pregnen-3β-ol-20-one
Progesterone	4-Pregnen-3,20-dione
Pregnanediol	5β-Pregnan-3α,20α-diol
Pregnanedione	5β-Pregnan-3,20-dione
Derivatives of cholane	
Cholic acid	5β-Cholanic acid-3α,7α,12α-triol
Chenodeoxycholic acid	5β-Cholanic acid-3α,7α-diol
Lithocholic acid	5β-Cholanic acid-3α-ol
Derivatives of cholestane	
Coprostane	5β-Cholestane
Cholesterol	5-Cholesten-3β-ol
Cholestenone	4-Cholesten-3-one
Kryptogenin	5-Cholesten-3β,26-diol-16,22-dione
Lanosterol	4,4,14α-Trimethyl-8,24(5α)-cholestadien-3β-ol
Cholestanol	5α-Cholestan-3β-ol
Desmosterol	5,24-Cholestadien-3β-ol
Ergosterol	(24S)-24-Methyl-5,7,22-cholestatrien-3β-ol
Stigmasterol	(24R)-24-Ethyl-5,22-cholestadien-3β-ol
Zymosterol	8,24,(5α)-Cholestadien-3β-ol

Table 1.4. *Some secondary trivial names of natural steroids*

Trivial names	Systematic names	Structural change
(Cortisone)	(4-Pregnen-17α,21-diol-3,11,20-trione)	+ 2H at C-11β
Hydrocortisone	4-Pregnen-11β,17α,21-triol-3,20-dione	+ 2H at Δ^4 ("normal" series)
Dihydrocortisone	5β-Pregnan-17α,21-diol-3,11,20-trione	+ 2H at C-3 & at Δ^4 ("normal" series)
Tetrahydrocortisone	5β-Pregnan-3α,17α,21-triol-11,20-dione	− 2H at Δ^1
Dehydrocortisone	1,4-Pregnadien-17α,21-diol-3,11,20-triol	+ 2H at C-11, − 2H at Δ^1
Dehydrohydrocortisone	1,4-Pregnadien-11β,17α,21-triol-3,20-dione	+ 2H at C-11 & at Δ^4 ("allo" series)
Allodihydrocortisone	5α-Pregnan-17α,21-diol-3,11,20-trione	
21-De(s)oxycortisone	4-Pregnen-17α-ol-3,11,20-trione	− 0 at C-21
(Progesterone)	(4-Pregnen-3,20-dione)	
11β-Hydroxyprogesterone	4-Pregnen-11β-ol-3,20-dione	+ 0 at 11β
(Androsterone)	(5α-Androstan-3α-ol-17-one)	
Epiandrosterone	5α-Androstan-3β-ol-17-one	Inversion of OH at C-3
Dehydroepiandrosterone	5-Androsten-3β-ol-17-one	Inversion of OH at C-3 & − 2H at Δ^5

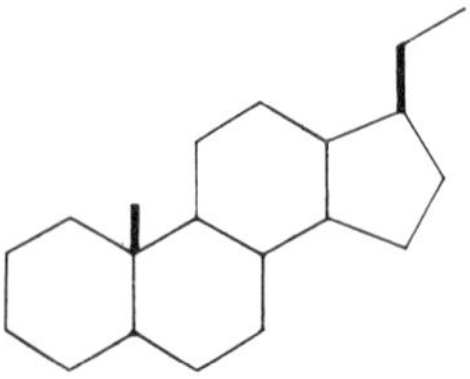

18-Nor-pregnane 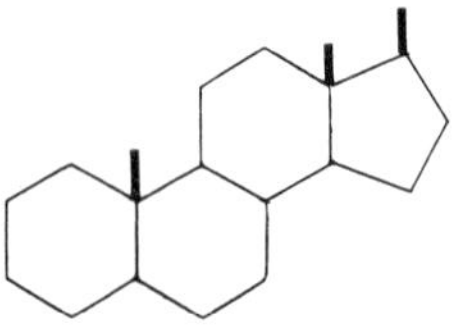   21-Nor-pregnane

Fig. 1.13. Side chain deletions.

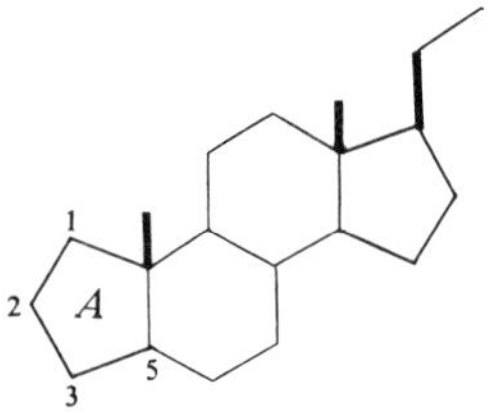

A-Nor-pregnane 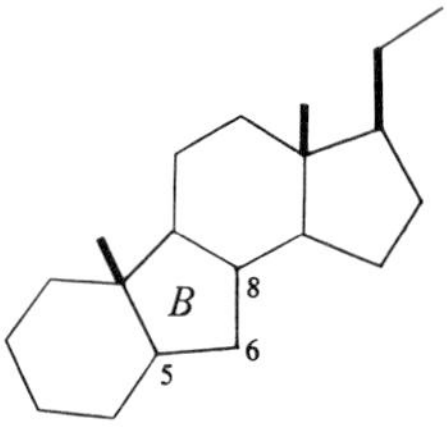   B-Nor-pregnane

Fig. 1.14. Ring contractions.

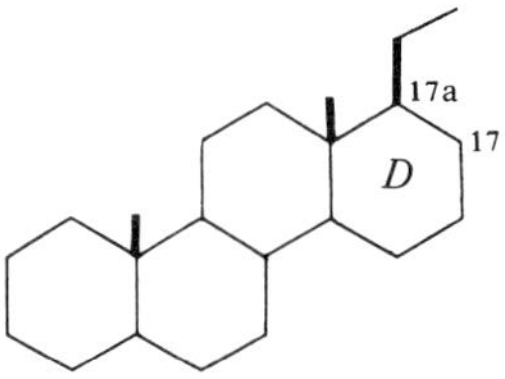

D-Homo-pregnane

Fig. 1.15. Ring addition.

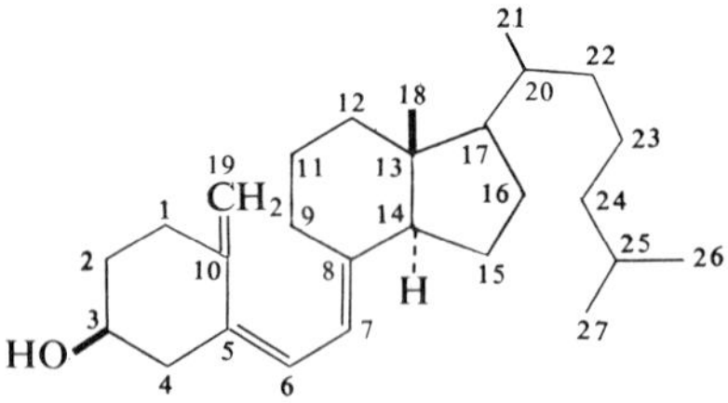

Cholecalciferol
9,10-Seco-5,7,10(19)-cholestratrien-3β-ol

Fig. 1.16. Ring cleavage.

VIII. SOME OTHER PREFIXES

1. D, L, *d* and *l*

The optical activity of a steroid may be described as *l* or (−) for laevorotatory (anti-clockwise) and *d* or (+) for dextrorotatory (clockwise). The racemate, *dl* or (±), is the inactive form. Cholesterol is laevorotatory and its biological reduction product coprostanol is dextrorotatory. The degree and direction of rotation is a distinctive physical property for identification purposes. Steroids can also be described as D or L (or DL which is the mixture of D and L) which describe its absolute configuration relative to D-glyceraldehyde. In steroids with substituents such as OH at a centre of a symmetry, α would correspond with L and β with D. A new asymmetric centre is created every time a monovalent substituent replaces hydrogen in a $C-CH_2-C$ group in the ring system. When both absolute configuration and optical activity are indicated, a compound may have the prefixes L(+), D(−), etc.

2. Cyclo-

When an additional ring is formed by means of a direct link between any two carbon atoms of the steroid ring system or the attached side chain, the name of the steroid is prefixed by "cyclo". This prefix is preceded by the numbers of the positions joined by the new bond and by the Greek letter (α, β or ξ) denoting the configuration of the new bond, unless that designation is already implied in the name.

3. *Ent- (enantio-)*

This prefix denotes inversion of all asymmetric centres from the naturally-occurring compound, including those due to named substituents, whether these are cited separately or are implied in the name. If there is stereochemical inversion at a minority of the asymmetric centres, whose configurations do not require to be specified in a name, the configuration of the hydrogen atoms or substituents at the affected bridgeheads, or the carbon chain (if any) at position 17, are stated by means of a prefix or prefixes α or β, each with its appropriate positional numeral, placed before the stem name, e.g.

ent-testosterone = *ent*-17β-hydroxy-4-androsten-3-one
5β, 9β, 10α-pregnane.

4. *Rac- (racemo-)*

Racemates are indicated by the prefix *rac-*.

5. *Rel-*

This indicates that the relative but not the absolute configuration at a particular asymmetric centre is known.

6. Abeo-

A compound that does not possess a steroid skeleton but may be considered formally to arise from a steroid by bond migration may be given the prefix of the form $x(y$-$z)$ abeo-, where x is a numeral denoting the unchanged end of the migrating bond, y is a numeral denoting the original position from which the other end of the bond has migrated, and z is a numeral denoting the new position to which the bond has moved.

7. Oxa-, aza-

These indicate hetero atoms in the steroid ring system, e.g. oxa- for oxygen, aza- for nitrogen.

IX. REACTIVITIES OF RING SUBSTITUENTS

As the interatomic distances between any pair of axial groups are small, those groups repel one another and any compound carrying an axial substituent is thermodynamically less stable than the corresponding compound carrying an equatorial substituent.

General rules regarding the stability and reactivity of equatorial and axial substituents are:

(a) if a substituent can be equilibrated (e.g. hydroxyl groups with sodium) the equatorial compound will predominate in the equilibrium mixture;

(b) for reactions which depend on the accessibility of the substituent, e.g. esterification and hydrolysis of esters, the equatorial substituent is less sterically hindered and reacts more rapidly than the axial. Due to steric hindrance the 17α-hydroxyl is more difficult to esterify than the 17β;

(c) for reactions which depend on the accessibility of a substituent H atom, e.g. oxidation of CHOH with chromic acid, equatorial H atoms react more rapidly than axial;

(d) for ionic elimination reactions, e.g. dehydration of hydroxy compounds with phosphorus oxychloride, the reaction proceeds most easily when an axial substituent eliminates with another axial group (probably H) on the adjacent carbon atom and on the other side of the molecule. This is because the four centres are in one plane;

(e) epoxide rings are opened by reagents, e.g. HCl, acetic acid, to give compounds with two axial substituents and by hydrogenation or lithium aluminium hydride to give the axial hydroxy compound;

(f) usually steroid molecules are attacked from the rear, e.g. hydrogenation of cholesterol gives the stanol in which the hydrogen at C-5 is in the rear (α). The front (or top) side of steroids is shielded by the angular methyl groups (C-18 and C-19) so that functional groups are more hindered to frontal attack. Especially hindered is the position at C-11 which makes the insertion of oxygen in the chemical synthesis of cortisol derivatives exceptionally difficult.

2

NEUROENDOCRINOLOGY AND SITES OF
STEROID BIOSYNTHESIS

I. THE STEROID CYCLE

At present steroid hormone production is believed to be initiated by the releasing factors of the hypothalamus of the brain which travel to the anterior lobe of the hypophysis (pituitary gland) in the portal blood stream of the pituitary stalk, where they cause the secretion of trophic hormone into the blood stream. The trophic hormone travels to the site of steroid synthesis, e.g. adrenal gland, ovary, testes, and stimulates the production of steroids which are released into the blood stream to travel to the target organ, e.g. kidney and skin. It is believed that steroids are transformed in the target cells and metabolites released into the blood. Steroids are further degraded and rendered inactive at special degrading sites, e.g. liver, and are then excreted. Steroids in blood represent a mixture of primary secretions, secondary metabolic products and metabolites produced by the target organs. The relative contributions of destructive metabolism and of metabolism by the target organs has not been determined, but the latter is thought to be small. There is a feedback inhibition system whereby no releasing factor is produced when the steroid blood levels are too high. The feedback inhibition occurs when excess active steroid is present in the blood reaching the hypothalamus. It is possible that inert steroid metabolites can be converted back to active substances that may influence the hypothalamus. The whole cycle may be represented as in Fig. 2.1.

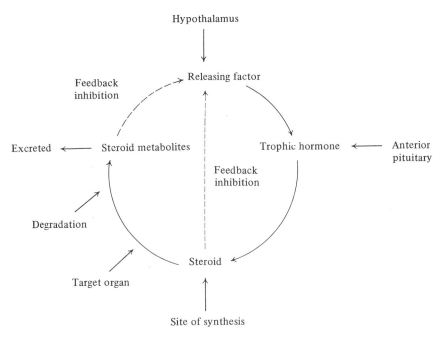

Fig. 2.1. The steroid cycle

Each type of steroid hormone is believed to have its own steroid cycle, the nomenclature of which is based on the organ of the site of synthesis, e.g. the corticosteroid cycle is initiated by the corticotrophin releasing factor, which causes the release of the (adreno-)corticotrophic hormone (corticotrophin or ACTH), which in turn stimulates the cortex of the adrenal gland to produce the corticosteroids. Similarly, luteotrophin releasing factor causes the release of the luteotrophic hormone, and this stimulates the corpus luteum of the ovary to produce its steroids. The evidence for feedback inhibition by androgens and estrogens is still not conclusive, although oral contraceptives are believed to act by suppressing the hypothalamic releasing factors.

A. LONG-FEEDBACK MECHANISM

The bulk of the evidence supports the idea that adrenocortical steroids act on the central nervous system rather than on the anterior pituitary to inhibit ACTH by the latter. It is believed that the median eminence is the receptor area for this feedback mechanism. The hypothalamus, rather than the pituitary, is also the site of the negative feedback action of sex steroids as intrahypothalamic implants of estrogen have been shown to produce gonadal atrophy in both sexes and the release of both FSH and LH is diminished. Estrogen has also been shown to exert a positive feedback effect on the hypothalamus of prepubertal female rats, puberty being advanced. These opposite effects may be due to small differences in the location of the implants but it seems that estrogen exerts a biphasic effect on LH secretion, stimulatory at first and inhibitory later.

B. SHORT-FEEDBACK MECHANISM

The secretion of ACTH appears to be regulated not only by the levels of blood corticoids but also by blood levels of ACTH itself. The receptor site appears to be the median eminence of the hypothalamus. Similar short-feedback mechanisms have been detected for LH and FSH. It is also believed that the pineal gland inhibits the synthesis and release of both FSH and LH.

II. NEUROENDOCRINOLOGY

A. THE HYPOTHALAMUS

The thalamus is the anterior portion of the brain stem and is a mass of grey matter at the base of the brain which projects into and bounds the third ventricle. The hypothalamus is the sub-thalamic region and forms the floor and part of the lateral wall of the third ventricle (Figs. 2.2, 2.3 and 2.4). Anatomically the hypothalamus can be divided into:

1. The sub-thalamic tegmental region.
2. The structures forming the floor of the third ventricle (the ventral hypothalamus).

(a) the posterior-perforated substance which is a small area of greyish matter;

(b) the mamillary bodies (the posterior hypothalamus) which are two round masses about the size of small peas, side by side in front of the posterior-perforated substance;

(c) the tuber cinereum which is a sheet of grey matter between the mamillary bodies behind and the optic chiasma in front. On each side it is continuous with the anterior-perforated substance but is separated from it on the basal surface of the brain by the optic tract. That part of the tuber

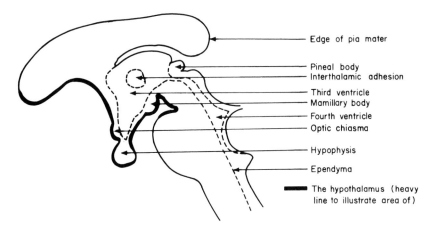

Fig. 2.2. Part of a median sagittal section through the human brain showing the position of the hypothalamus.

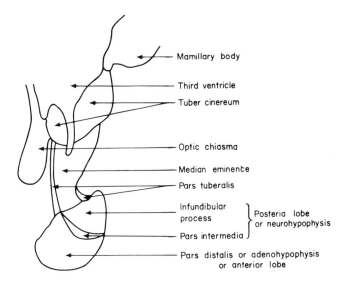

Fig. 2.3. The human pituitary gland and part of the hypothalamus.

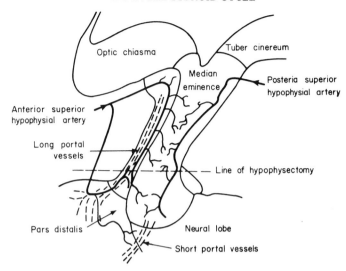

Fig. 2.4. The portal blood system of the pituitary stalk.

cinereum which is related to the pars tuberalis of the hypophysis is termed the median eminence (the anterior hypothalamus);

(d) the infundibulum which projects down from the undersurface of the tuber cinereum (which is covered by the tuberal part of the hypophysis);

(e) the hypophysis or pituitary gland. Although anatomically part of the hypothalamus, this structure is usually considered a separate entity;

(f) the optic chiasma.

3. The anterior part of the lateral wall of the third ventricle, below and in front of the thalamus.

B. THE HYPOPHYSIS

The hypophysis is a reddish-grey, ovoid body about 12 mm by 8 mm connected to the median eminence of the tuber cinereum by the pituitary stalk or pars tuberalis which surrounds the infundibulum and covers the tuber cinereum. The gland itself consists of an anterior lobe (adenohypophysis) and a posterior (neural) lobe which are of different embryological origins. The posterior lobe, infundibulum and median eminence are frequently called the neurohypophysis. The anterior lobe is larger and is marked by a narrow cleft, or, more frequently in the adult, by a row of colloid-containing vesicles. Between the two lobes is the pars intermedia. Man and some of the higher apes are the only species where the anterior and posterior lobes of the hypophysis are adherent. In other animals there is a cleft or lumen between the anterior lobe and the pars intermedia which is adherent to the infundibulum as shown in Fig. 2.5 for the rat.

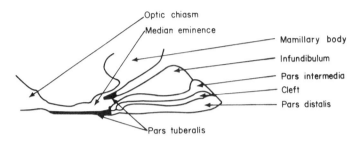

Fig. 2.5. The pituitary gland of the rat.

C. RELEASING FACTORS

It is not known which parts of the hypothalamus synthesize the releasing factors, although the mechanism is believed to be similar to that for oxytocin and vasopressin. Some neurones have developed secretory functions to such an extent that they have become morphologically distinguishable from other nerve cells and are called neurosecretory cells. They have dendrites, axis cylinders and Nissl bodies. Visible granules appear in the perikaya. The complex formed by the axons and close association of vascular structures serves as a storage and release centre for the neurohormones of which the best known is the neural lobe of the pituitary. The hypothalamic releasing factors are synthesized as electron dense particles in the cell body of neuronal cells and become secretory droplets which travel down the main process of the neurone together with canaliculi until they are secreted from the end of the neuronal cell. The hypothalamic nerve tracts which contain the releasing factors end in the median eminence very close to the capillaries of the primary plexus formed from the incoming hypophysial arteries (Fig. 2.4). The releasing factors enter the blood which flows on to coalesce into the long portal veins of the pars tuberalis. On entering the anterior lobe of the hypophysis, the portal vessels break up into sinusoids and the releasing factors pass into the cells. In the case of oxytocin and vasopressin the neurones which synthesize these compounds pass right down the median eminence and into the posterior (or neural) lobe. Oxytocin and vasopressin are thus secreted, but not synthesized, by the neural lobe.

The following releasing factors have been identified and partially characterized:

CRF   = corticotrophin releasing factor;
LH-RH (LRF) = luteinizing hormone (or luteotrophin) releasing factor;
FSH-RF = follicle-stimulating hormone releasing factor;
TRF   = thyrotrophin releasing factor;
SRF   = somatotrophin releasing factor;
PIF   = prolactin inhibiting factor.

The last is so called because the factor related to the secretion of prolactin appears to act by an inhibitory process. SRF and prolactin also do not participate in the usual feedback inhibition system and the central nervous system is believed to regulate their secretion. There is also evidence for the secretion by the pineal gland of factors which inhibit the secretion of trophic hormones.

D. TROPHIC HORMONES OF THE ADENOHYPOPHYSIS

The anterior lobe of the pituitary gland is very vascular and consists of epithelial cells arranged in trabeculae, irregular masses or alveoli separated by thin-walled sinusoidal vessels and reticular tissue. Histochemically there are three basic cell types—acidophils and basophils which contain granules and the chromophores which do not. In the human adenohypophysis there are zones of acidophils and zones of basophils. Basophil zones may not contain a large number of basophils but have less acidophils. It is believed that each trophic hormone is secreted by its special type of cell in the adenohypophysis and the following sub-groups have been identified in man.

1. Acidophils

These cells stain with acidophilic dyes and their granules are negative to the PAS (periodic acid–Schiff) stain for glycoprotein. Their granules are believed to consist almost entirely of protein only.

(a) Somatotrophs

These are the ordinary acidophils or alpha-cells which stain well with gold, i.e. they are aurantiphil. They form a large proportion of the total cells and are concentrated in the posterior-lateral regions. Fluorescent antibody labelling has shown that they secrete somatotrophin (i.e. growth hormone, GH). They stain orange with Herlant's tetrachrome stain (orange G, erythrosin, aniline B and acid alizarin blue).

(b) Lactotrophs

These are the minor acidophils or epsilon-eta cells. These are erythrophil, i.e. they stain red with Herlant's tetrachrome stain. Epsilon cells are present in the

2*

non-pregnant state while during pregnancy they show the presence of more active and numerous granules and are called eta cells. The epsilon cells of some publications correspond to the eta cells of others and much confusion exists in the literature. In man these cells are mammotrophic but a prolactin (or lactogenic hormone) separable from somatotrophin has not yet been found. In other species their secretion is luteotrophin, i.e. the luteotrophic hormone, LTH.

2. Neutrophils

(a) Corticotrophs

The neutrophil cells do not stain with acidic or basic dyes and are weakly PAS positive. These are the gamma cells and are often found in groups forming acini. They occur also in the intermediate zone and have been identified as secreting corticotrophin, i.e. the adrencorticotrophic hormone, ACTH.

3. Basophils

These cells stain with basophilic dyes and their granules are strongly positive to the PAS stain for glycoprotein. Sub-groups can be identified by differential staining with basic dyes and for the different types of glycoproteins. These cells have been described as the mucoid group while the PAS negative cells are serous in type.

(a) Thyrotrophs

These are the blue beta cells, theta cells, cyanophils, AF_1, AlB_1 or S_2 cells according to the method of staining. AF is aldehyde-fuchsin which stains the theta and zeta cells dark purple, the delta cells blue and the gamma cells pale blue. AlB refers to the alcian blue stain, used in conjunction with PAS, which stains these cells blue. They are most variable in size and shape, the larger ones having an irregular and angular outline, and they have been identified as secreting thyrotrophin, i.e. the thyroid-stimulating hormone, TSH.

(b) Gonadotrophs

These are the delta cells, cyanophils, AlB_{2-3} or S_1 cells according to the method of staining. They are lightly granulated, small, round or oval cells found mainly in the acidophil-rich zones. In man it has not yet been possible to distinguish the two theoretical types of gonadotrophs but in the rat the distinction between the folliculotrophs, which secrete follicle-stimulating hormone, FSH, and the interstitiotrophs which secrete the luteinizing hormone, LH, sometimes called the interstitial cell-stimulating hormone, ICSH, depends on the distribution of the granulation in the cytoplasm. The folliculotrophs have coarsely flocculant granules while the interstitiotrophs have more uniformly dispersed granules. There is very little difference in their staining properties.

(c) Melanotrophs

These are the zeta cells, amphophils, AF_2, purple beta or R cells according to the method of staining. They are the most numerous and conspicuous of the basal cells and are the only cells which "invade" the neural lobe. They are present in the intermediate zone and secrete melanotrophin, i.e. the melanophore (or melanocyte)-stimulating hormone, MSH. This is sometimes called intermedin. The R cells are so called because their PAS positive granules are not extracted with performic acid. The S-cell granules are extracted with performic acid. S_1 cells stain a pure phthalocyanine blue while S_2 cells stain a deep purplish-blue with this dye. Table 2.1 summarizes the different types of cells. The pars intermedia contains small agranular cells interspersed with basophils, the zeta cells or melanotrophs which secrete MSH.

Of these trophic hormones, only FSH, LH, prolactin and ACTH are concerned with the control of steroid biosynthesis. FSH, LH and prolactin are known collectively as the pituitary gonadotrophins. The trophic hormones are released into the sinusoids of the anterior lobe of the hypophysis which collect into the

Table 2.1. *Cell types and secretions of the adenohypophysis and pars intermedia*

Functional name	Alternative name(s)	Secretion
Somatotroph	Alpha cells	Somatotrophin = growth hormone = GH
Lactotroph	Epsilon or eta cells	Luteotrophin = luteotrophic hormone = LTH≡ prolactin = lactogenic hormone
Corticotroph	Gamma cells	Corticotrophin = adreno-corticotrophic hormone = ACTH
Thyrotroph	Theta cells	Thyrotrophin = thyroid-stimulating hormone = TSH
Gonadotroph	Delta cells	Gonadotrophins
Folliculotroph		Follicle-stimulating hormone = FSH
Interstitotroph		Luteinizing hormone = LH≡ interstitial cell-stimulating hormone = ICSH
Melanotroph	Zeta cells	Melanotrophin = melanocyte-stimulating hormone = MSH intermedin

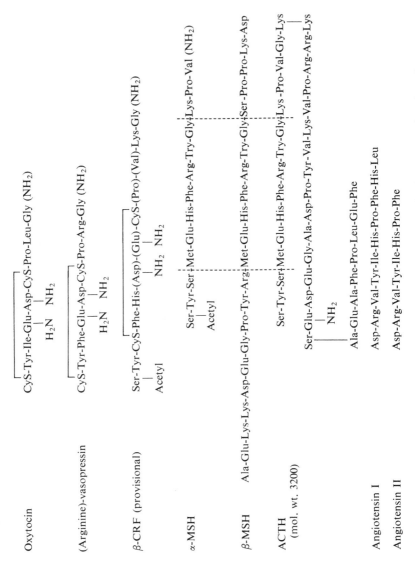

Fig. 2.6. Structure of the polypeptide human releasing factors, trophic hormones and angiotensins.

branches of the hypophysial veins and so into the general blood stream. The same gonadotrophins are present in the pituitary glands of both sexes but the hypothalamus is sexually dimorphic and this results in different patterns of pituitary release. The female type of hypothalamus releases LH and FSH cyclically.

E. STRUCTURE OF RELEASING FACTORS AND TROPHIC HORMONES

The releasing factors are believed to be small peptides similar in structure to oxytocin and vasopressin (Fig. 2.6). Corticotrophin releasing factor (CRF) appears to exist in at least five forms and a tentative structure has been assigned to one of them. Oxytocin and vasopressin are bound to proteins neurophysin I and II, respectively, of molecular weight 25,000-30,000 when stored in their microvesicles.

ACTH and MSH are also peptides, though rather larger (Fig. 2.6). The two chains of MSH have a large peptide portion in common with the peptide chain of ACTH and it is often difficult to measure the relative activities of the two hormones in biological tests as ACTH has some MSH activity and vice versa. The gonadotrophins FSH and LH are glycoproteins. A recent analysis of both human FSH and LH gave 78% and 60% protein respectively. FSH is higher in aspartate, glutamate, glycine, alanine, phenylalanine, lysine and histidine and lower in proline, valine, tyrosine and arginine. The carbohydrate portion consisted of:

	LH	FSH
N-Acetyl-neuraminic acid (a sialic acid	1.4	5.2
Hexose	11.0	11.6
Hexosamine	3.1	9.1
Protein	60.0	78.0
Total	75.5	103.9

F. HYPOPHYSECTOMY AND PITUITARY STALK SECTION

Hypophysectomy implies the complete ablation of the entire pituitary gland but the median eminence of the tuber cinereum and most or all of the infundibular stem, both constituting parts of the neurohypophysis, are left in place as is that part of the pars tuberalis situated outside the hypophysical capsule. The pars distalis, pars intermedia and part of the pars tuberalis of the adenohypophysis and the infundibular process of the neuro hypophysis is all

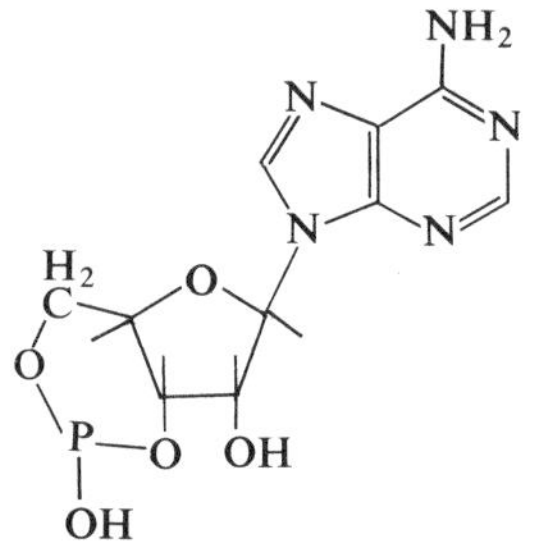

Fig. 2.7. Cyclic-3′,5′-adenosine-monophosphate.

that can be removed. Laboratory animals prepared in this way, especially rats, are used in many routine assays of hormones and can survive for a normal life span provided they are kept free of stress and infection. The effects of hypophysectomy in laboratory animals are:

1. atrophy of the gonads and arrest of their hormonal activities as indicated by the atrophic condition of accessory and secondary sex organs;
2. atrophy of the thyroid glands and substantial decrease in metabolic rate;
3. atrophy of the adrenal cortices, a substantial decrease in glucocorticoid activity and a reduction in aldosterone production;
4. loss of weight. The volume of food ingested is much reduced and the use of more highly concentrated food pellets is often recommended;
5. arrest or retardation of body growth and splanchromicria (abnormal smallness of the viscera).

As all the anterior pituitary hormones are absent, all of which exert actions essential to the regulation of general metabolism, the animals must make a quick adjustment of the rates and pathway of metabolism.

Pituitary Stalk Section is a term which should be used only for procedures which result in the separation of the pituitary gland from all structures contained in the stalk. There is usually a massive haemorrhage, especially in the rat, which causes necrosis. However, the hypophysical portal vessels regenerate very quickly unless measures are taken at the time of operation to prevent this. In rats an appreciable amount of well vascularized anterior hypophysial tissue remains in spite of the haemorrhage, although there is considerable impairment of the hormonal activities of the pituitary gland.

In man, hypophysectomy or pituitary stalk section are sometimes carried out as palliative treatments for advanced carcinoma of the breast with widely disseminated metastases, for intractable diabetes mellitus and for Cushings' syndrome of pituitary origin. It is necessary to give cortisone replacement therapy from immediately after the operation, thyroid replacement therapy after 1-2 months and sometimes pitressin to control thirst and polyuria. Atrophy of the gonads takes place.

G. TROPHIC HORMONES IN BLOOD

ACTH is found on Cohn's blood fractions II and III, i.e. in the α-globulins and β-lipoproteins, and is present as a complex of higher molecular weight. FSH and LH activities have been found in all fractions but FSH appears to be especially concentrated in fractions V and VI while LH is mainly in fractions II and III.

H. CYCLIC-3',5'-AMP

Certain fast-acting hormones, e.g. adrenalin in liver and muscle, ACTH in adrenal cortex, LH in corpus luteum, are known to stimulate the synthesis of cyclic-3',5'-AMP (Fig. 2.7). In liver and muscle the response is the degradation of glycogen to glucose-1-phosphate by phosphorylase which exists in two forms a and b. This is so for both tissues although the enzymes are different. Phosphorylase a is much more active than the b form, from which it is derived by phosphorylation with ATP. This activating phosphorylation is catalysed by phosphorylase kinase and is facilitated by cyclic-3',5'-AMP which is formed from ATP by adenyl cyclase. This latter enzyme is situated in the cell membrane and is stimulated by adrenalin. There is evidence that LH stimulates steroidogenesis in the corpus luteum via cyclic-3',5'-AMP formation. It is probable that its specificity is due to the specificity of the adenyl cyclase present in each target tissue. It is possible that LH and FSH stimulate steroidogenesis in the testes and ovaries respectively, also via cyclic-3',5'-AMP formation.

III. SITES OF STEROID BIOSYNTHESIS AND METABOLISM

A. SUMMARY

The principal sites of biosynthesis of steroids in the human body, together with their characteristic spectrum of steroids produced, is shown in Table 2.2.

B. ADRENAL GLANDS

These are two small flattened bodies of a yellowish colour situated immediately above and in front of the upper end of the kidney. Each gland consists of an outer cortical portion which is rich in lipids and contains no chromaffin tissue and a thin inner medullary portion. In man it is not uncommon to find small

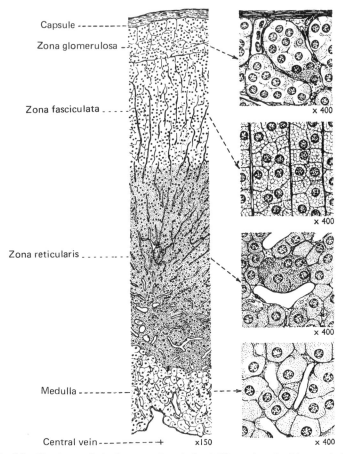

Fig. 2.8. Histology of the human adrenal gland (*Reproduced with permission from "A Student's Histology" 2nd edition 1965, by H. S. D. Garven, E. & S. Livingstone Ltd., Edinburgh and London*).

masses of tissue identical with the adrenal cortex in the neighbourhood of the gland or in other situations (e.g. spermatic cord, epididymus and the broad ligaments of the uterus) and these are called "cortical bodies". The right adrenal gland is pyramidal and the left is semilunar and usually larger. Each gland weighs about 5 g and is about 50 mm high, 30 mm wide and 10 mm thick. The gland is contained in a thick collagenous capsule which contains a rich plexus of arteries from which branches pass into the gland.

The mammalian adrenal gland appears to have a higher blood flow rate than any other tissue, derived from as many as fifty small arteries coming from the aorta, the inferior phrenic and renal arteries. The zona glomerulosa has an abundant blood supply from a subcapsular plexus and capillaries run down into

Table 2.2. *Sites of steroid biosynthesis*

Site	Type of steroid produced
Adrenal cortex	Corticosteroids Glucocorticosteroids, e.g. cortisol, cortisone, corticosterone Mineralocorticosteroids, e.g. aldosterone Some androgens, e.g. dehydroepiandrosterone A small amount of estrogens and progestogens
Testis	Androgens A small amount of estrogens
Ovary	Estrogens A small amount of androgens Progestogens
Placenta	Progestogens Estrogens Chorionic gonadotrophin Placental lactogen
Skin	Cholesterol Vitamin D Steroid hormone metabolites
Liver	Cholesterol metabolism to bile acids Steroid hormone metabolites
Kidney	Steroid hormone metabolites

the cortex between the columns of cells in the zona fasciculata to supply the zona reticularis. A single large vein emerges from the gland but a considerable part of the drainage of the gland may take place via the numerous small veins leaving the capsule. It has been customary to consider those steroids found in a greater concentration in the adrenal vein than in arterial blood to be true secretory products of the gland.

The medulla, which is of different embryological origin, consists of groups and columns of chromaffin cells permeated by wide venous sinusoids together with nerve cells. These cells produce adrenalin and noradrenalin which pass from the cells directly into the sinusoids which open into the supravenous vein.

The cortex consists of three zones of cells, (Fig. 2.8). The outer zone immediately beneath the capsule is the zona glomerulosa which consists of short columnar cells arranged in groups or columns. The cytoplasm is weakly basophilic and contains abundant mitochondria and dense endoplasmic reticulum. This zone produces the mineralocorticosteroid, aldosterone, and is much broader and constitutes most of the cortex. There is no sharp dividing line between the zona glomerulosa and the zona fasciculata. The cells of the latter

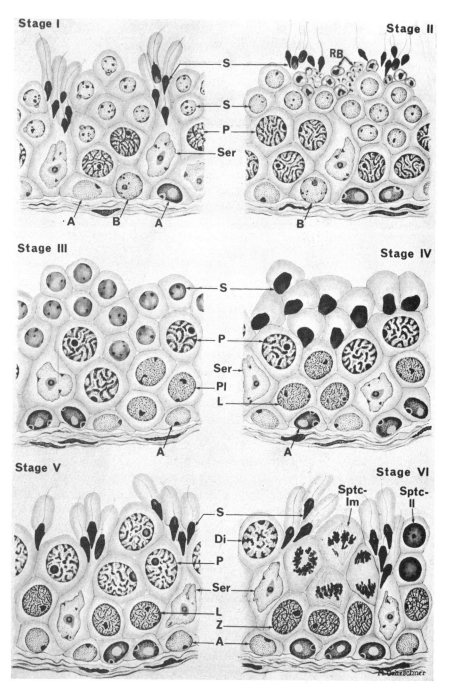

Fig. 2.9. (a) Histology of the human testis, the stages of spermatogenesis. (From Ham and Leeson, 1965.)

Key to Fig. 2.9(a)

Ser = nucleus of Sertoli cell;
A = type A spermatogonia;
B = type B spermatogonia;
PL = preleptotene primary
    spermatocytes;
L = leptotene primary spermatocytes;
Z = zygotene primary spermatocytes;
P = pachytene primary spermatocytes;

Di = diplotene primary spermatocytes;
Sptc-Im = primary spermatocytes in
    division;
Sptc-II = secondary spermatocytes in
    interphase;
S = spermatids at various steps in
    spermiogenesis;
RB = residual bodies.

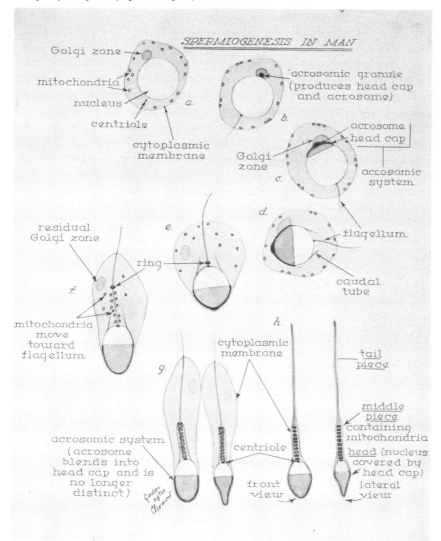

Fig. 2.9. (b) Histology of the human testis, the maturation of spermatid to spermatozoön. (From Ham and Leeson, 1965.)

are large and polyhedral with basophilic cytoplasm and contain numerous lipid droplets and large amounts of phospholipids and cholesterol with few mitochondria. As the lipid globules are removed in paraffin section histology these cells have been called "clear cells". The change to the "compact cells" of the innermost zona reticularis is abrupt. These cells are arranged in alveoli separated by thin-walled prominent sinuses and are poor in lipid and rich in mitochondria.

It is believed that the cells of the zona fasciculata and zona reticularis function as a single unit, the outermost cells being in a resting state, ready with their store of cholesterol for steroid biosynthesis. Under the stimulus of ACTH these cells rapidly produce steroids and become the compact cells of the zona reticularis. The two combined inner zones synthesize the glucocorticosteroids, the androgens and the estrogens of the adrenal cortex. Histochemical investigations have shown that 3β- and 17α-hydroxy-steroid dehydrogenase activities are greater in the outer zona fasciculata and it would appear that these outer cells synthesize cortisol and its metabolite, cortisone, to a greater extent than the inner cells of the zona reticularis. The adrenal cortex can store up to 7% of its weight as cholesterol and appears to synthesize corticosteroids only on demand as the amount of steroids stored is only about the amount secreted in three minutes. The adrenal cortex contains very high concentrations of ascorbic acid but its precise role in the biochemical reactions occurring has still to be elucidated.

The biosynthesis of aldosterone is not under the exclusive control of ACTH but is controlled from the kidney by the renin-angiotensin system. Renin is an enzyme which is released into the general circulation by the kidney and which hydrolyses the leucine-leucine bond of angiotensinogen (Fig. 2.6), a polypeptide of unknown origin circulating in the plasma. The angiotensin I so produced is further hydrolysed by a peptidase to produce angiotensin II, which is the compound which controls aldosterone production by the adrenal cortex. It is also believed that glomerulotrophin, a substance isolated from the pineal gland similar in structure to melatonin, may also assist in the control of aldosterone secretion.

The adrenal cortex, but not the medulla, is essential for life. Adrenalectomy results in an increased release of ACTH from the pituitary. A series of metabolic disturbances are produced which are identical with those appearing in patients with Addisons' disease, e.g. muscular weakness, hypoglycemia, reduced blood pressure and body temperature, renal failure. Exposure to stress, e.g. trauma, cold, heat, infections or exercise is likely to prove fatal. Life can be maintained by the administration of cortisone.

C. TESTES

The glandular part of a testis consists of 200-300 lobules each of which contain one to three convoluted seminiferous tubules which are supported by

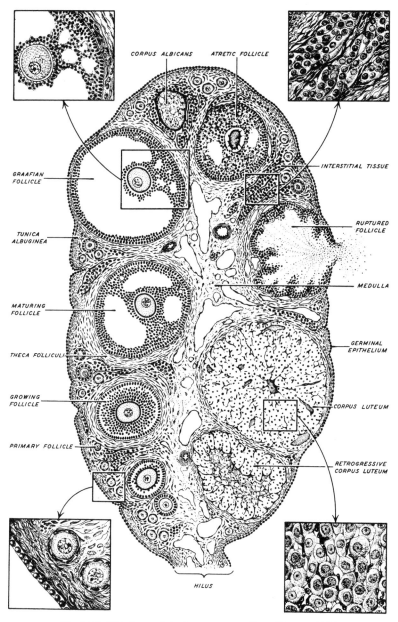

Fig. 2.10. Histology of the human ovary (from Turner, 1966.)

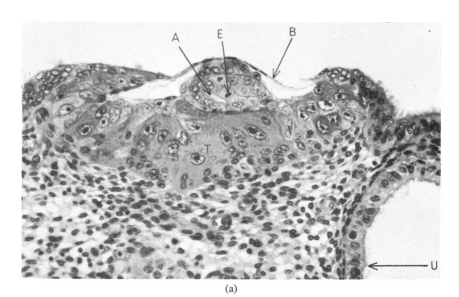

(a)

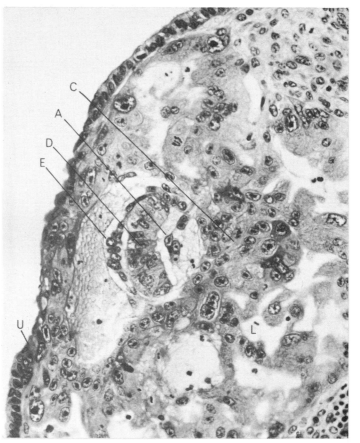

(b)

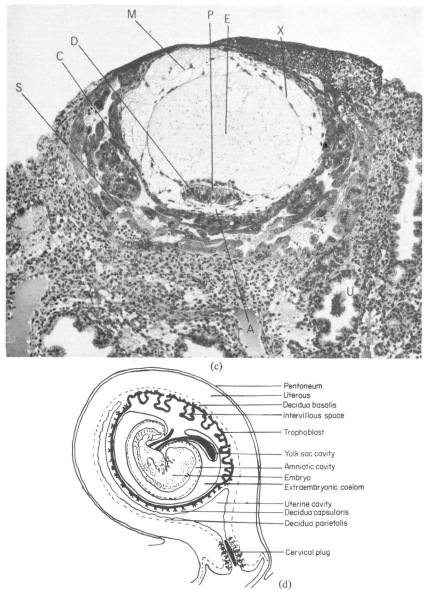

(c)

Pentoneum
Uterous
Decidua basalis
Intervillous space

Trophoblast

Yolk sac cavity
Amniotic cavity
Embryo
Extraembryonic coelom

Uterine cavity
Decidua capsularis
Decidua parietalis

Cervical plug

(d)

Fig. 2.11. Structure of the placenta. (a). Human blastocyst at $7\frac{1}{2}$ days gestation (x 300). Uterine gland (U), outer wall of blastocyst (B), trophoblast (T), embryonic disc (E) and amniotic cavity (A) are shown. (b). Human embryo at 9 days gestation (x 300). Uterine epithelium (U), trophoblastic lacunae (L), endoderm (E), embryonic disc (D), amniotic cavity (A) and cytotrophoblast (C) are shown. (c). Human embryo at about 12 days gestation (x 100). Extraembryonic mesoblast (M), amnion (A), primitive endoderm (P), embryonic disc (D), cytotrophoblast (C), syncytotrophoblast (S), exocoelomic cavity (E), utrine gland (U), and Heuser's (exocoelomic) membrane (X) are seen. (All from Assali, N. S. ed. "Biology of Gestation", Vol. 1", Academic Press, New York, 1968.) (d). Schematic diagram at about 4 weeks (from G. Bourne, "The Human Amnion and Chorion", Lloyd-Luke Medical Books Ltd., London, 1962.)

loose connective tissue interspersed with groups of interstitial cells which contain yellow pigment granules. Each tube has a basement membrane and then three layers of cells—spermatogonia, spermatocytes and spermatids which become spermatozoön (Fig. 2.9). Interspersed are supporting or Sertoli cells which are elongated and columnar, projecting inwards from the basement membrane. The interstitial cells (Leydig cells) are large polyhedral cells lying in the connective tissue between the seminiferous tubules and comprise the endocrine system of the testis. They contain fats, phospholipids and cholesterol and are very rich in ascorbic acid. The interstitial cells secrete the testicular androgens and are influenced by the luteinizing hormone (LH) (which is identical with the interstitial cell-stimulating hormone, ICSH) and by FSH. The Sertoli cells are believed by some workers to secrete estrogens and to be under the control of the follicle-stimulating hormone (FSH), while others believe that the testicular estrogens are secreted by Leydig cells and that the Sertoli cells provide nourishment for the spermatids with which they are intimately associated. The function of FSH in males is to cause the growth of the seminiferous tubules and to maintain spermatogenesis.

D. OVARIES

(a) Structure

In mature nulliparous women the ovaries are almond shaped, about 3 cm long, 1.5 cm wide and 1 cm thick and are arranged vertically. The surface of the ovary is covered by the germinal epithelium. There is a thick cortex which contains the ovarian follicles and corpora lutea. In the centre is the richly vascular medulla. The interstitial framework or stroma of the cortex consists of reticular connective tissue fibres and numerous spindle-shaped cells. Immediately beneath the germinal epithelium, the connective tissue of the cortex is condensed to form a delicate tunica albuginea (Fig. 2.10). The stroma of the ovary is now recognized as a distinct endocrine organ responsible for the synthesis of the ovarian androgens, while the follicles synthesize estrogens.

(b) Menstrual cycle

The development of cells in the ovary follows a cyclical pattern which governs the menstrual cycle. The following phases may be distinguished (day 1 being the first day of menstrual bleeding):

(i) The proliferative or follicular phase, days 6-14. The ovarian cortex contains numerous primary follicles each consisting of a large central cell, the oogonium, surrounded by a single layer of small cubical or flattened cells. Each month some of these primary follicles develop to form vesicular or Graafian follicles, one of which usually matures and ruptures (ovulation). The primary follicle develops by multiplication of the follicular cells to form several layers surrounding a cavity, the antrum, which contains fluid. The antrum divides the follicular cells into two

groups, the outer set forming the membrana granulosa and the inner set, which surrounds the ovum, forming the cumulus ovaricus. The membrana granulosum secretes estrogens.

The stromal cells of the cortex form a sheath, the theca, around the follicle which becomes differentiated into an inner part, the cellular tunica interna, and an outer part, the fibrous tunica externa. The tunica externa becomes well developed and constitutes the thecal gland. The cells of the tunica interna also secrete estrogens.

The follicular phase takes place under the stimulus of FSH and later LH. The main action of FSH in the female is to stimulate the young ovarian follicles to develop multiple layers of granulosa cells and to form antra. When FSH acts alone in hypophysectomized females, LH being absent, these follicles do not reach full size and do not secrete estrogen. LH acts synergistically with FSH to promote the secretion of estrogens by follicles undergoing maturation to cause ovulation. Pure LH alone administered to hypophysectomized females has no conspicuous effect on the ovarian follicles. Ovulation occurs when the balance between FSH and LH has swung sufficiently in favour of the latter. Secretion of progesterone begins just before ovulation from the follicle which is destined to release an ovum.

(ii) Ovulation, day 14. The oogonium becomes converted into a primary oocyte and later divides by meiosis into a secondary oocyte and a first polar body. When the fully developed follicle, which is about 10 mm in diameter, ruptures the secondary oocyte is extruded surrounded by follicular cells of the cumulus ovaricus. Other developing follicles degenerate and the cells of their tunica interna form the interstitial cells of the ovary where they secrete some endogenous estrogen.

(iii) Progestational or luteal or secretory phase, days 15-28. After ovulation, the wall of the Graafian follicle collapses and becomes folded. The cells of the membrana granulosa become greatly increased in size and a yellow carotenoid pigment (lutein) is formed in their cytoplasm. These are luteal cells and form the major part of the corpus luteum. Smaller paraluteal cells, derived from the cells of the tunica interna, also lie between the luteal cells. Blood capillaries grow in from the vessels in the tunica interna and a small blood clot occurs in the centre of the corpus luteum. The luteal cells produce progesterone and both luteal and paraluteal cells produce some estrogens. This phase takes place under the stimulus of LH. In rats and mice prolactin is also necessary for the maintenance of the corpora lutea and for their secretion of progestogens, but in the majority of mammals, e.g. man, rabbits and guinea pigs, prolactin is not luteotrophic. The function of prolactin is for the initiation and maintenance of lactation. At present human prolactin has not been separated from growth hormone. The abrupt termination of the release of progesterone from the corpus luteum at the end of the cycle is the main determinant of the onset of menstruation.

(iv) Menstruation, days 1-5. After about 12-14 days, the corpus luteum degenerates forming fibrous tissue, the corpus albicans.

E. PLACENTA

In man, it is probable that the second meiotic division, forming the ovum and the second polar body, takes place only after fertilization and occurs in the uterine tube. The ovum lies within its zona pellucida, which is a thick transparent envelope, which in turn is surrounded by follicular cells from the cumulus ovaricus which form the corona radiata. The first polar body usually divides and the three polar bodies are embedded in the zona pellucida.

After fertilization, the zygote starts to divide forming a mass of cells, the morula, in which fluid accumulates. On the fourth or fifth day after ovulation (about 72 h after fertilization), the zygote has been converted into a blastocyst consisting of fifty-eight cells, five of which are destined to form the foetus and fifty-three of which are destined to form the trophoblast which is the embryonic epithelium which encloses all embryonic structures and forms the embryonic side of the placenta. In the blastocyst, the trophoblast forms the outer epithelium which encloses a single fluid cavity and to which the embryonic cells are joined.

Implantation of the blastocyst normally begins on the seventh day after fertilization and occurs by deep or interstitial embedding in the stroma of the endometrium. Implantation depends on the changes in the endometrium which result in the formation of the decidua which is the mucosa of the pregnant uterus and which has nourishing functions. That part of the blastocystic trophoblast which invades the endometrium forms a thick plaque which differentiates into the inner cytotrophoblast and the outer syncytiotrophoblast. The cytotrophoblast, or Langhans cells, is cellular with large nuclei which have prominent nucleoli, large mitochondria and few Golgi bodies. The cytoplasm contains numerous free ribosomes but little endoplasmic reticulum. It is now believed that these cells have a purely growth and differentiation function serving to form the syncytiotrophoblast by rapid cellular proliferation and coalescence of the daughter cells. Electron microscopy has shown that the syncytiotrophoblast is a true syncytium, i.e. there is a mass of cytoplasm, in the form of a sheet, which is enclosed in a single continuous plasma membrane and contains many nuclei. It is now regarded as the endocrinologically and morphologically mature form of the trophoblast and contains a well-developed endoplasmic reticulum and Golgi bodies together with numerous free ribosomes. Many of the secretory granules present consist of protein while others contain mostly lipid. Immunofluorescence has led to the belief that the syncytiotrophoblast is a multifunctional endocrine organ which secretes human chorionic gonadotrophin (HCG), human placental lactogen (HPL) and the steroid hormones of the placenta. The syncytiotrophoblast is in direct contact with maternal blood and is relatively thick in early placental development, thinning progressively throughout pregnancy. The secretory granules migrate into the microvillous border of the syncytium and are discharged into the intervillous space by pinocytosis. HCG has both FSH and LH activity and stimulates the corpus luteum to increase to about 2.5 cm diameter at which size it remains until near the end of pregnancy, secreting progesterone and estrogens. HCG is a glycoprotein with a high carbohydrate content. At some time during the third month of pregnancy (counting from the last menstrual period), the developing placenta begins to synthesize and excrete large quantities of estrogens and progesterone, and the corpus luteum is no longer essential for the continuation of pregnancy. The histology of the early placenta is shown in Fig. 2.11.

F. SKIN

The skin (Fig. 2.12) is an organ which covers the whole of the outside of the body and its structure and function varies with the area of the body covered. The epidermis is separated from the dermis by a basement membrane containing polysaccharides and reticulin. Above the basement membrane is a single layer of basal cells of the epidermis, the stratum basale, which are columnar and have deeply basophilic cytoplasm. Mitotic figures are often seen in these cells and the rest of the epidermis is populated by cells which have arisen from this basal or germinal layer by cell division, one of the daughter cells migrating through the various layers of the epidermis until being shed from the surface of the skin. In man this process takes about 30 days. Interspersed between the basal cells and the basement membrane are the melanocytes which synthesize melanin. These cells possess several dendrites and the melanin granules are passed along these into every basal cell of the epidermis where they take up a position over the top of the nucleus and serve to prevent radiation damage to these cells, e.g. by sunlight.

Above the basal layer are about six layers of squamous cells which form the stratum spinosum. They become flattened towards the surface and gradually contain more tonofibrils of keratin as they progress towards the surface. The metabolism of these cells is gradually turned over completely to the manufacture of keratin and they lose most other normal cell functions. Above the stratum spinosum is the granular layer, or stratum granulosum, the cells of which are usually one to three layers thick, diamond shaped and filled with "keratohyalin granules" which are deeply basophilic and which are believed to complete the keratinization process by cementing keratin fibrils and tonofibrils together. The skin of the palms and soles, which has a thicker layer of outer keratin, has a stratum lucidium, or clearer layer, between the stratum granulosum and the usual next layer, the stratum corneum or horny layer. The thickness of the horny layer varies from 0.02 mm on the inside of the arm to 0.5 mm on the sole and consists of dead cells which have lost their nuclei and are filled with keratin.

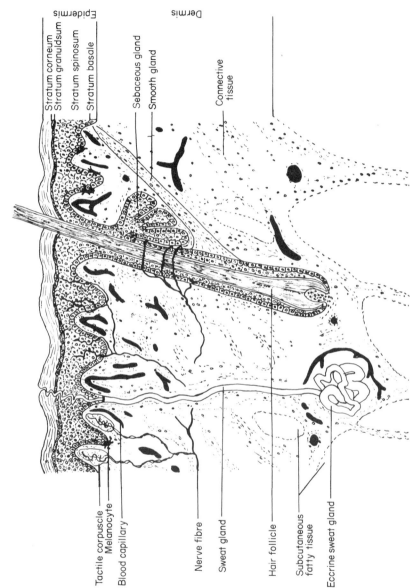

Fig. 2.12. Structure of the human skin (from Montagua, W. (1965). "The Skin", *Scientific American* **212**, 55-66).

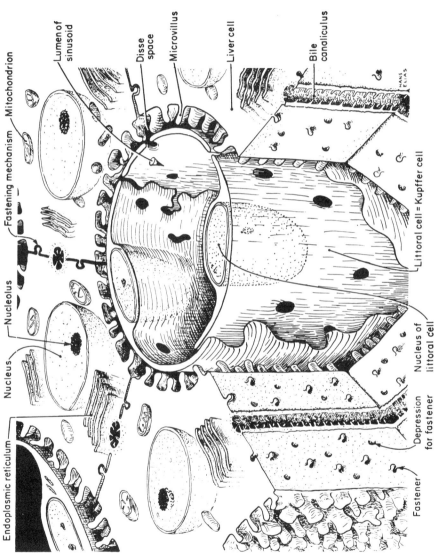

Fig. 2.13. Structure of the liver (from Rouiller, 1963).

They are held together by an intercellular cement and are gradually lost from the surface of the skin.

Below the basement membrane is the dermis which is connective tissue formed by collagen, reticulin and elastin fibres, interspersed with a variety of cell types. The most common cells present belong to the reticulo-histocyticfibro-blastic group. The fibroblasts synthesize collagen fibrils which are condensed into the collagen fibres of the dermis after secretion from the cells.

Interspersed between the cells of the epidermis and dermis are sweat glands, sebaceous glands and hair follicles. The sebaceous glands are important in steroid biosynthesis and metabolism. They are present everywhere on the skin except on the palms and soles and are especially concentrated on the forehead, lower face, chest and back (the acne areas) and the scalp (the dandruff area). The sebaceous glands secrete the sebum which contains fatty acids, squalene and cholesterol with its esters and derivatives. The sebaceous glands are not endocrine glands like the adrenals, ovaries and testes, which discharge steroids as granules from their cells, but are holocrine glands in that the cells break down to release their contents.

The skin surface film consists of a mixture of the sebum, sweat and the breakdown products of the stratum corneum, forming an emulsion. The emulsifying agents are cholesterol, lecithin and long chain alcohols of the cetyl alcohol type. The components of the oil phase are cholesterol esters, long chain alcohol esters, squalene, glycerides and fatty acids, while the water and salts of the sweat constitute the aqueous phase. It is believed that this emulsion can be either oil-in-water or water-in-oil according to the relative proportions of each phase present at any given time. Most of the cholesterol on the skin surface comes from the desquamating keratinized cells. Cholesterol and squalene make up 30% of the total surface film in man. Palms and soles which lack sebaceous glands have a surface film containing much cholesterol and little squalene while this is reversed on the face. The cholesterol of the desquamating cells is synthesized mainly in the cells of the epidermis, although some is made in the dermis.

Cholesterol is the principal sterol of higher animals and besides being abundant in the skin and nerves is found to some extent in nearly all bodily structures. It is usually accompanied by traces of dihydrocholesterol (choles-tanol) and 7-dehydrocholesterol. Internal epithelial structures, especially the aorta and the intestine, also show appreciable cholesterol content. In the skin, cholesterol of the epidermial cells is the precursor of vitamin D.

G. LIVER

The liver is responsible for most of the metabolism of cholesterol and the steroid hormones. This organ can be defined as a *continuous* mass of paren-chymal cells tunnelled by vessels through which venous blood flows on its way from the intestines to the heart. The parenchymal partitions between these vessels form a system or walls of muralium which are one cell thick (Fig. 2.13). The spaces between the parenchymal walls are all continuous with each other and form a labyrinth which pervades the entire organ. Thus the entire liver is one single plate of cells. The specialized capillaries of the liver, called sinusoids, are suspended in the spaces and enter almost exclusively the central veins. The bile canaliculi are formed by two grooves in the contact surfaces of two adjoining liver cells. Bile drains via these canaliculi into ductules, intrahepatic ducts, hepatic duct and enters the small intestine via the gall bladder. Certain bile constituents, especially the bile salts, are reabsorbed from the small intestine into the portal veins and returned to the liver, whence they are again excreted in the bile.

In man, the bulk of the metabolites of steroid hormones appear in the urine, but prior to urinary excretion they are in part excreted in the bile and reabsorbed from the gut. For the estrogens and progesterone, relatively rapid excretion into bile represents an important method of inactivation. Over half the estrogen metabolites and a third of the progesterone metabolites appear in bile shortly after the administration of radioactive parent hormones. Metabolites of corticosterone and testosterone are excreted into bile to a lesser extent and the excretion of cortisol metabolites into bile is slight. Most of these metabolites are reabsorbed, with the possible exception of progesterone.

3

PATHWAYS OF BIOSYNTHESIS AND METABOLISM
OF STEROIDS

I. SUMMARY

Figure 3.1 shows a summary of the pathways of biosynthesis and metabolism of the steroids and indicates the location of more detailed pathways in Figs. 3.2-3.20.

II. BIOSYNTHESIS OF CHOLESTEROL

A. BIOSYNTHESIS OF SQUALENE FROM ACETATE

The biochemical reaction which initiates steroid biosynthesis is the enzymatic reduction by 2H transfer from reduced nicotinamide-adenine dinucleotide phosphate (NADPH) to S-3-hydroxy-3-methylglutaryl coenzyme-A (Fig. 3.2). This reaction is not easily reversible and produces R-mevalonic acid. The

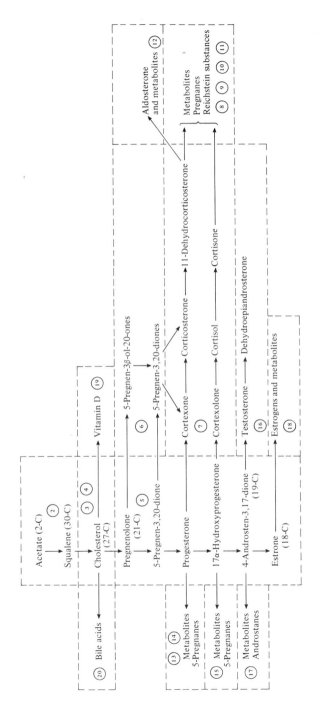

Fig. 3.1. Summary of biosynthesis and metabolism of steroids in animal tissues (the numbers in circles refer to the figure number which shows the detailed pathways and the numbers in brackets indicate the number of carbon atoms present).

3

S-3-hydroxy-3-methyl glutarate is produced by the usual condensation of three molecules of acetate with the aid of coenzyme-A, ATP and the enzymes acid coenzyme-A ligase or succinyl coenzyme-A: 3-oxo-acid coenzyme-A transferase followed by β-hydroxymethylglutaryl-coenzyme-A synthetase which occurs prior to lipid biosynthesis. So far as is known mevalonic acid is produced by no other pathway, nor is it used for anything except the biosynthesis of steroids, other terpenoids and some alkaloids. Only the R-form gives rise to these compounds, the S-form being metabolically inert. An alternative minor pathway to mevalonic acid may be from malonyl-coenzyme-A. A pathway from leucine via glutaconyl coenzyme-A has also been established.

Mevalonate becomes phosphorylated in two kinase steps, ATP being the phosphate donor. The mevalonyl pyrophosphate formed is degraded with the aid of ATP to give 3-methyl-3-butenyl pyrophosphate, ADP, inorganic phosphate and CO_2. The oxygen atom from the tertiary hydroxyl group is found in the inorganic phosphate after the reaction. The enzyme is an anhydrodecarboxylase. Stereochemically the process is a *trans*-elimination (not a dehydration followed by a decarboxylation) and this type of reaction has not been found elsewhere in enzyme chemistry.

Next, 3-methyl-3-butenyl pyrophosphate undergoes a prototropic shift into 3-methyl-2-butenyl pyrophosphate with the aid of isopentenyl pyrophosphate isomerase. This is one of the few reversible reactions in the series. The elimination of a proton is stereospecific, the hydrogen atom Hc being the one eliminated. The effect is to change a compound which has a relatively unreactive phosphoryl group and a nucleophilic double bond to a compound which is a highly reactive electrophilic allyl pyrophosphate.

The enzyme prenyltransferase catalyses the condensation of three molecules of 3-methyl-3-butenyl pyrophosphate into farnesyl pyrophosphate as shown in Fig. 3.2 with the elimination of pyrophosphate. Each condensation reaction is believed to proceed in two steps: the *trans*-addition of the allylic unit and of an electron donating group and the *trans*-elimination of the electron donating group and of a hydrogen ion. The formation of the new carbon-carbon bond is accompanied by the complete inversion of configuration of the allylic carbon atom. It is this head-to-tail condensation together of 5-carbon units which has become known as the isoprene rule (isoprene is $CH_2=CH(CH_3)-CH=CH_2$). Naturally occurring terpenoid compounds tend to have either ten (monoterpenes), fifteen (sesquiterpenes), twenty (diterpenes), twenty-five (sesterterpenes), thirty (triterpenes), or forty (carotenoids) carbon atoms.

Two molecules of farnesyl pyrophosphate are then condensed together to form squalene, which is triterpene. (An example of a non-steroidal C-30 triterpene is α-amyrin (see Fig. 10.3).) A hydrogen atom, Hc, is removed from one but not the other of the farnesyl pyrophosphate molecules and is replaced with a H from NADPH. The enzyme is called squalene synthetase.

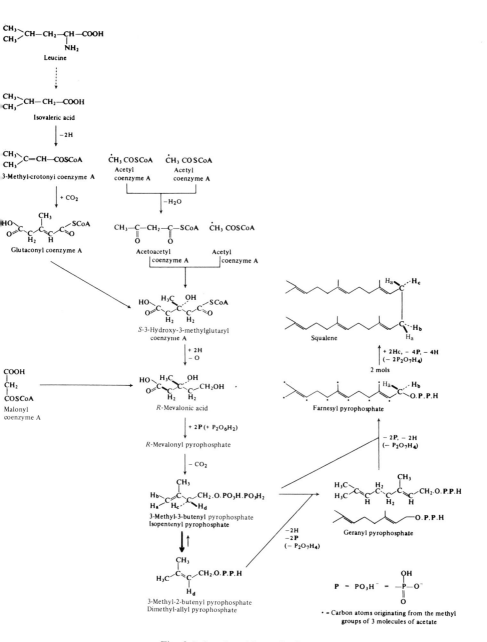

Fig. 3.2. Squalene biosynthesis.

B. CYCLIZATION OF SQUALENE TO LANOSTEROL

In animals and yeasts it has been firmly established that lanosterol is the triterpene that is converted to cholesterol and ergosterol respectively. In the higher plants and algae there is good evidence that cycloartenol is the product of cyclization of squalene. Molecular oxygen and TPNH are required for the first stage of the cyclization step and a monoepoxide, 2,3-oxidosqualene is formed. The cyclization can be represented as beginning with the uptake of one H and ending with expulsion of another (Fig. 3.3). The enzyme for this second stage, 2,3-oxidosqualene cyclase, has been isolated from liver microsomes. The stereochemical change is attributed to a specific type of folding imposed by the enzyme upon the long hydrocarbon chain and the stereochemistry of the final product is also due to a series of stereospecific rearrangements following cyclization, e.g. the methyl groups at C-18 and attached to C-14, together with the hydrogen atoms at C-13 and C-17, undergo a concerted *trans*-migration. There are two 1,2-methyl shifts, the methyl group at C-8 of the intermediate cation going to C-14 and that at C-14 going to C-13 to form the C-18 methyl group of lanosterol.

C. DEGRADATION OF LANOSTEROL TO CHOLESTEROL

This process is shown in Figs. 3.3 and 3.4. The essential steps are the removal of three ring methyl groups (the *gem*-dimethyl group at C-14 and the α-methyl group at C-14), together with the addition of 2H at C-24 and the shift of the ring double bond from C-8 to C-5. The main pathway is believed to be via zymosterol, 7,24(5α)-cholestadien-3β-ol and desmosterol, i.e. the three methyl groups are removed first, the ring double bond shifts, and then 2H is added at C-24. If these reactions take place in a different order, the other intermediates shown in Fig. 3.4 are produced. An important alternative pathway appears to be via zymosterol and lathosterol. The carbon atoms of the methyl and carboxyl groups of the original three molecules of acetate can be traced through to their final positions in cholesterol as shown. Cholesterol is believed to be the principle starting molecule for steroid hormone biosynthesis in animals but desmosterol and lathosterol may also be utilized in significant quantities.

The mechanisms of the reactions involved in the conversion of lanosterol to cholesterol are still being elucidated. It is believed that CH_2 at C-14 is removed first via oxidation to carboxyl and the loss of the hydrogen atom from C-15, together with one from the carboxyl group. Carbon dioxide is then eliminated to give 4,4'-dimethyl-cholesta-8,14,24-trien-3β-ol, to which 2H is readded to form 4,4'-dimethyl-cholesta-8,24-dien-3β-ol.

Each removal of a CH_2 group from C-4 requires the prior removal of 2H from the adjacent ring CH.OH group to form a keto group. The removal of CH_2 then takes place in three oxidation steps, which require molecular oxygen, i.e. oxidation to aldehydic and carboxylic derivatives and then the elimination of

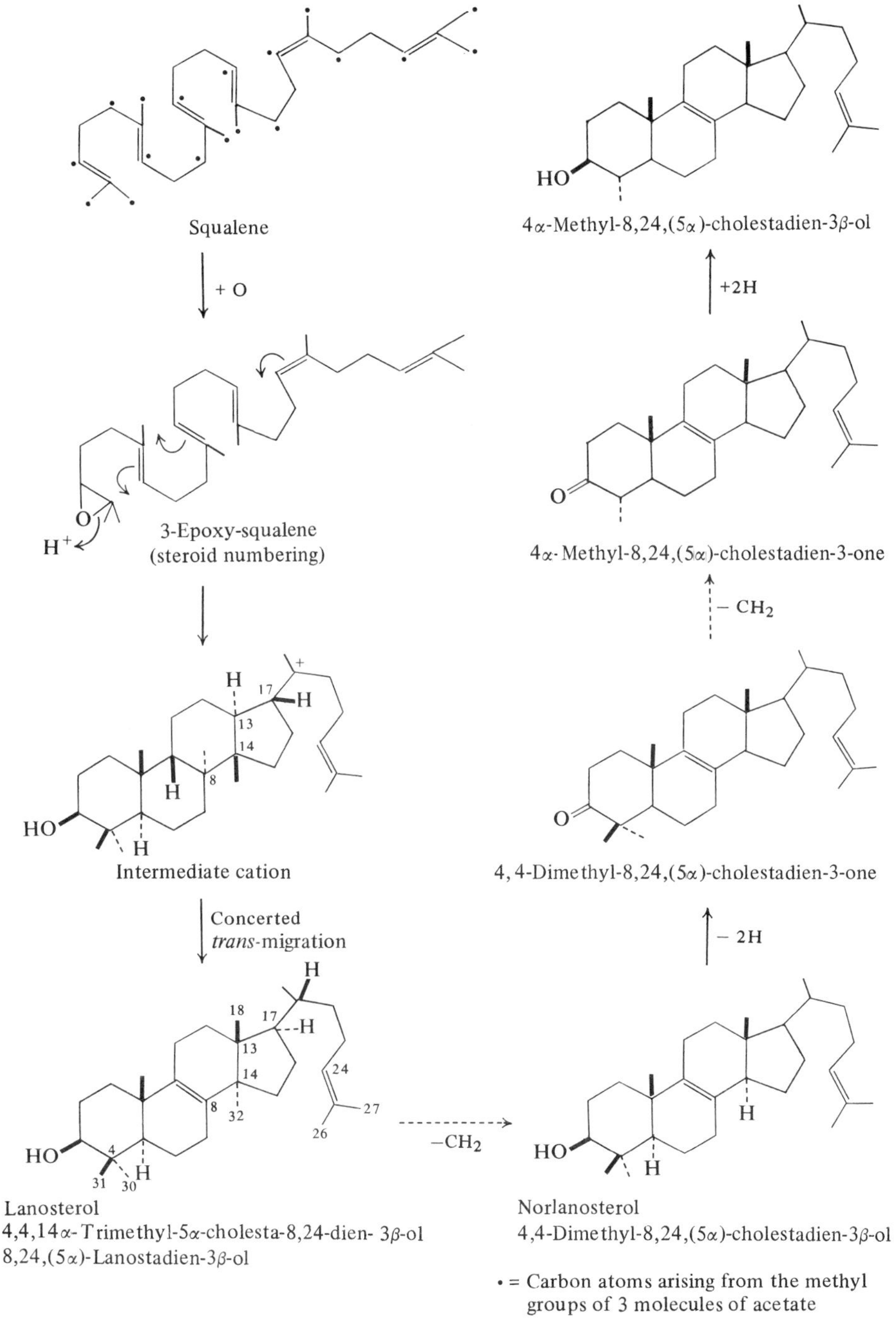

Fig. 3.3. Squalene to cholesterol-Part 1.

Squalene

$+ O$

3-Epoxy-squalene
(steroid numbering)

H^+

Intermediate cation

Concerted
trans-migration

Lanosterol
4,4,14α-Trimethyl-5α-cholesta-8,24-dien-3β-ol
8,24,(5α)-Lanostadien-3β-ol

$-CH_2$

Norlanosterol
4,4-Dimethyl-8,24,(5α)-cholestadien-3β-ol

• = Carbon atoms arising from the methyl
groups of 3 molecules of acetate

$-2H$

4,4-Dimethyl-8,24,(5α)-cholestadien-3-one

$-CH_2$

4α-Methyl-8,24,(5α)-cholestadien-3-one

$+2H$

4α-Methyl-8,24,(5α)-cholestadien-3β-ol

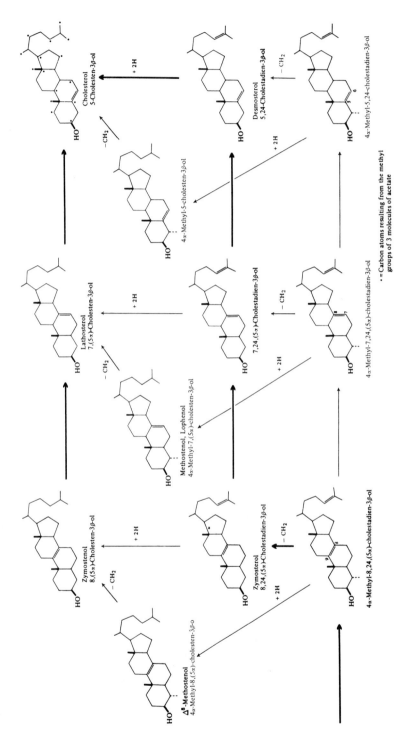

Fig. 3.4. Squalene to cholesterol-Part 2.

* = Carbon atoms resulting from the methyl groups of 3 molecules of acetate

Cholesterol
5-Cholesten-3β-ol

Desmosterol
5,24-Cholestadien-3β-ol

4α-Methyl-5,24-cholestadien-3β-ol

4α-Methyl-5-cholesten-3β-ol

+ 2H

− CH₂

− CH₂

+ 2H

Lathosterol
7,(5α)-Cholesten-3β-ol

7,24,(5α)-Cholestadien-3β-ol

4α-Methyl-7,24,(5α)-cholestadien-3β-ol

Methostenol, Lophenol
4α-Methyl-7,(5α)-cholesten-3β-ol

+ 2H

− CH₂

+ 2H

− CH₂

Zymostenol
8,(5α)-Cholesten-3β-ol

Zymosterol
8,24,(5α)-Cholestadien-3β-ol

4α-Methyl-8,24,(5α)-cholestadien-3β-ol

Δ⁸-Methostenol
4α-Methyl-8,(5α)-cholesten-3β-o

+ 2H

− CH₂

− CH₂

+ 2H

carbon dioxide. The 3β-hydroxyl group is then reformed by the readdition of 2H. It is believed that the β-methyl group is removed first. The intermediate 3-ketones in these reactions are not shown in Fig. 3.4.

The shift of the ring double bond from C-8 to C-5 takes place in two steps, the first being an anaerobic isomerase reaction to convert the Δ^8-sterol to the Δ^7-sterol. Conversion to the Δ^5-sterol requires molecular oxygen, hydroxylation probably occurring at C-6β. A *trans*-diaxial elimination of H_2O could then produce the known intermediate (between 7,24(5α)-cholestadien-3β-ol and desmosterol) of 7-dehydrocholesterol (5,7,24,(5α)-cholestatrien-3β-ol, i.e. a 5,7-dienol). Subsequent reduction to the Δ^5-sterol requires TPNH.

III. DEGRADATION OF CHOLESTEROL TO CORTICOIDS, ANDROGENS AND ESTROGENS

A. FORMATION OF PREGNENOLONE FROM CHOLESTEROL

Cholesterol is converted to pregnenolone by enzyme systems present in adrenocortical mitochondria and there is evidence that 20α-hydroxycholesterol and 20α,22R-dihydroxycholesterol are intermediates as shown in Fig. 3.5. The supply of pregnenolone for steroid biosynthesis appears to be rate limiting and it is reasonable to regard the conversion of cholesterol to pregnenolone as a control point for the whole steroid biosynthetic process. The stimulation of corticosteroid biosynthesis by ACTH takes place between cholesterol and pregnenolone and the precise point appears to be the 20α-hydroxylation of cholesterol which is the slow rate-limiting step. Thus, ACTH reduces the store of cholesterol and its esters in the tissue which synthesizes steroid. A single enzyme, 20α,22-hydroxylase seems to be responsible. The splitting of the side chain of 20α,22R-dihydroxycholesterol to form pregnenolone and isocaproic aldehyde (isolated as isocaproic acid) is mediated by the enzyme 20α,22-C-27-desmolase (pregnenolone synthetase). The mechanism appears to be an initial enzymatic removal of a hydride ion from the C-20α hydroxy group, then a double shift of electrons with the expulsion of a proton from the C-22 hydroxyl group. The entire process probably occurs in a concerted action with breakage of the 20-22 carbon-to-carbon bond.

B. 17α,20-C-21-DESMOLASE AND 10,19-DESMOLASE

Figure 3.5 shows that the essential steps for the biosynthesis of androgens and estrogens from pregnenolone is the action of two further desmolase enzymes. The androgen series is initiated by 17α,20-C-21-desmolase which splits acetaldehyde (isolated as acetate) from 17α-hydroxyprogesterone. (Androgens may also be synthesized from pregnenolone and 17α-hydroxypregnenolone but these are probably minor pathways.) The mechanism of action appears to be similar to that of 20α,22-C-27-desmolase and also requires NADPH and mole-

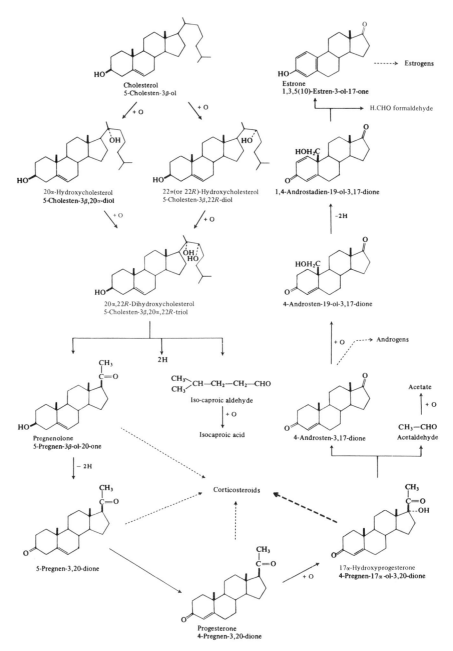

Fig. 3.5. Main pathway of steroid hormone biosynthesis from cholesterol.

cular oxygen. There is evidence for a 17H,20-C-21-desmolase which splits progesterone without prior conversion to 17α-hydroxyprogesterone.

The essential step for estrogen biosynthesis appears to be 19-hydroxylation of 4-androstan-3,17-dione followed by the action of 10,19-desmolase (estrogen synthetase) with the elimination of formaldehyde. There is evidence that the 1β-hydrogen atom is eliminated preferentially in the aromatization process.

IV. BIOSYNTHESIS AND METABOLISM OF CORTICOSTEROIDS
A. BIOSYNTHESIS OF CORTISONE AND 11-DEHYDROCORTICOSTERONE

The adrenal corticosteroids are formed from pregnenolone, 5-pregnen-3,20-dione, progesterone and 17α-hydroxyprogesterone as shown in Figs. 3.6 and 3.7. The main pathway is believed to be pregnenolone → 5-pregnen-3,20-dione → progesterone → 17α-hydroxyprogesterone → cortexolone → cortisol → cortisone, with the principal secondary pathway being from progesterone → cortexone → corticosterone → 11-dehydrocorticosterone. The principal steroids occurring in excess in adrenal vein blood are:

1. cortisol;
2. cortisone;
3. 11-dehydrocorticosterone;
4. cortexolone;
5. corticosterone.

The principal corticoid synthetic products of adrenal cortex are cortisol and corticosterone, with minor amounts of cortexolone. Cortisone and 11-dehydrocorticosterone are probably inert metabolites. Many other mammals, e.g. rat, mouse, rabbit, produce mainly the 11-oxo-compounds. The complexities of the pathways in Figs. 3.6 and 3.7 are due to alternative sequences of the same basic enzymatic reactions. The enzymes involved with examples of their actions are:

1. Δ^5-3β-hydroxy-steroid dehydrogenase
e.g. pregnenolone → 5-pregnen-3, 20-dione;

2. Δ^5-Δ^4-isomerase
e.g. 5-pregnen-3, 20-dione → progesterone.

Previously these two enzymes were thought to be identical as the oxidation of the 3β-hydroxyl group is much slower than the transfer of a proton from C-4 to C-6. The latter reaction was thought to be spontaneous but the enzyme responsible has now been separated from the dehydrogenase. The reaction is irreversible:

3. 17α-steroid hydroxylase
e.g. progesterone → 17α-hydroxyprogesterone;

4. 21-steroid hydroxylase
e.g. 17α-hydroxyprogesterone → cortexolone
e.g. progesterone → cortexone;

5. 11β-steroid hydroxylase
e.g. cortexolone → cortisol
e.g. cortexone → corticosterone.

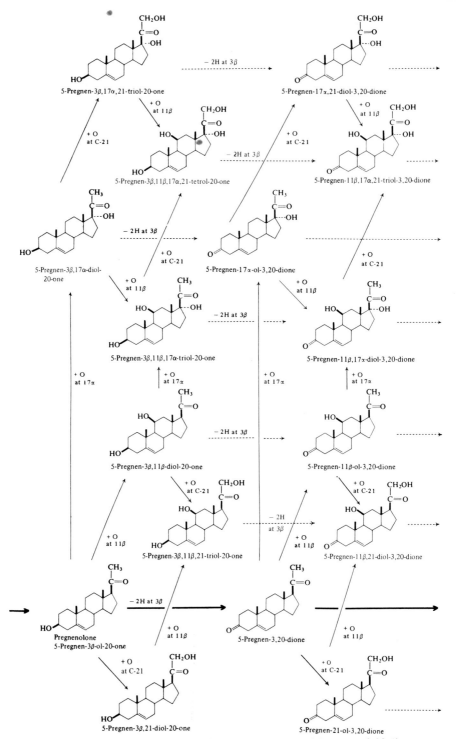

Fig. 3.6. Corticosteroid biosynthesis from pregnenolone and 5-pregnen-3,20-dione.

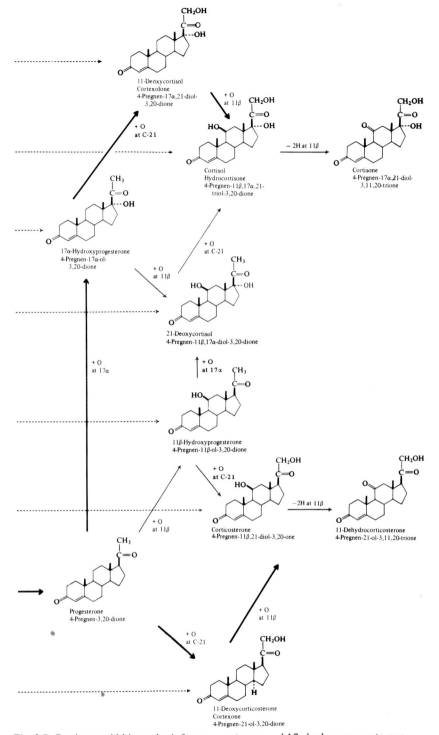

Fig. 3.7. Corticosteroid biosynthesis from progesterone and 17α-hydroxyprogesterone.

These three hydroxylases require NADPH and molecular oxygen. The 17α- and 21-hydroxylases are associated with the adrenal microsomal fractions and the 11β-hydroxylase with the adrenal mitochondrial fraction. The 17α- and 11β-hydroxylases are stereospecific in that only one of the possible two hydroxy compounds is produced. This is a constant feature of steroid biosynthesis and metabolism, as is the retention of configuration. Progesterone may be hydroxylated in a variety of positions, but a definite sequence appears to be obligatory in man, e.g. 17α-hydroxylation may not follow 21-hydroxylation. When 21-hydroxylation precedes 11β-hydroxylation some corticosterone is formed:

> 6. 11β-steroid dehydrogenase
> e.g. cortisol → cortisone
> e.g. corticosterone → 11-dehydrocorticosterone

This oxidative enzyme appears to be in the microsomal fraction and requires NADP.

B. THE REICHSTEIN SUBSTANCES AND CORTICOSTEROID METABOLITES

Figures 3.8-3.11 show the further biosynthesis and metabolism of the corticosteroids by the addition of 2H at Δ^4 to form the 5α- and 5β-pregnanes, mediated by Δ^4-reductases. In general, Δ^4-5α-reductase occurs in the adrenal glands and produces 5α-pregnanes by a stereospecific process. These are the Reichstein substances, named after the scientist who discovered them in the adrenal gland. (There are two further series of compounds named after Kendall and after Wintersteiner, but the three systems overlap considerably.) These substances are minor metabolic products of no biological importance, although they have the flat ring structure of the allo series. A list is given in Table 3.1.

Δ^4-5β-Reductase occurs in the liver and produces the 5β-pregnanes, also stereospecifically. These compounds and their metabolites appear in the urine. The 5β-pregnanes belong to the normal series and represent the inert metabolites. It is believed that there are Δ^4-5α-reductases and Δ^4-5β-reductases specific for each substrate. The reduction of the 4-5 double bond in liver appears to determine the rate at which the steroids are inactivated. The reaction is irreversible, NADPH is the H donor and fluctuations in liver NADPH concentrations *in vivo* appear to be great enough to alter the rate of steroid double bond reduction. There appears to be more activity in female livers. Cortisol and aldosterone go mainly to the 5β-pregnanes, as does progesterone but not quite so exclusively. Corticosterone and testosterone form the 5β- and 5α-pregnanes in approximately equal amounts.

The 5α and 5β-pregnanes undergo further reduction, mediated by the following enzymes:

> 1. 3α- and 3β-dehydrogenases (working in reverse). These are different stereospecific enzymes which reduce the 5α- and 5β-pregnanes to the

Table 3.1. *Reichstein, Kendall and Wintersteiner substances found in the adrenal glands*

	Reichstein	Kendall	Wintersteiner
5α-Pregnane-3β,11β,17α,20β,21-pentol	A	D	A
5α-Pregnane-3α,11β,17α,21-tetrol-20-one	C	C	D
5α-Pregnane-3β,11β,17α,21-tetrol-20-one	V		
5α-Pregnane-3β,17α,21-triol-11,20-dione	D	G	B
4-Pregnene-11β,17α,20β,21-tetrol-3-one	E		
4-Pregnene-17α,20β,21-triol-3,11-dione	U		
4-Pregnene-11β,17α,21-triol-3,20-dione (cortisol)	M	F	
4-Pregnene-17α,21-diol-3,11,20-trione (cortisone)	F	E	F
5α-Pregnane-3β,17α,20β,21-tetrol	K		
5α-Pregnane-3β,17α,21-triol-20-one	P		
5α-Pregnane-3β,11β,21-triol-20-one	R		
5α-Pregnane-3β,21-diol-11,20-dione	N	H	
4-Pregnene-17α,21-diol-3,20-dione (cortexolone)	S		
4-Pregnene-20β,21-diol-3,11-dione	T		
4-Pregnene-11β,21-diol-3,20-dione (corticosterone)	H	B	
4-Pregnen-21-ol-3,11,20-trione (11-dehydrocorticosterone)		A	
5α-Pregnane-3β,17α,20β-triol	J		
5α-Pregnane-3β,17α,20α-triol	O		
5α-Pregnane-3β,17α-diol-20-one	L		G
4-Pregen-21-ol-3,20-dione	Q		

3-hydroxy compounds, producing unequal mixtures of 3α- and 3β-hydroxy groups.

e.g. dihydrocortisol → urocortisol, producing more of the 3α-hydroxy compound, allo-dihydrocortisol → Reichstein V and Reichstein C. More of Reichstein V, i.e. the 3β-hydroxy compound is produced.

2. 20α- and 20β-dehydrogenases (working in reverse).

e.g. urocortisol → cortol and β-cortol, Reichstein V → Reichstein A and Reichstein epi-A. When acting on 5β-pregnanes, this enzyme produces more of 20α-hydroxyl compound, i.e. cortol. When acting on 5α-pregnanes, this enzyme produces more of the 20β-hydroxyl compound, i.e. Reichstein A.

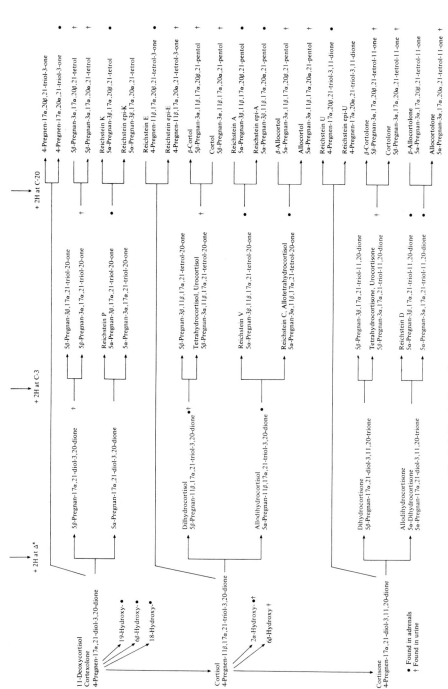

Fig. 3.8. Metabolism of cortexolone, cortisol and cortisone.

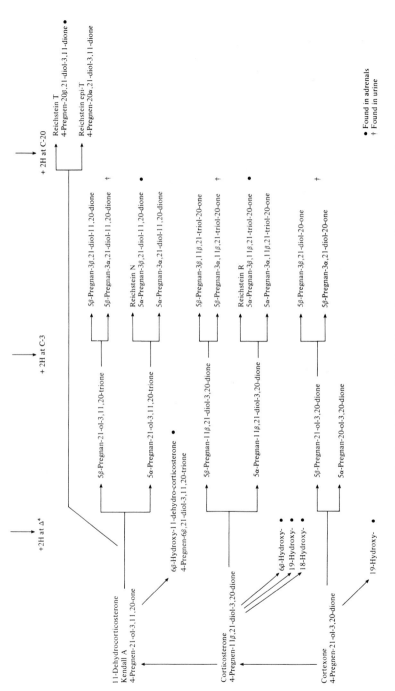

Fig. 3.9. Metabolism of 11-dehydrocorticosterone, corticosterone and cortexone.

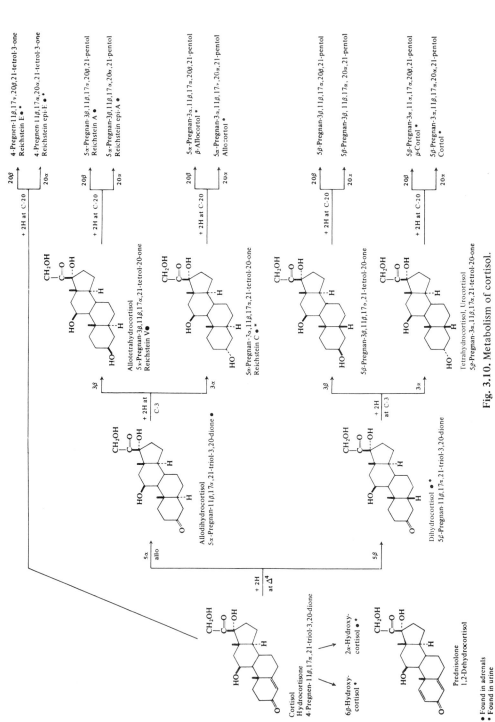

Fig. 3.10. Metabolism of cortisol.

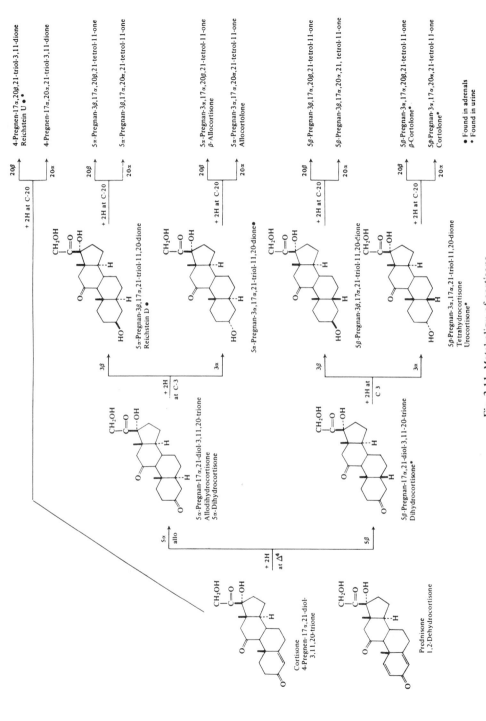

Fig. 3.11. Metabolism of cortisone.

The adrenal glands also contain 6β-hydroxy-, 19-hydroxy- and 18-hydroxy-steroid hydroxylases.

In the liver the principle hydroxy-steroid dehydrogenases and oxo-reductases act on the 3-ketone, 11β-hydroxyl, 17β-hydroxy and 20-ketone groups. By convention when the reduction is reversible, the enzyme is called a dehydrogenase and when it is irreversible it is called an oxo-reductase. The reduction of a 3-ketone produces almost exclusively the 3α-hydroxy derivative usually preceded by reduction of the 4-5 double bond but substituents at C-2 and C-6 increase the liability of 3-ketone reduction to occur prior to 4-5 double bond reduction. The enzyme occurs in the microsomal fraction, is NADH dependent and of low substrate specificity. Reduction of the 20-ketone group is irreversible. Up to a third of the urinary metabolites of cortisol and progesterone are 20-hydroxy-derivatives, mainly 20α. The 20-oxo-reductase is also present in kidney and muscle which requires NADPH. Most of the corticosteroid metabolites are excreted in urine conjugated as the glucuronosides.

C. BIOSYNTHESIS AND METABOLISM OF ALDOSTERONE

Figure 3.12 shows the pathways to aldosterone. The main pathway appears to be progesterone → 11-deoxycorticosterone → corticosterone → 18-hydroxy-corticosterone → aldosterone. However, all the precursors can undergo 18-hydroxylation, which is the essential step. Aldosterone biosynthesis takes place in different cells of the adrenal gland to those involved in the synthesis of the other corticosteroids described previously. It is not under the exclusive control of ACTH but is controlled by the kidneys, via the renin-angiotensin system. Urinary metabolites of aldosterone are shown in Figs. 3.12 and 8.2.

D. METABOLISM OF PROGESTERONE AND 17α-HYDROXY-PROGESTERONE

Figures 3.13-3.15 show the essential steps in this process, which are the same as the metabolic processes of the corticosteroids, namely production of mainly the 5β-pregnanes, the 3α-hydroxy-compounds and the 20α-hydroxy-compounds. The principle urinary metabolites are pregnanolone, pregnanediol and pregnanetriol. The metabolism of progesterone and 17α-hydroxyprogesterone in extrahepatic, non-endocrine tissues, e.g. uterus, appears to be different, the main metabolites being 5α-pregnanes with 3α- and 20α-hydroxyl groups.

V. BIOSYNTHESIS AND METABOLISM OF THE ANDROGENS

Figures 3.16 and 3.17 show the pathways involved from 4-androsten-3,17-dione which is formed by desmolase action from 17α-hydroxyprogesterone. Similar desmolase actions can occur from pregnenolone, when the product is dehydroepiandrosterone, and from 5-pregnen-3,17-dione. These two alternative pathways of androgen biosynthesis have been shown to exist in adrenals, testes, ovaries, the theca and granulosa cells of the human follicle, and in the ovarian

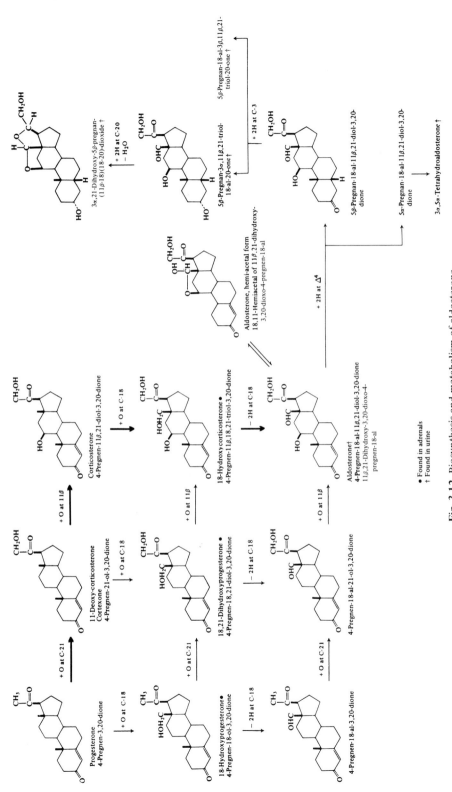

Fig. 3.12. Biosynthesis and metabolism of aldosterone.

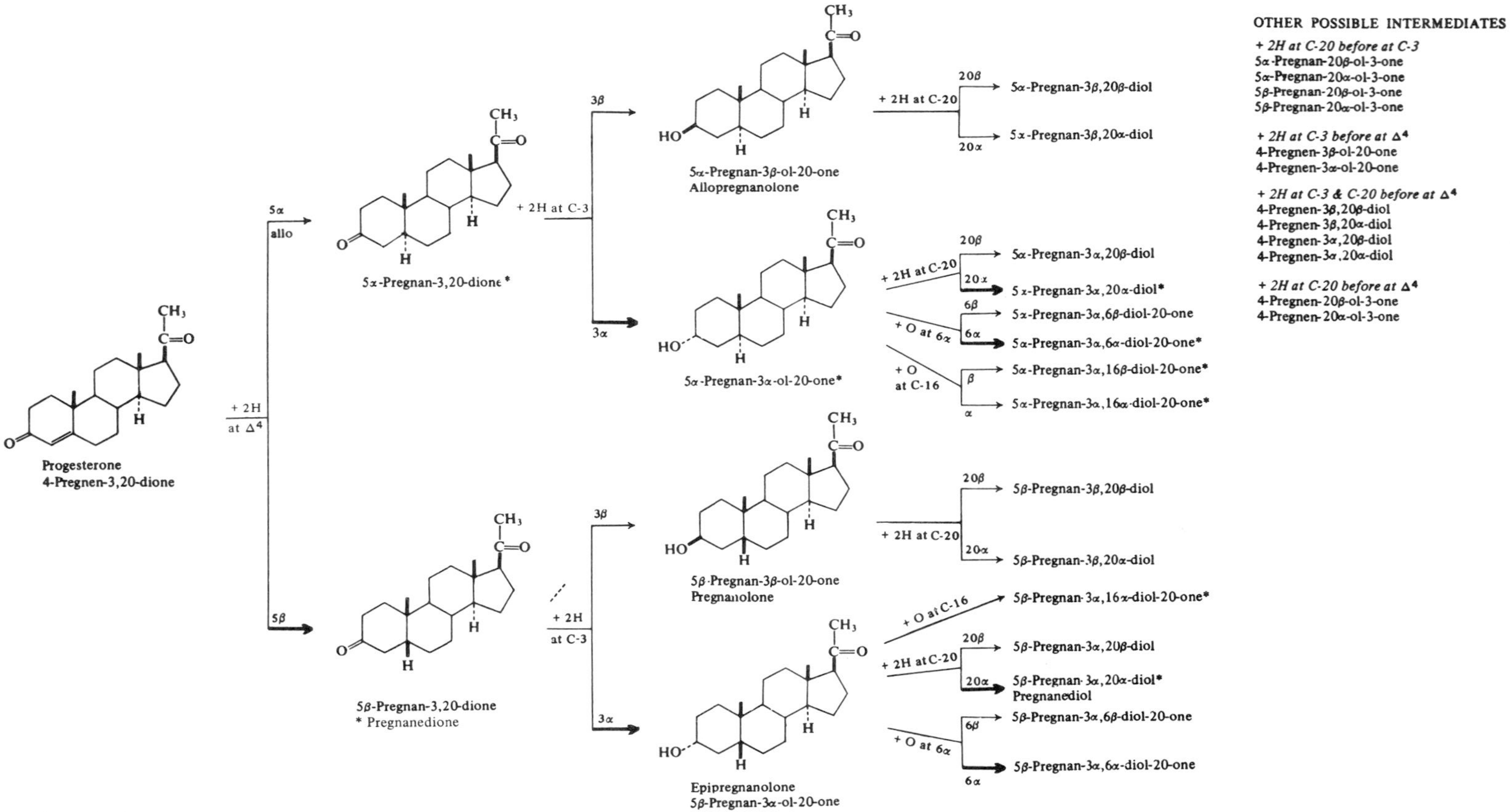
Progesterone
4-Pregnen-3,20-dione
+ 2H
at Δ4
5α
allo
5β
5α-Pregnan-3,20-dione *
5β-Pregnan-3,20-dione
* Pregnanedione
+ 2H at C-3
3β
3α
5α-Pregnan-3β-ol-20-one
Allopregnanolone
5α-Pregnan-3α-ol-20-one*
5β-Pregnan-3β-ol-20-one
Pregnanolone
Epipregnanolone
5β-Pregnan-3α-ol-20-one
+ 2H at C-20
20β
20α
5α-Pregnan-3β,20β-diol
5α-Pregnan-3β,20α-diol
5α-Pregnan-3α,20β-diol
5α-Pregnan-3α,20α-diol*
+ O at 6α
6β
6α
5α-Pregnan-3α,6β-diol-20-one
5α-Pregnan-3α,6α-diol-20-one*
+ O
at C-16
β
α
5α-Pregnan-3α,16β-diol-20-one*
5α-Pregnan-3α,16α-diol-20-one*
5β-Pregnan-3β,20β-diol
5β-Pregnan-3β,20α-diol
+ O at C-16
5β-Pregnan-3α,16α-diol-20-one*
5β-Pregnan-3α,20β-diol
5β-Pregnan-3α,20α-diol*
Pregnanediol
5β-Pregnan-3α,6β-diol-20-one
5β-Pregnan-3α,6α-diol-20-one
OTHER POSSIBLE INTERMEDIATES
+ 2H at C-20 before at C-3
5α-Pregnan-20β-ol-3-one
5α-Pregnan-20α-ol-3-one
5β-Pregnan-20β-ol-3-one
5β-Pregnan-20α-ol-3-one
+ 2H at C-3 before at Δ4
4-Pregnen-3β-ol-20-one
4-Pregnen-3α-ol-20-one
+ 2H at C-3 & C-20 before at Δ4
4-Pregnen-3β,20β-diol
4-Pregnen-3β,20α-diol
4-Pregnen-3α,20β-diol
4-Pregnen-3α,20α-diol
+ 2H at C-20 before at Δ4
4-Pregnen-20β-ol-3-one
4-Pregnen-20α-ol-3-one

* Found in urine

Fig. 3.13. Metabolism of progesterone.

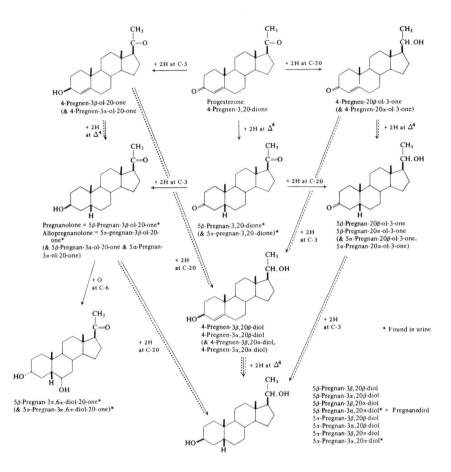

Fig. 3.14. Metabolism of progesterone showing all the theoretical intermediates.

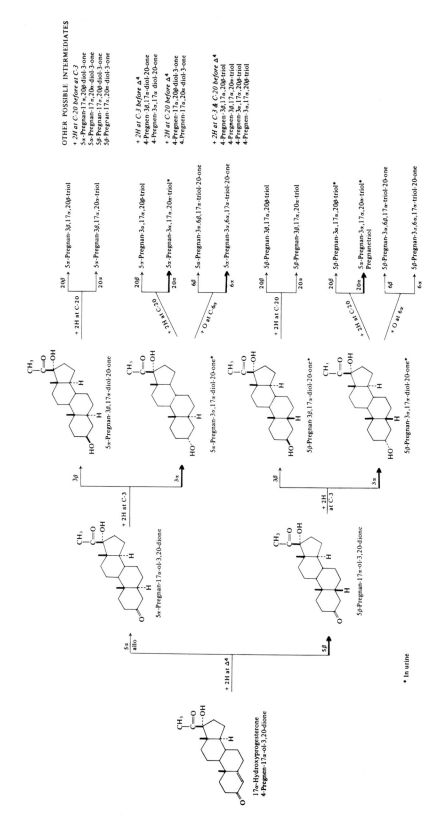

Fig. 3.15. Metabolism of 17α-hydroxyprogesterone.

stroma. In contrast, only the first pathway seems to be involved in the biosynthesis of estrogens in the corpus luteum of the human. The bulk of the dehydroepiandrosterone is secreted as the sulphate but this conjugate is formed reversibly. The adrenal androgens have an 11β-hydroxy group, being products of desmolase action on cortisol. The principal androgens secreted by the adrenal cortex are androstenedione and 11β-hydroxyandrostenedione. The adrenals also secrete quite large amounts of dehydroepiandrosterone sulphate which acts as an androgen precursor and itself has an activity of 10% of that of testosterone. Recently an enzyme has been discovered in the calf testis which is capable of converting cholesterol directly to dehydroepiandrosterone and 2-methylheptan-6-one without the intermediate formation of pregnenolone. The cholesterol side chain is cleaved between C-17 and C-20.

In man there are two pathways of testosterone metabolism. One involves primarily the oxidation of the 17β-hydroxy group by a 17β-hydroxysteroid dehydrogenase to produce androstenedione which is further reduced to 5α- and 5β-androstanedione and then to androsterone, isoandrosterone and 5β-androsterone. These are excreted in the urine as sulphates and glucuronosides. The second pathway involves a direct reduction of testosterone by specific Δ^4-3-ketosteroid 5α- and 5β-reductases and a specific 3α-hydroxysteroid dehydrogenase. The end products are 5α- and 5β-androstanediols which are conjugated with glucuronic acid. The relative importance of the two pathways depends on the activity of the specific enzymes known to be present in hepatic and extrahepatic tissues (prostate, skin, etc.). Dihydrotestosterone is possibly a more potent androgen than testosterone and may be the biologically active androgen.

VI. BIOSYNTHESIS AND METABOLISM OF THE ESTROGENS

Figure 3.18 shows the pathways to and from estrone. The main pathway from 4-androsten-19-ol-3,17-dione appears to be via 1,4-androstadien-19-ol-3,17-dione, i.e. Δ^1-reductase action takes place before 10,19-desmolase action. However, 19-nor-4-androsten-3,17-dione remains as an alternative pathway to estrone and estradiol. Metabolism in the liver is mainly hydroxylation at C-2, C-6 and C-16 with estrone as the principal substrate. No reduction of the aromatic rings appears to take place.

VII. STEROID DEHYDROGENASES AND HYDROXYLASES

From the preceding metabolic pathways it can be seen that the principal reactions involved in steroid biosynthesis and metabolism are the addition or removal of 2H by dehydrogenases and the addition of molecular oxygen by hydroxylases. Two complete sets of stereospecific enzymes exist—those in the steroid-synthesizing tissues which make the steroids, and those in the steroid-degrading tissues, mainly the liver and kidney, which degrade the same steroids.

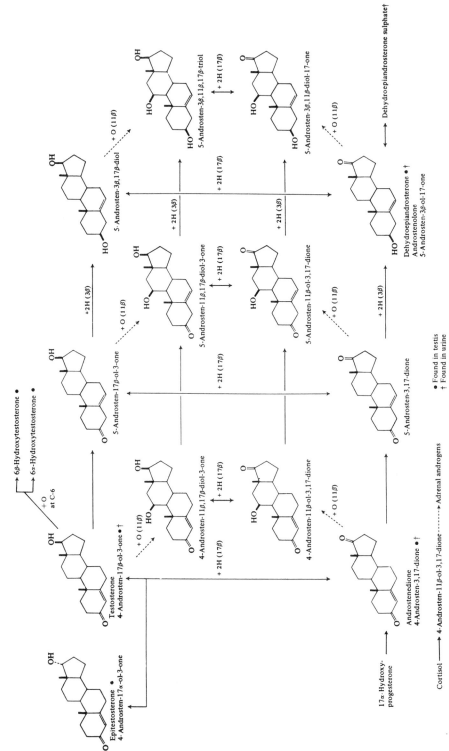

Fig. 3.16. Biosynthesis of androgens (androstenes).

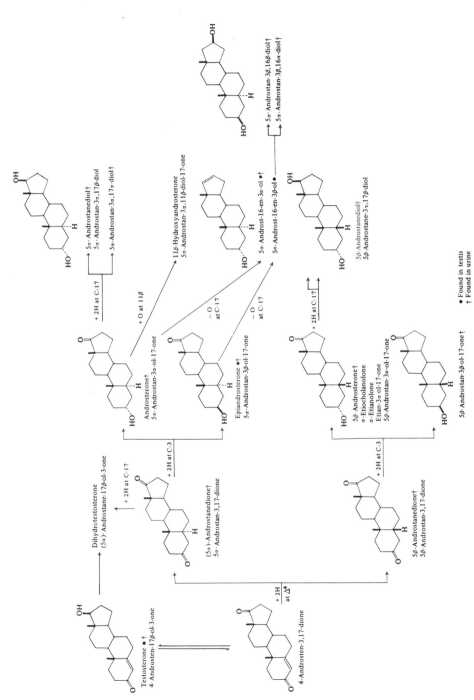

Fig. 3.17. Metabolism of the androgens (androstanes).

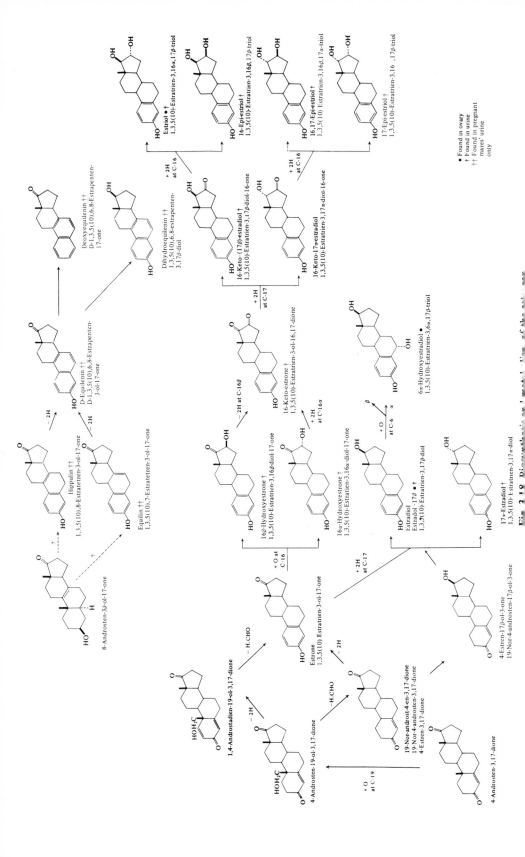

Deoxyequilenin ††
D-1,3,5(10),6,8-Estrapenten-17-one

Estriol • †
1,3,5(10)-Estratrien-3,16α,17β-triol

16-Epi-estriol †
1,3,5(10)-Estratrien-3,16β,17β-triol

16,17-Epi-estriol †
1,3,5(10)-Estratrien-3,16β,17α-triol

17-Epi-estriol †
1,3,5(10)-Estratrien-3,16 ,17β-triol

Dihydroequilenin ††
1,3,5(10),6,8-estrapenten-3,17β-diol

16-Keto-(17β)-estradiol †
1,3,5(10)-Estratrien-3,17β-diol-16-one

16-Keto-17α-estradiol
1,3,5(10)-Estratrien-3,17α-diol-16-one

+ 2H at C-16

+ 2H at C-16

D-Equilenin ††
D-1,3,5(10),6,8-Estrapenten-3-ol-17-one

Hippulin ††
1,3,5(10),8-Estratetren-3-ol-17-one

Equilin ††
1,3,5(10),7-Estratetren-3-ol-17-one

− 2H

2H

8-Androsten-3β-ol-17-one

16-Keto-estrone †
1,3,5(10)-Estratrien-3-ol-16,17-dione

− 2H at C-16β

+ 2H at C-16α

+ 2H at C-17

16β-Hydroxyestrone †
1,3,5(10)-Estratrien-3,16β-diol-17-one

16α-Hydroxyestrone †
1,3,5(10)-Estratrien-3,16α-diol-17-one

6α-Hydroxyestradiol •
1,3,5(10)-Estratrien-3,6α,17β-triol

β
+ O at C-6
α

+ O at C-16

+ 2H at C-17

Estradiol-17β • †
1,3,5(10)-Estratrien-3,17β-diol

17α-Estradiol †
1,3,5(10)-Estratrien-3,17α-diol

Estrone
1,3,5(10)-Estratrien-3-ol-17-one

− H.CHO

− 2H

1,4-Androstadien-19-ol-3,17-dione

− H.CHO

19-Nor-androst-4-en-3,17-dione
19-Nor-4-androsten-3,17-dione
4-Estren-3,17-dione

4-Estren-17β-ol-3-one
19-Nor-4-androsten-17β-ol-3-one

+ O at C-19

4-Androsten-19-ol-3,17-dione

4-Androsten-3,17-dione

• Found in ovary
† Found in urine
†† Found in pregnant mares' urine only

Fig. 2.19 Biosynthesis and metabolism of the estrogens

The pathway for electron transport in steroid 11β-hydroxylation and probably also in 18, 20 and 22-hydroxylations in adrenal mitochondria is:

$$\text{NADPH} \rightarrow \text{F}_{PT} \rightarrow \text{NHFe-P} \rightarrow \text{cytochrome P450} \xrightarrow[\substack{\text{Steroid} \\ O_2 \\ 2H^+}]{} \text{hydroxysteroid} + H_2O.$$

This pathway is believed to be connected to the respiratory chain by an energy-linked nicotinamide nucleotide transhydrogenase. Also, under certain conditions, an energy-linked reversal of electron transport in the respiratory chain contributes reducing equivalents to the hydroxylating enzymes via the nicotinamide nucleotide transhydrogenase. In adrenal mitochondria the steroid hydroxylating pathway and the respiratory chain are believed to be inter-related as:

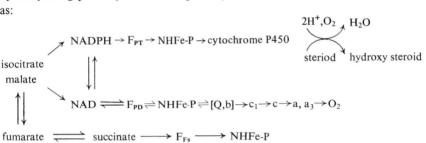

where F_{PT} = NADPH-specific flavoprotein dehydrogenase and NHFe-P = a non-haem iron protein. P450 must cycle between reduced and oxidized forms in order to activate successive molecules of O_2 required for hydroxylation. A possible explanation is shown below:

$$\text{P450Fe}^{2+}\!\!-\!\!O_2 \xrightleftharpoons{O_2} \text{P450Fe}^{2+} \xrightleftharpoons{CO} \text{P450Fe}^{2+}\text{CO}$$

e^-

hydroxysteroid
$+H_2O$ P450Fe^{3+}

$2H^+$
e^- steroid

$\text{P450Fe}^{3+}\!\!-\!\!E_1\!\!-\!\!S$ $\text{P450Fe}^{3+}\!\!-\!\!E_1\!\!-\!\!S$

O_2^- O_2

$\text{P450Fe}^{2+}\!\!-\!\!E_1\!\!-\!\!S$

CO

$\text{P450Fe}^{2+}\!\!-\!\!E_1\!\!-\!\!S$
$|$
CO

The non-haem iron protein (NHFe-P) supplies electrons (e^-) to $P450Fe^{3+}$ via the hydroxylating pathway, allowing reduced P450 to react with either O_2 or CO. Steroid substrate (S) then reacts with oxidized P450 only. Additional specific enzymes (E_1, E_2, etc.) have been postulated to interact with either the $P450Fe^{3+}$ complex or the steroid before its interaction with $P450Fe^{3+}$. Automatic oxidation of reduced P450 could take place at several points in the cycle. Carbon monoxide interferes with the cycle by competition with O_2. It is assumed that an intracomplex transfer of the first electron occurs (shown by the reoxidized form of P450 with the incompletely reduced oxygen attached) so that the second reducing equivalent from NHFe-P can be accepted. One oxygen atom is transferred to the appropriate site on the steroid, while the other, having received the two electrons, accepts two protons from the medium and is split off from water. The cycle is now complete and can be repeated since free, oxidized P450 has been regenerated.

The hydroxylation steps have the characteristic of the "mixed function oxidases" in that there are two substrates (NADPH and the steroid) both of which are oxidized. Molecular oxygen is the source of hydroxyl oxygen, and hydrogen in the steric position to be hydroxylated is displaced. The NADPH reduces a flavoprotein, which may be a dehydrogenase. The flavoprotein reduces a ferridoxin-like non-haem protein which has been called adrenodoxin and this in turn reduces a haemprotein, cytochrome P450. At this stage one atom of molecular oxygen is reduced to water by the reduced cytochrome P450 and the other is involved in the steroid hydroxylation.

VIII. CONJUGATION

Steroids are often excreted as the sulphates or glucuronosides. In liver, two systems for the formation of sulphates appear to exist, one for the estrogens and one for the 3β-hydroxysteroids. The sulphokinases appear to utilize $3'$- phospho-adenosine-$5'$-phosphosulphate (PAPS) as sulphate donor and require ATP and Mg. Glucuronosides are formed from the active glucuronoside donor, uridine diphosphoglucuronic acid, and are catalysed by a glucuronosyl transferase present in liver microsomes. Uridine diphosphate is liberated.

In addition to excretion in the urine and circulation in the blood, steroid sulphates have been found in many organs of the body. All endocrine glands which can synthesize steroids, can also sulphate steroids, especially the adrenal gland. Dehydroepiandrosterone sulphate is an important secretory product of the adrenals in both males and females. It is now believed that circulating steroid sulphates are not inert metabolic products but have important biological effects. Dehydroepiandrosterone sulphate is metabolized without prior cleavage of the sulphate moiety and appears in the urine as $3\beta,17\beta$-dihydroxyandrost-5-ene-3-sulphate, the 3,17-disulphate, 16α-hydroxydehydroepiandrostene sulphate, and

3β,17β,16α-trihydroxyandrost-5-ene-3-sulphate. It is also believed to be synthesized in small amounts directly from cholesterol sulphate via pregnenolone sulphate and 17α-hydroxypregnenolone sulphate. Dehydroepiandrosterone sulphate from the adrenals is also an important precursor of estrogens during pregnancy, via androstenedione and testosterone. These conversions occur mainly in the placenta.

IX. VITAMIN D

In animals the provitamins D are partly absorbed from food and partly formed within the body. A carniverous diet supplies cholesterol and 7-dehydrocholesterol directly although these are also synthesized in the body, especially the stratum granulosum of skin. A vegetable diet supplies ergosterol and 22,33-dihydroergosterol, all of which are of plant origin, although significant quantities of ergosterol are obtained from hens eggs. Vitamin D is also obtained directly by eating liver, fish, eggs and drinking milk but the amounts obtained in this way are small compared with the total requirement and the body has to rely on the manufacture of vitamin D in the skin, from provitamin, by exposure to the sun (Fig. 3.19). Excess vitamin D is stored in the liver. Ingested cholesterol is converted to some 7-dehydrocholesterol as it crosses the intestinal wall and is thus found there in quantities as large, or larger, than in skin. It is not certain how much of the 7-dehydrocholesterol in skin is synthesized there and how much has come from the intestine.

The provitamins D absorb strongly over the whole region from 300 mμ-230 mμ and it takes 9.3×10^3 quanta of light to produce one International Unit of vitamin D_2 from ergosterol (1 IU $\equiv$ 0.025 mg cholecalciferol). A normal infant requires about 1000 IU per day to prevent ricketts. In skin, the melanin and the stratum corneum filter out light in the far and near ultraviolet especially in the darker races, which are thus more prone to ricketts. The erythema spectrum is 290-320 mμ, while the tanning spectrum is from 300-660 mμ with a peak at 420-460 mμ. When the quanta used for vitamin D biosynthesis are less energetic, more of them are required. It is believed that provitamin D is activated by absorption of a quantum of light and can return to the ground state either as lumisterol, tachysterol or vitamin D. On prolonged illumination lumisterol is itself activated and transformed into tachysterol and vitamin D, while tachysterol is also activated and converted to vitamin D. Tachysterols and lumisterol are given a subscript which defines their precise structure in terms of the particular vitamin D into which they are transformed. The reaction proceeds beyond vitamin D to form toxisterols and suprasterols of ill-defined structure. Human skin contains 4-18 IU vitamin D per cm^2. Nomenclature depends on the use of the prefix "seco" which shows fission of a ring with the addition of a hydrogen atom at each terminal group thus created. The original steroid numbering is retained.

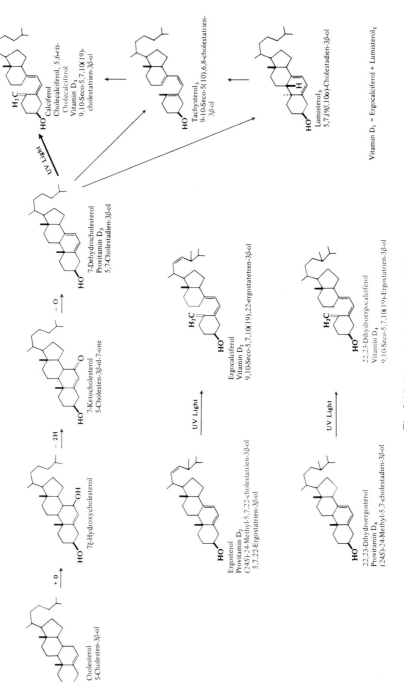

Fig. 3.19. Biosynthesis of Vitamin D.

Vitamin D₁ = Ergocalciferol + Lumisterol₂

X. BILE SALTS

These are produced uniquely by liver cells. The primary bile acids in human bile are cholic acid and chenodeoxycholic acid, with traces of allocholic acid and $3\alpha,7\alpha,12\alpha$-trihydroxycoprostanic acid (Fig. 3.20). Intestinal Micro-organisms introduce deoxycholic acid, which makes up 20% of the total bile acids, together with small amounts of lithocholic acid and ursodeoxycholic acid. All but a trace of the bile acids are present as conjugates with taurine or glycine. As the biliary pH is 7.5-8.0 these conjugates are present as ions $R-\underset{\underset{O}{\parallel}}{C}-NH-CH_2-COO^-$ and

$R-\underset{\underset{O}{\parallel}}{C}-NH-CH_2-CH_2-SO_3^-$. The principal cations are Na^+ and K^+, with Na^+

predominant. The proportion of glycine and taurine conjugates is variable. The six predominant bile salts are thus glycocholate, taurocholate, glycochenodeoxycholate and taurochenodeoxycholate, with lesser amounts of glycodeoxycholate and taurodeoxycholate (as shown in Table 3.2). They also occur in faeces.

Table 3.2. *Bile salts in man*

Sodium glycodeoxycholate	15%
Sodium taurodeoxycholate	5%
Sodium glycocholate	30%
Sodium taurocholate	10%
Sodium glycochenodeoxycholate	30%
Sodium taurochenodeoxycholate	10%

A large variety of other bile acids have been detected in faeces and are mainly derivatives of 5β-cholanic acid, e.g.

3-oxo-	3,12-dioxo-
$3\alpha,12\beta$-dihydroxy-	3β-7α-dihydroxy-
$3\beta,12\alpha$-dihydroxy-	3α-hydroxy-7-oxo-
$3\beta,12\beta$-dihydroxy-	3-oxo-7α-hydroxy-
3α-hydroxy-12-oxo-	$3\alpha,7\beta,12\alpha$-trihydroxy-
3β-hydroxy-12-oxo-	$3\beta,7\alpha,12\alpha$-trihydroxy-
3-oxo-12α-hydroxy-	

These compounds are believed to be synthesized by micro-organisms. In an adult man about 0.8 g of bile salts is made from cholesterol in 24 h. The main metabolic pathway appears to be via 7α-hydroxycholesterol to the 5β-cholestanes (coprostanes). The main derivatives have an additional hydroxyl at C-12α. There is evidence that the cholic acid nucleus (coprostan-$3\alpha,7\alpha,12\alpha$-triol) is formed before the side chain is oxidized. This takes place first by an hydroxylation at C-26, which is regarded as the C atom derived by biosynthesis from the β-methyl group of mevalonic acid. The $-CH_2OH$ group at C-26

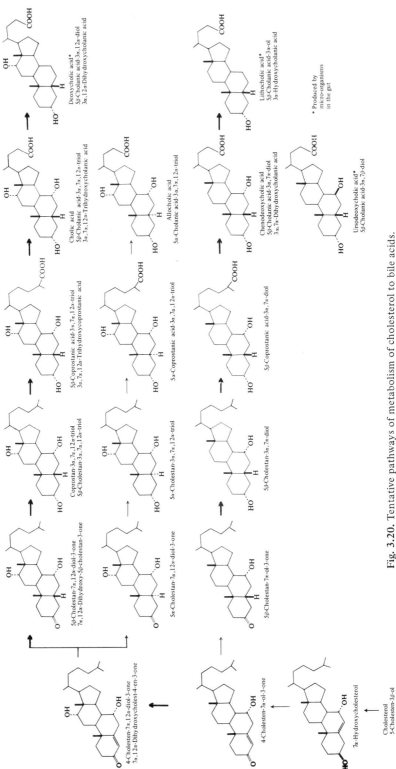

Fig. 3.20. Tentative pathways of metabolism of cholesterol to bile acids.

becomes further oxidized to $-COOH$ giving $3\alpha,7\alpha,12\alpha$-trihydroxycoprostanic acid which is cleaved by a mitochondrial enzyme to give cholic acid and propionyl-coenzyme-A ($CH_3-CH_2-CO.S.CoA$). The mechanism of conjugation is known to be with the aid of coenzyme-A and ATP to form cholyl-CoA, AMP and pyrophosphate. The cholyl CoA then conjugates with glycine or taurine with the release of CoA.SH.

Not all the ingested and unwanted cholesterol is metabolized by the liver, significant quantities escaping into the bile, and hence the faeces, unchanged. In the faeces, cholesterol undergoes a variety of metabolic reactions mediated by micro-organisms. The principle metabolite is coprostanol (= coprosterol = 3β-hydroxy-5β-cholestane) together with its 3α-hydroxy-epimer (epicoprostanol). These sterols are present mainly as the free alcohols.

4

4

TARGET ORGAN EFFECTS–A. ESTROGENS AND PROGESTOGENS

I. INTRODUCTION

The manner in which hormones select target sites and activate intracellular biosynthetic patterns is not known. Target organs sequester the appropriate hormone from the general circulation, or from the intracellular fluid, and some organs concentrate a given hormone to a greater extent than others. Most steroid hormones are active in extremely minute amounts. The facts that hormones localize in specific organs and are concentrated and retained by these organs suggest the existence of specific "receptor" substances in target cells capable of recognizing a particular hormone; some of these receptors have now been isolated.

The difference between estrogens, progestogens, androgens and anabolic steroids appear to lie in the target organs rather than in the effect produced. All types of steroid hormone stimulate their particular type of target cell to "grow", e.g. to divide, to synthesize protein, and to secrete. The similarity between the effects of the estrogens and androgens is particularly marked as both stimulate their particular target organs to become larger by the division of cells and the accumulation of the bulk of cytoplasm. Both males and females possess androgens and estrogens and the appropriate target organs, although in different proportions, e.g. androgens secreted by the female adrenal cortex stimulate the growth of the clitoris, whereas the larger amounts of androgens secreted by the male adrenal cortex and testes together stimulate the growth of the penis. Similarly small amounts of estrogens secreted by the male adrenal cortex are responsible for breast development in males.

It is now well established that a number of growth and developmental hormones regulate the protein synthetic activity of their target cells at some level at which the ribosome is involved, but fail to influence amino acid incorporation when added *in vitro* to cell-free systems. At the same time there is a rapid stimulation of RNA synthesis *in vivo* and it has been shown that some or all of the RNA formed under the influence of hormones is important for the hormonal regulation of growth and protein synthesis. The present hypothesis is that hormones modulate protein synthesis through a selective regulation of messenger RNA synthesis. Hormonal regulation of RNA synthesis can be demonstrated by the higher activity of RNA polymerase in isolated nuclei and it has now been established that all classes of nuclear RNA are influenced by steroid hormones. The abrupt increase of cytoplasmic protein synthesis stimulated in the target cell by many hormones does not occur until the hormone-induced ribosomes begin to accumulate in the cytoplasm, e.g. the effect of estrogen on uterine growth is very rapid. Most growth and developmental hormones probably alter the biosynthetic activity of their target cells at multiple steps of both the transcriptimal and translational processes. So far the primary site of action of growth and developmental hormones has not been identified, but the current hypothesis is that multiple biological actions are all derived from a unique interaction at a single site, e.g. some permeability control mechanism. A part of estrogen action involves very rapid adjustment of permeability of the uterus towards nucleotides and amino acids.

The regulation of gene activity is believed to be based on the induction of enzymes by substrates (Fig. 4.1). The structure of the enzyme to be induced is determined by a structural gene present on the genome. At the end of the genome is an "operator gene" which is governed by a "regulator gene". The product of the regulator gene is believed to be a specific protein whose function is to block the operator gene and so prevent the read-out of the genetic information. On the other hand, the repressor is able to form a complex with the inducer of the enzyme. This complex does not act as a blocking agent and the read-out of the genetic information is initiated. The mRNA is produced from the

DNA and then the induced protein (enzyme) is synthesized on the ribosomes. Steroid hormones can act as inducers of specific enzymes. Examples of enzyme induction by steroids are tryptophan pyrrolase and tyrosine-α-ketoglutarate transaminase by cortisol and DOPA-decarboxylase by ecdysone. Cortisol, estradiol, testosterone, aldosterone and progesterone have all been shown to increase RNA polymerase activity in suitable target tissues.

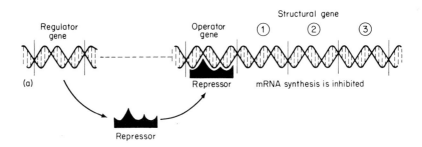

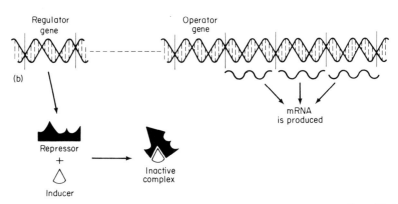

Fig. 4.1. Regulation of gene activity by operator and regulator genes. (From Karlson, 1968.)

II. EFFECTS OF ESTROGENS

Estrogens are compounds responsible, with other hormones, for the development and maintenance of female sexual organs and secondary sexual characteristics and also for the maintenance of the menstrual, or estrous, cycle and pregnancy. These effects may be divided into genital and non-genital. The major role of estrogens is to control the growth and function of the uterus. Other genital growth effects are on the ovaries, cervix, fallopian tubes, vagina, external genitalia and breasts. They are necessary for the development of both the duct and secretory systems of the breast and the increase in size, pigmentation and mobility of the nipple in pregnancy. Estrogens exert a pronounced proliferative effect on all tissues arising from the Müllerian duct system. Increased mitotic division produces rapid tissue growth in the endometrium, vaginal epithelium, fallopian tubes and endocervix. They appear to alter the physico-chemical properties of ground substance, e.g. the adhesion between collagen fibres, so that the uterine cervix, which has a high collagen content, stretches with great ease in late pregnancy, but not in the non-pregnant female.

Extra genital effects of estrogens are:

1. General development and maintenance of the secondary sexual characteristics, namely fat deposition on breast and hips to give the typical female contours; limitation of pubic hair to give the typical inverted triangle shape; vocal cord development to produce the higher pitch and lighter timbre; psyche formation; skin texture of a soft, fine and non-greasy type; general hair growth and texture.

2. Estrogens are mildly anabolic and increase the retention of nitrogen and sodium. Other minerals, e.g. calcium and phosphorus are also retained and this promotes the deposition of calcium in bone matrix and hastens the closure of the epiphyses. Retention of sodium leads to a retention of water which is shown most markedly in the skin and subcutaneous fat. This occurs to its highest degree immediately premenstrually and is believed to be partly responsible for the premenstrual tension syndrome which is characterized by depression, headaches and edema. Premenstrual weight gain can be as much as 2-3 lb.

3. Estrogens are mildly vasodilator and stimulate the peripheral circulation. This leads to "hot flushes".

4. Feedback inhibition of gonadotrophin secretion by the pituitary.

5. Styptic effect on uterine haemorrhage.

6. General proliferative effect and re-epithelialization of epithelial tissues which is particularly marked in nasal and buccal mucosa. The occurrence of sterile ulcers on the buccal mucosa and the gingiva can often be associated with the menstrual cycle.

Estrogens are synergistic with androgens in all the extra-genital effects of both hormones and are antagonistic to androgens in all genital effects in the female. Estrogen effects are modified by progesterone and the presence of estrogens in small amounts ensures the full effectiveness of progesterone.

III. EFFECTS OF PROGESTERONE

Progesterone appears to be the only important physiological (pro)gestogen. It interacts strongly with estrogens in its effects on tissues. Sometimes the two types of substances supplement each other and at other times they are antagonistic. The primary target for progesterone is the uterine endometrium upon which it exerts a strong secretory effect provided the tissue has been previously under the influence of estrogen. If this is not so, progesterone has little or no effect on the endometrium. Progesterone also has a secretory effect on the vaginal epithelium and endocervix.

Progesterone is primarily the hormone of pregnancy and is essential for the initial establishment and the continuation of pregnancy. It plays an essential role in establishing a thick layer of tissues richly supplied with blood and glycogen, providing ideal conditions for the nidation of a fertilized ovum and the sustenance of that ovum until such time as complete nidation allows for maternal nourishment. During pregnancy, the main purpose of progesterone is believed to be to reduce the muscle tone of the uterus, possibly by direct diffusion from the placenta. Any hormone which appears in the blood may simply be an overflow. There is a general relaxation of smooth muscle, e.g. atonic dilation of the ureter, reduced motility of the stomach and colon (producing constipation) and reduced vascular tone. It is thought that progesterone renders smooth muscle unresponsive to oxytocin, which is a peptide released by the posterior pituitary, and stimulates the contraction of uterine smooth muscle. This is the "progesterone block".

During pregnancy and to a minor degree during the progestational phase of the menstrual cycle, progesterone acting in conjunction with estrogen, brings about the proliferation of the acini of the mammary glands. Towards the end of pregnancy the acini fill with secretion and vascularization of the glands increases. At parturition the influence of estrogen and progesterone is withdrawn, the breast cells differentiate into secretory units and lactation begins. The fall in progesterone secretion occurs just before the onset of labour and is accompanied by a rise in oxytocin secretion which causes uterine contractions.

The main extragenital effect of progesterone is thermogenic. There is an increase in body temperature of 0.5 to 1°F (Fig. 4.2). Careful temperature

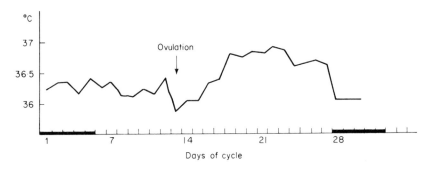

Fig. 4.2. A normal morning temperature curve.

measurements taken preferably rectally, immediately on waking, before rising, drinking or smoking can be used as a simple and precise means of assessing the occurrence and time of ovulation. In a normal cycle, the temperature remains fairly constant until ovulation when there is a slight drop followed by a rise which lasts for 9-13 days. The optimum fertile period is believed to precede the temperature rise by about 2 days. The temperature rise is usually sharp but is often stepwise or gradual. There is a fall in temperature prior to menstruation. If conception occurs the body temperature remains raised to about midpregnancy when it declines to normal, possibly due to the antagonistic action of estrogen. Other extragenital effects of progesterone are the promotion of water excretion and a weak styptic effect on uterine haemorrhage.

IV. CYCLIC EFFECTS OF ESTROGENS AND PROGESTERONE

A. MENSTRUAL CYCLE

1. Uterus

(a) Endometrium

The endometrium lines the uterine cavity and consists of two major layers— a basal or regenerative layer and a functional or decidual layer. It undergoes profound changes under the influence of estrogens and progestogens (Fig. 4.3).

(i) Proliferative or follicular phase, days 6-14. The most general effect of estrogens is to promote tissue growth, the most pronounced being in the accessory sexual tissues, e.g. uterus. Firstly the surviving epithelial cells in the glands move and rearrange to cover the bare areas of tissue. The frequency of endometrial mitoses during the follicular phase can be correlated with the action of estrogens. The lining of uterus becomes thickened and highly vascularized. The small arteries become tortuous and corkscrew. The glands of the mucous membrane elongate and glycogen appears in the gland cells but they do not secrete. By ovulation the endometrium is 2-4 mm thick.

(ii) Ovulation. There are no conspicuous changes in the endometrium.

(iii) Progestational or luteal or secretory phase, days 15-28. Under the influence of both estrogens and progestogens, the endometrium differentiates into a tissue which can fulfil the requirements of an embryo ready to implant. The stroma becomes highly vascularized and edematous and the size of the cells increase causing the endometrium to reach a maximum thickness of 4-8 mm shortly before the end of the cycle. The glands become further corkscrew in shape and actively secrete glycogen into the uterine cavity. The folded glandular epithelium has a characteristic jagged outline. The intervening connective tissue becomes closely packed with cells.

Days of cycle	Menstruation	Proliferative phase	Secretory phase	Pseudo-decidual phase	Predicidual phase
Normal	1-5	5-15 {quicker to develop	15-26		26-28
Combined type } oral	1-5	5-10 {quicker to develop	10-15	15-26	26-28
Sequential type } contraceptive	1-5	5-20 slower to develop	20-26		26-28

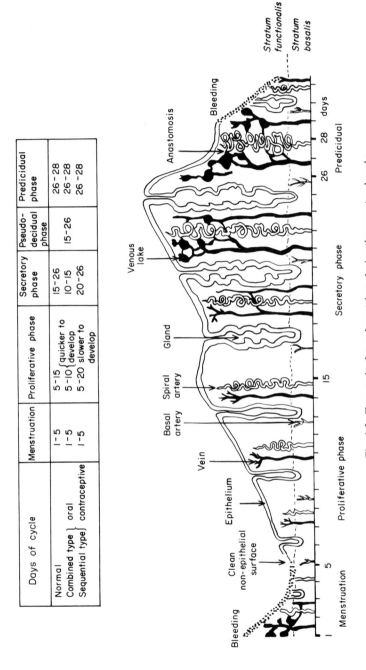

Fig. 4.3. Changes in the endometrium during the menstrual cycle.

If a blastocyst is not implanted (at about day 21) degenerative changes are seen. Predicidual cells form solid sheaths below the surface epithelium, leukocytes invade the tissue, necrotic changes occur in the stroma and the uterine glands involute.

(iv) Menstruation, days 1-5. The endometrium shrinks due to dehydration causing the coiling of the spiral arteries to be intensified. These arteries become constricted within the basal layer causing venous stasis and ischaemia. Preliminary bleeding from the surface of the endometrium through diapedesis, rupture of arteriols and disruption of venous return is followed by decimation of the stroma and separation from the basal layer. Lytic enzymes break down the stromal tissue, destroy clotted blood, fibrinogen and prothrombin. The estimated blood loss is about 30-40 ml. After menstruation the endometrium is thin, about 1 mm thick and poorly vascularized. Only the basal parts of the endometrial glands remain.

For a total blood loss of 40 ml, the average iron loss is 0.6 mg per day during menstruation, in addition to the normal loss via the skin, intestines and urine of 0.5-1.0 mg per day. The average daily consumption of iron in the United Kingdom is 14.2 mg and the mean absorption 6.5%, giving a mean intake of 0.82 mg per day. The average woman is in a delicate state of iron balance and iron-deficiency anaemia is not uncommon. In the normal menstrual cycle serum iron falls immediately prior to menstruation and is lowest during menstruation. This is thought to be due to diversion of plasma iron into tissue stores by estrogen. Women taking oral contraceptives have a mean serum iron significantly higher than women not taking oral contraceptives.

(b) Myometrium

This consists of two layers of muscle separated by a vascular layer. During the proliferative phase the muscle fibres lengthen and contractions are frequent and of small amplitude. In the progestational phase the myometrium becomes soft and spongy and the uterus softer and larger. The frequency of contractions is less and their amplitude increased. These contractions are believed to be one of the causes of painful menstruation (dysmenorrhea) which is a common feature of ovulatory cycles only.

2. Cervix

The cervix consists mainly of connective tissue with some muscle fibres and numerous acemose glands. The epithelium of the internal aspect (endocervix) is of the ciliated columnar type. The endometrium of the cervical part of the uterus is not shed in menstruation. The glandular secretion of cervical mucus is stimulated by estrogen and inhibited by progesterone. The condition of the cervical mucus is a more sensitive indicator of estrogen activity than the endometrium or the vaginal epithelium (Fig. 4.4). After menstruation the mucus

4*

94

(a)

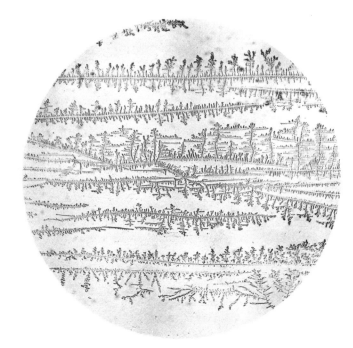

(b)

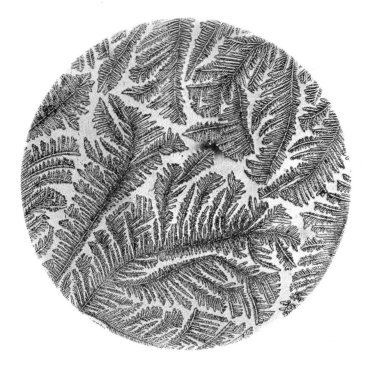

(c)

(d)

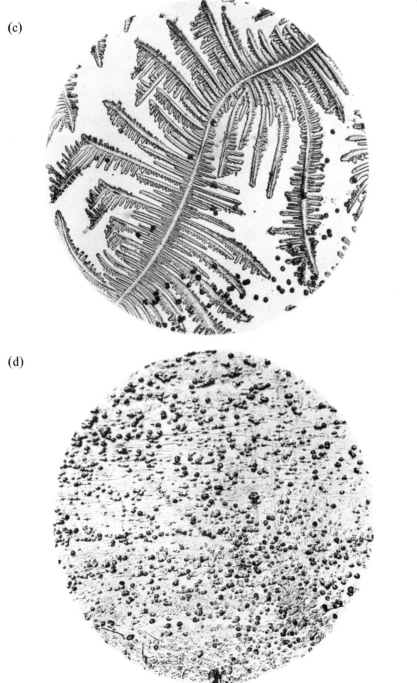

Fig. 4.4. Cervical mucus in the menstrual cycle. (a) Day 8, (b) day 10, (c) day 13, (d) day 19. (From MacDonald, 1967.)

is scanty and a dried smear shows minimum crystallization. By the eighth day the quantity of mucus and the amount of crystallization are beginning to increase. By mid-cycle (ovulation) the mucus is profuse, clear and watery, being about ten times the quantity after menstruation. Crystallization of a dried smear is at its maximum, producing the characteristic fern or palm leaf pattern. The mucus is rich in carbohydrate and protein and is highly alkaline (pH 8-9). The maximum secretion precedes the rise in basal body temperature by 1-3 days and is associated with minimum viscosity and maximum sperm penetration. The "spinnbarkeit" of the mucus is also maximal (i.e. the mucus can be drawn out into an elastic thread). On about the nineteenth day there is a sharp decrease in the amount of mucus, a considerable increase in viscosity and in cellularity. The degree of crystallization falls sharply. In normal pregnancy the dried smear shows a clear cellular pattern resembling the premenstrual period. The cells are mainly leukocytes with a few squamous and columnar cells. Similar but less pronounced changes have been noticed in saliva and nasal mucus in women during the menstrual cycle. It has been postulated that the increase in dental decay and gingival disease commonly observed in pregnancy may be related to changes in the glycoprotein content of the saliva.

3. Vagina

Changes in the vagina mirror those in the uterus although the interpretation of vaginal smears in women is much more difficult than in laboratory animals (Fig. 4.5). In the proliferative phase, the vaginal smear shows large, flat, slightly keratinized cells with small darkly staining (pyknotic) nuclei and acidophilic cytoplasm. The small amount of fluid in the vagina becomes acid (pH 4-4.5) due to the conversion of glycogen present to lactic acid by bacilli. In the secretory phase, the cells are polygonal, the nuclei elongated and the cytoplasm basophilic. There is less glycogen in the vaginal secretion and the pH drops to about 6.5-7.

4. Fallopian tubes

In the proliferative phase there is a growth of ciliated and non-ciliated columnar epithelial cells and an increase in peristaltic contractions from about four per minute to about ten per minute after ovulation. In the secretory phase the ciliated epithelial cells regress and the non-ciliated cells show secretory activity while contractions wane. It is believed that the secretion of the cells of the fallopian tubes play an important part in achieving fertilization, either by coating the ovum with a glycoprotein or by causing capacitation of sperm. The albumin coating of a hen's egg and a glycogen coating of a rabbit's ovum are laid down in the fallopian tubes.

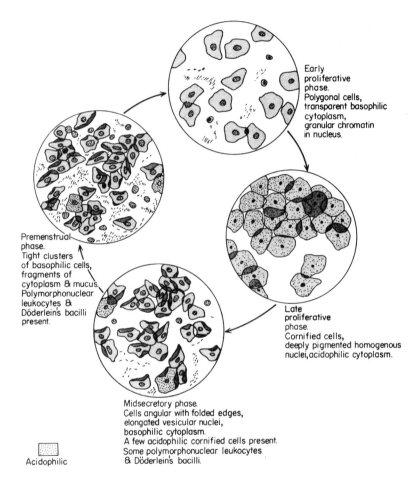

Fig. 4.5. Vaginal cells in the menstrual cycle. (From the Ciba Collection of Medical Illustrations, 1965.)

B. ESTROUS CYCLE

1. Introduction

Monoestrous animals complete a single estrous cycle annually, a long anestrous period separating the heats. Polyestrous animals complete two or more cycles annually. Ovulation is the dominant event in the estrous cycle and usually occurs during estrus, but in a few species, e.g. cow, it occurs after the end of estrus. In most mammals ovulation occurs "spontaneously" preceded by a short period of very rapid follicular growth while in others, e.g. rabbit and cat, ovulation is only induced by coitus or a comparable stimulation of the uterine cervix. The induced ovulators generally remain in continuous heat, the ovary being characterized by large follicles for long periods and preovulatory growth of the follicles and ovulation occur after coitus. Also with induced ovulators there are occasional intervals during which the female is not receptive to the male. At these times there is massive atresia of the vesicular follicles. Some domestic animals, e.g. cows and mares, occasionally show "quiet heat" when only sexual receptivity is lacking from the other signs of heat. Wild animals tend to reproduce at certain seasons, when environmental factors are optimal, but often lose this effect after domestication, e.g. wild rats, rabbits and cattle exhibit definite breeding seasons while their domestic or laboratory counterparts do not. Domestic breeds of sheep have an elongated and sometimes nearly continuous breeding season, contrary to their wild state.

2. The rat

Laboratory rats, mice, hamsters and guinea pigs are polyestrous. The estrous cycle of the rat is completed in 4-5 days depending on the environment and is roughly divided into four stages:

(a) Estrus (heat)

This is the period of heat, and copulation is only permitted during this time which lasts 9-15 h. Under the influence of FSH and estrogen a dozen or more ovarian follicles grow rapidly. The uteri undergo progressive enlargement, many mitoses are present and the superficial epithelial layers of the vaginal mucosa become squamous and cornified. These cells are exfoliated and their presence in vaginal smears indicates estrus. Ovulation occurs during estrus which is the phase of increased estrogen secretion.

(b) Metestrus (the postovulatory phase)

This period lasts 10-14 h. The ovaries contain corpora lutea and small follicles and the uteri have diminished. The vaginal smear shows a mixture of cornified and nucleated epithelial cells with an infiltration of leukocytes. In mammals which have short estrous cycles, e.g. rats and mice, the luteal or progestational phase, which occurs at the end of metestrus in other animals, is so abbreviated that the uteri do not undergo changes associated with the action of progesterone.

(c) Diestrus (resting phase)

This period in rats lasts 60-70 h during which functional regression of the corpora lutea occur. The uteri are small and the vaginal mucosa thin, and invaded by leukocytes. The vaginal smear consists almost entirely of leukocytes.

(d) Proestrus (the preovulatory or follicular phase)

There is a functional involution of the corpora lutea and preovulatory swelling of the follicles. Nucleated epithelial cells occur singly or in sheets in the vaginal smear.

It has been postulated that very low levels of estrogens coming from immature follicles, stimulate the pituitary to augment its release of FSH. When the blood estrogen becomes high due to full-grown ovarian follicles, it acts to prevent greater release of FSH and to promote the release of LH which causes the preovulatory swelling. Ovulation occurs when LH is in the ascendency and there is an immediate fall in circulating estrogens. The ruptured follicle becomes transformed into a corpus luteum which becomes functional under the influence of prolaction. Removal of the ovaries leads eventually to involution and atrophy of the reproductive tract and associated estrogen-maintained structures. Table 4.1 shows the length of the estrus cycle in some other polyestrous domesticated animals. Figure 4.6 shows the ovarian, endometrial and vaginal cycle in the cow.

Table 4.1. *Reproductive cycles in polyestrous domestic animals*

Animal	Breeding Season	Length of cycle (interval) between heats), average and range (days)	Length of estrus, average and range	Length of pregnancy, average and range (days)
Mare	Spring	22 (16-30)	6 (2-11) days	336 (329-346)
Ass	Spring	23 (13-31)	6 (2-14) days	365
Cow	All year	21 (18-24)	16 (8-30) h	282 (274-291)
Ewe	Autumn	$16\frac{1}{2}$ (14-20)	35 h (1-3) days	150 (140-160)
Goat	Autumn	21 (15-24)	$2\frac{1}{2}$ (2-3) days	151 (140-160)
Sow	All year	21 (18-24)	2-3 (1-5) days	113 (110-116)
Rat	All year	5	10-20 h	22 (21-23)
Guinea pig	All year	15	6-12 h	62
Mouse	All year	5	10-20 h	19
Golden hamster	Spring	4	12 h	16

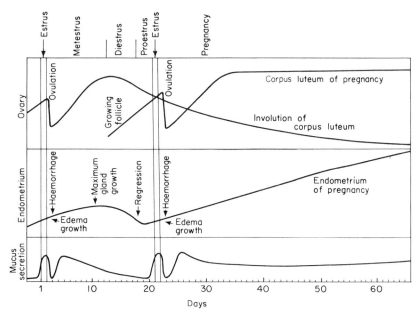

Fig. 4.6. The ovarian, endometrial and vaginal cycles of the cow. (From Dukes, 1965.)

3. The dog

Ovulation is spontaneous and there are generally two estrous periods a year, i.e. the dog is polyestrous. Proestrus lasts about 10 days and estrus 6-10 days. Ovulation typically occurs during early estrus and copulations may be permitted for 6-8 days afterwards. Loss of blood from the vagina occurs during proestrus and sometimes extends throughout estrus. This arises by leakages from engorged vessels in the uterus and is not analogous to the menstrual bleeding of primates. After estrus there is a luteal phase of about 60 days and then a period of pseudopregnancy in which the reproductive tract and mammary glands are developed as in pregnancy. Pseudopregnancy, or metestrus, lasts about 3 months, followed by anestrus which lasts about 2 months. Pregnancy lasts about 60 days. The estrus cycle of the fox is very similar, with a gestation period of about 52 days.

4. Induced ovulators

Rabbits, ferrets and cats are induced ovulators (Table 4.2). In the rabbit the ovaries contain follicles in all stages of development and atresia and cyclical changes in physiology and behaviour are difficult to detect. After a sterile mating, pseudopregnancy is induced which lasts about 18 days in the rabbit. Coitus appears to cause the release of LH from the hypophysis within an hour

Table 4.2. *Reproductive cycles of some induced ovulators*

	Length of pregnancy, average and range (days)	Age at puberty
Rabbit	31 (30-32)	About 6 months
Ferret	42	
Cat	64 (58-71)	Very variable, 7-12 months

and ovulation occurs about 10 h later. Under domestic conditions cats generally breed twice a year, anestrus occurring during October, November and December. Cats are polyestrus, showing recurrent estrus at 14-day intervals, in the breeding seasons lasting 3-6 days. Copulation during estrus induces ovulation 26-27 h later.

C. PUBERTY AND MENOPAUSE

Until the age of 8 years in girls gonadal function is insignificant. At about the age of 9 years the body build begins to alter, the ovaries enlarge and the production of follicular hormones increases. Puberty lasts from about 10-16 years, the menarche occurring in the middle of this period. At the beginning of puberty follicular rupture does not occur and hence neither corpora lutea nor progesterone are formed. Early menstrual periods are usually anovulatory, although they indicate the cyclical function of the hypothalamic-anterior-pituitary-ovarian axis. The increase in size of the adrenal cortex is an important part of female puberty and there is increasing secretion of glucocorticoids, mineralocorticoids and adrenal androgens. Ovulation usually begins 2-3 years after the menarche.

The climacterium begins with the failure of ovulation and ends with the body's adaptation to a state in which the ovaries are almost without function. After ovulation fails, follicular hormone is still produced and endometrial bleeding persists for a time and then ceases altogether (the menopause). Women with an early menarche, e.g. at 12 years, tend to have a late menopause, for example at 50 years, while menarche at 19 years is associated with menopause at 45 years. There is a much higher urinary excretion of gonadotrophins in menopausal and post-menopausal women. The secretion of androgenic adrenal hormones decreases rapidly after about 65 years, but the secretion of mineralo-corticoids and glucocorticoids remains unchanged. Many organs and tissues undergo gradual atrophy after the menopause, especially the former target tissues, e.g. genital organs, breast, bone matrix (producing osteoporosis) and skin. All anabolic processes slow down while catabolic processes continue at the same rate.

V. ESTROGENIC POTENCY: BIOLOGICAL ASSAY

A. UNITS

When substantially pure estrone and estradiol became generally available, the animal unit of potency became obsolete. Now 1 unit of estrone or estradiol benzoate, determined biologically, may be taken as identical with 0.1 μg of either substance measured by some other non-biological method of analysis. The potency of existing and new estrogens can only be assayed by biological methods, all of which have serious limitations. Entirely dissimilar results may be obtained with the same method when minor modifications are introduced, e.g. changing the solvent for the estrogen or varying the number of injections. When different methods are used, enormous variations in results occur.

B. METHODS

1. Allen-Doisy test

This is the most widely used assay of oestrogenic activity and is based on the induction of vaginal cornification in rodents. While both rats and mice have been used, the mouse is the animal of choice. The ratio of the mouse unit to the rat unit varies from 1.5 to 1.8. Immature female mice are spayed shortly after weaning. They are unsuitable for use for about 2 weeks. To maintain sensitivity of the tissues to estrogens it is customary to "prime" them at about 6-week intervals with 1 μg of a potent estrogen. While the same mice can be repeatedly used for assay purposes, at least 2 weeks between assays ensures the absence of carry over effects. In a typical test, at least two doses of test and control oestrogen are given to separate groups of twenty mice. The route of administration is usually subcutaneous but most routes give some response. The median effective dose by intravaginal injection is about 0.0003 μg estrone. Usually two or four doses are given on days 1 and 2 of the assay. On days 3 and 4 vaginal smears are taken by metal spatula. The smears are then stained, washed and scored for the degree of cornification. The relative potency is then determined by comparison of the concentrations necessary to produce estrus in more than 50% of the animals. Table 4.3 shows some typical results. Estradiol (-17β) is

Table 4.3. *Some estrogenic potencies on the Allen-Doisy test*

	μg/Rat unit	Rat units/mg	I.U./mg
Estradiol (-17β)	0.1	12,000	120,000
17α-Ethinylestradiol	0.1		
Estrone	0.8	1000	10,000
Estradiol-17α	4		
Estriol	10	150	1500

revealed as the most potent natural estrogen. Potency ratios of estradiol, estrone and estriol of 1000:100:1 have been quoted.

2. Vaginal mitosis and epithelial thickness tests

Up to certain dose levels, estrogens stimulate the mitosis of vaginal epithelial cells and increase the epithelial thickness. At very high doses the effect is not dose related and in fact the reverse effects may appear. Young, ovariectomized mice are used, previously primed 2 weeks before with a single dose of 1 μg of estrogen. The estrogen under test is administered directly into the vagina in a small volume of water. About 7 h later 0.1 μg of colchicine is given, which blocks the completion of all mitoses then in progress. The animals are killed, their vaginas sectioned and a series of sections examined for numbers of mitoses and thickness of epithelium. This test is much more sensitive than the Allen-Doisy test, the median effective dose being 0.00003 μg estrone.

3. Uterine weight test

Estrogens stimulate both the growth of the uterus and its water uptake. The latter is a rapid effect taking only a few hours, while the former takes several days. If estrogens are injected daily into groups of young spayed female rats and the uteri are collected after four days treatment, a considerable increase in weight is apparent compared to controls. While the effect is dose related, it is not specific for estrogens as both androgens and progestogens also increase uterine weight. There is a linear relationship between the logarithm of the dose and the effect. Some relative potencies are shown in Table 4.4. A similar assay

Table 4.4. *Rank estrogenic potencies by the uterine weight method*

Diethylstilbestrol dipropionate	14.37
Estradiol 17-cypionate	11.09
Estradiol benzoate	10.75
Estradiol dipropionate	10.00
Ethinylestradiol	9.72
Benzestrol	9.28
Diethylstilbestrol	8.76
Estrone	8.59
Estradiol	8.02
Dienestrol	7.73
Promestrol dipropionate	6.83
Diethylstilbestrol dipalmitate	6.60
Sodium estrone sulphate	4.00
Monomestrol	3.26
Hexestrol	2.48
Estriol	2.26
Control	1.00

using increase in weight of chick oviduct has been described. More specific is the rapid water uptake of the uterus in response to estrogens. If the uteri are removed from young female rats only 6 h after estrogen administration a quite marked increase in weight, due almost entirely to water, can be detected. Again the response is dose related.

4. Placental isocitrate dehydrogenase test

Extracts of human, term placentae contain an NAD-dependent isocitrate dehydrogenase that is stimulated by estrogens (though not by estriol). As the activity of the enzyme can easily be followed spectrophotometrically at 340 mμ by increase in NADH$_2$, the effects of added estrogens can be assayed. The major difficulties of this assay are first, that non-steroidal oestrogens are inactive, and secondly that some androgens and corticoids also have a stimulatory action.

C. NON-STEROIDAL AND SYNTHETIC ESTROGENS

The potency of estrogens in man depends on their mode of administration and their molecular structure. Estradiol is almost inactive when given by mouth, estrone must be given in five times the oral dose compared with the injected dose, while estriol is about equally potent either orally or by injection. Estradiol can be given by injection of a sterile suspension in water but better results are obtained by intramuscular injection of an ester in a suitable oil. Typical esters used are the 3-benzoate, 3-cypionate (cyclopentylpropionate), 3,17-dipropionate, 17β-undecenoate and the 17β-n-valerate (Fig. 4.7). These compounds form a depot from which the active estrogen is released. Their potency is similar to that of estradiol.

Orally active estrogens are now more widely used than depot estrogens. The oldest, stilbestrol (diethylstilbestrol), is a synthetic non-steroidal estrogen which is readily absorbed from the gastrointestinal tract, 1 mg by mouth being equivalent to 0.05 mg estradiol benzoate by injection. Less active derivatives are benzestrol, dienestrol and hexestrol. These structures are shown in Fig. 4.7. The most active oral estrogen is (17α-)ethinylestradiol which is about twenty-five times more potent than stilbestrol. Other potent oral estrogens are mestranol, which is more potent than estradiol, chlorotrianisene, which has long acting effects because of storage in adipose tissue and is better classed as a proestrogen, and methallenestrol. Estrone may be given orally with advantage as piperazine estrone sulphate or as "conjugated estrogen", "Premarin", which is a preparation from pregnant mares' urine containing mainly sodium estrone sulphate.

Many weakly estrogenic substances have been isolated from plants but are not used therapeutically. Their isoflavone structure may be considered not unlike the structure of estradiol. Genistein occurs in Australian strains of subterranean clover and has been the cause of poor fertility and abortion in sheep due to suppression of pituitary gonadotrophins. Daidzein occurs in soya beans where it

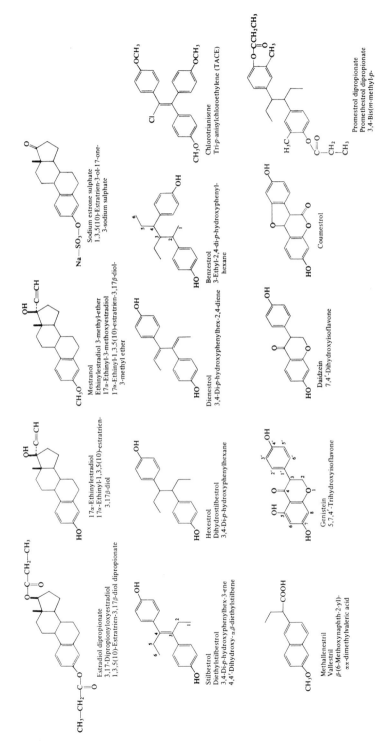

Fig. 4.7. Synthetic and non-steroidal estrogens.

exists as the 7-glucoside. Both these compounds are only about 5×10^{-6} as potent as diethylstilbestrol, but white clover contains coumestrol which is about thirty times more potent but still only $1/1000$ as potent as estradiol.

VI. PROGESTATIONAL POTENCY: BIOLOGICAL ASSAY

A. METHODS

1. Clauberg-McPhail test

Bioassays for progesterone are complicated by the responding tissues requiring preliminary or auxiliary treatment with estrogen. This is a variant of the original Corner and Allen method which used adult female rabbits spayed at the proper stage of follicle ripening after mating. The Clauberg test uses immature female rabbits weighing 750-950 g. They are primed with 150 IU estrone daily by subcutaneous administration for 6 days prior to the assay to produce the suitable endometrium. The animals are usually dealt with in groups of five. All animals in each group receive the same dose (by a given route) of the test substance, and the substance is usually tested over a wide dose range. At the end of the test period the uteri are removed, sectioned and the degree of endometrial proliferation estimated on a five-point scale. A dose-response curve can then be drawn for the substance under test and the ED_{50} calculated (the effective dose required to produce a standard response in 50% of the animals tested), and compared with that of a standard compound, usually progesterone. Many androgens give a positive test result and the method is relatively insensitive.

2. McGinty test

Like the first test this is also conducted on oestrogen-primed immature rabbits. However, on the first day of the test the uterus is exposed by laparotomy and the upper middle segment of each uterine horn is ligated. Care is taken not to disturb the vascular supply to the horns. Progesterone, or a test substance, is now injected into the ligated lumen and the lower ligature drawn tight immediately after injection. The vehicle used as solvent for the test substance is injected as a control into the opposite ligated uterine horn. The rabbits are killed 3 days after the operation, the uterine horns removed, sectioned and scored for endometrial response as before. The test is very sensitive (0.1-0.05 μg progesterone).

3. Pincus-Werthessen test

Mature rabbits are mated and then spayed 18 h later. Progesterone, or the test substance, is given subcutaneously on the second, third and fourth days after mating. On the fifth day the rabbits are killed and ova washed from the uterus for examination. The diameter of each ovum is measured (excluding albumin coating). A section of the uterus is also examined and the ratio of glandular proliferation (G) to total mucosa (M) is determined by the use of a planimeter on a traced, projected section. A combined index of ovum diameter and the ratio G:M is directly proportional to the progesterone dose. The method is extremely laborious but does appear to give good results in skilled hands. A modification of the method by Pincus and Miyake uses estrogen-primed immature rabbits and only the G:M ratio is calculated.

4. Lutwak-Mann test

Using oestrogen-primed immature rabbits it has been demonstrated that the carbonic anhydrase content of the uterine endometrium increases logarithmically with the dose of progestogen over a wide dose range. It is consequently possible to use this enzyme method alongside many of the previous tests and so obtain a double assessment of the test substance.

5. Hooker-Forbes test

Using ovariectomized mice it can be shown that progestogens injected into the lumen of a ligated uterine segment induce an hypertrophy of the stromal nuclei of the endometrium. The test is exceedingly sensitive needing as little as 2×10^{-10} g of progesterone. Because of this sensitivity a micrometer syringe is needed for accurate administration. The minimal interval between ovariectomy and the test is 18 days. The animal is killed 2 days after the injection of the progestogen. In examining uterine sections for effects on stromal nuclei, the latter must be distinguished from the nuclei of glandular cells which are not affected by progestogens. To do this usually requires detailed examination of serial sections. While the test is highly sensitive (0.0002 μg progesterone) it is time-consuming and requires skilled technicians to interpret the slides. Discrepancies in assays of particular compounds between laboratories are common.

6. Astwood test

Adult female rats in oestrus are given electrical cervical stimulation. Four days later the animals are ovariectomized and at the same time the endometrium of one uterine horn is traumatized by scratching with a needle the entire internal length. Progestogens are then injected for 3 days and the animals killed on the fourth day. The degree of swelling of the deciduoma formed along the site of traumatization is assessed by comparison with similar deciduoma in intact and untreated control animals. Alternately, the diameter of the traumatized horn can be measured and similarly correlates with the progesterone dose. Variations to this test include induction of deciduoma by intro-uterine injection of histamine.

7. Maintenance of pregnancy

If pregnant animals are spayed, the foetus aborts. The pregnancy can be maintained by exogenous progesterone above certain levels. It is consequently possible to compare a test compound with progesterone in this assay. Unfortunately there appear to be marked species and even strain differences in this assay. The stage of the pregnancy is also critical, and the assay has been little used. An analogous assay uses the inhibition of progestogens of oxytocin-induced abortion.

B. STRUCTURE

Table 4.5 shows some relative progestational potencies and Fig. 4.8 some progestational structures. It is seen that synthetic progestogens fall into three distinct categories—derivatives of progesterone, e.g. megestrol, chlormadinone; derivatives of testosterone, e.g. ethisterone; and derivatives of 19-nor-testosterone (4-estrene), e.g. norethisterone, norethynodrel, lynestrenol, and ethynodiol. The last group have strong structural features in common with the steroidal estrogens. Many of the compounds have androgenic and anabolic activities as well as their progestational activities and those used in oral contraceptives have been selected for their relative lack of androgenic and anabolic activities as well as their good progestational potency. One of the most interesting compounds is dydrogesterone as it is a retro-progesterone derivative, i.e. there is inversion of the ring substituents at C-9 and C-10. This compound is claimed to cause feedback inhibition of gonadotrophin secretion but not to inhibit ovulation.

VII. CONTRACEPTIVE EFFECTS OF ESTROGENS AND PROGESTOGENS

A. TYPES AVAILABLE

Three distinct types of hormone contraceptive are in widespread use. All regimens are arranged to give a regular 28-day cycle.

1. Combined preparation

Each tablet contains an estrogen and a progestogen and one is taken daily for 20-22 days, followed by a space of 5-6 days. The start is made on the fifth day of a normal cycle. Table 4.6 shows the six combinations of estrogen and progestogen at present available. Recent trends have been to lower the concentration of one or both compounds and hence lower the cost, when extended trials have shown the lower amounts to be effective. Some combinations are strongly progestogenic, e.g. Anovlar with a low incidence of "break-through" bleeding (2-3%), while others are weakly progestogenic, e.g. Ovulen with a high incidence of "break-through" bleeding (4-40%).

2. Sequential or serial preparation

A tablet containing estrogen alone is taken for 14-16 days, then another type of tablet containing both estrogen and progestogen is taken for 5-7 days (Table

Table 4.5. *Progestational activity in the Clauberg assay, subcutaneously in the rabbit, relative to progesterone*

4-Pregnen-3,20-dione	(progesterone)	1
4-Pregnen-3,19,20-trione		0.1
4-Pregnen-17α-ol-3,20-dione	(17α-hydroxyprogesterone)	0
4-Pregnen-17α-ol-3,20-dione acetate	(17α-hydroxyprogesterone acetate)	10
4-Pregnen-17α-ol-3,20-dione caproate	(17α-hydroxyprogesterone caproate)	2^a
6α-Methyl-4-pregnen-3,20-dione	(6α-methylprogesterone)	5
6α-Methyl-4-pregnen-17α-ol-3,20-dione acetate	(medroxyprogesterone acetate)	10-20
21-Fluoro-6α-methyl-4-pregnen-17α-ol-3,20-dione acetate	(21-fluoromedroxyprogesterone acetate)	50
9α-Bromo-4-pregnen-11β,17α-di-ol-3,20-dione 17, acetate		5
21-Fluoro-6α-methyl-4-pregnen-17α-ol-3,20-dione acetate		50
4-Pregnen-2-acetofuran-16α, 17α-diol-3, 20-dione		32-64
17α-Bromo-6α-fluoro-1,4-pregnadien-3, 20-dione		10
3,5-Pregnadien-3-ol-20-one cyclopentyl ether	(quingesterone)	10
6-Chloro-4,6-pregnadien-17α-ol-3, 20-dione acetate	(chlormadinone acetate)	50
17α-Ethinyl-4-androsten-17β-ol-3-one	(ethisterone)	0.3
17α-Ethinyl-4,6-androstadien-3β, 17-diol		0^b
17α-Ethinyl-4-estren-17β-ol	(lynestrenol)	1
17α-Ethinyl-4-estren-17β-ol-3-one	(norethisterone)	0.5
17α-Ethinyl-4-estren-17β-ol-3-one acetate	(norethisterone acetate)	30^a
17α-Ethyl-4-estren-17β-ol-3-one	(norethandrolone)	5-10
4-Estren-17β-ol-3-one		0
17α-Ethinyl-4-estren-17β-ol-3-one caproate	(norethisterone caproate)	60^a
17α-Ethinyl-4,6-estradien-17β-ol-3β-ol acetate		1
17α-Ethyl-5 (10)-estren-17β-ol-3-one		0.25
17α-Ethinyl-5 (10)-estren-17β-ol-3-one	(norethynodrel)	0.25

[a] Long acting
[b] Oral administration.

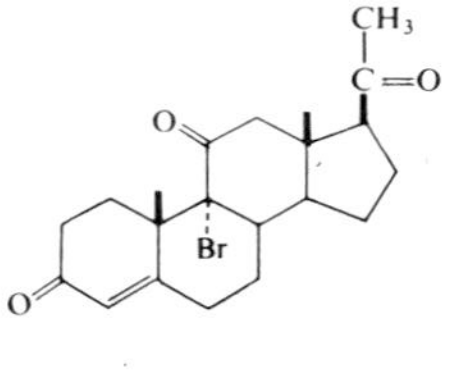

Angesterone acetate
6α-Methyl-4-pregnen-17α-ol-20-one acetate

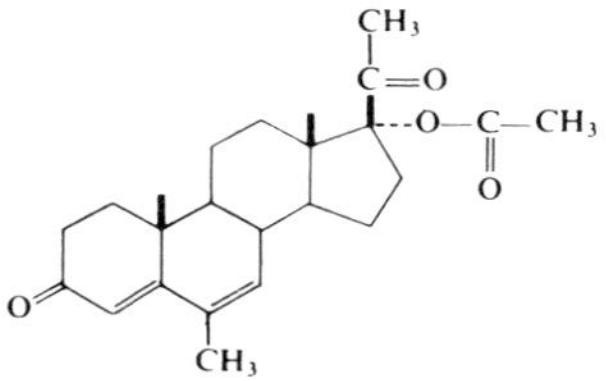

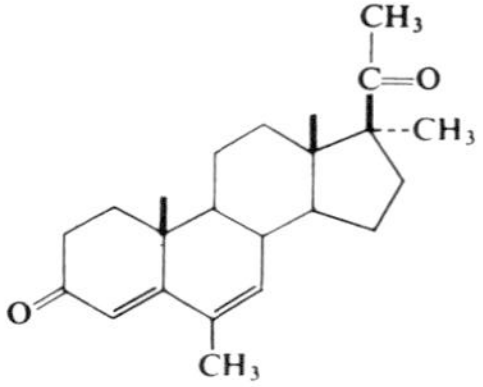

Metrogestone, Medrogestone
6,17-Dimethyl-4,6-pregnadiene-3,20-dione

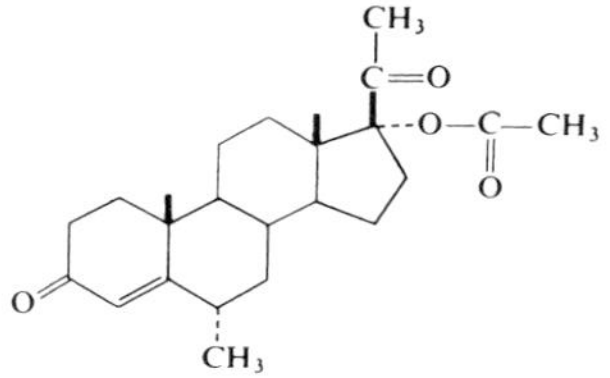

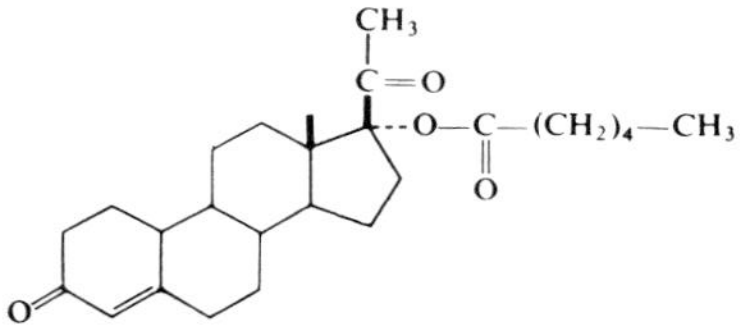

Medroxyprogesterone acetate
Depo-provera
6α-Methyl-17α-acetoxyprogesterone, (MAP)
6α-Methyl-4-pregnen-17α-ol-3,20-dione
acetate

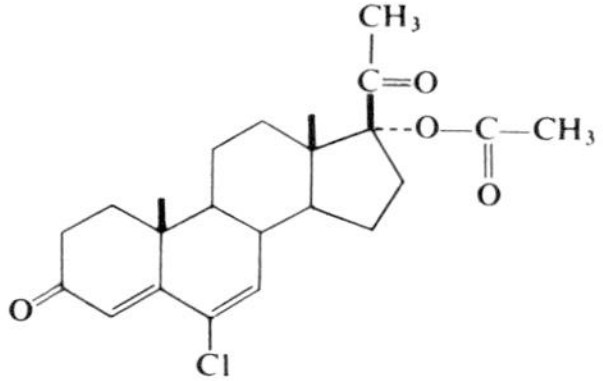

Chlormadinone acetate, (CAP)
6-Chloro-4,6-pregnadien-17α-ol-
3,20-dione acetate

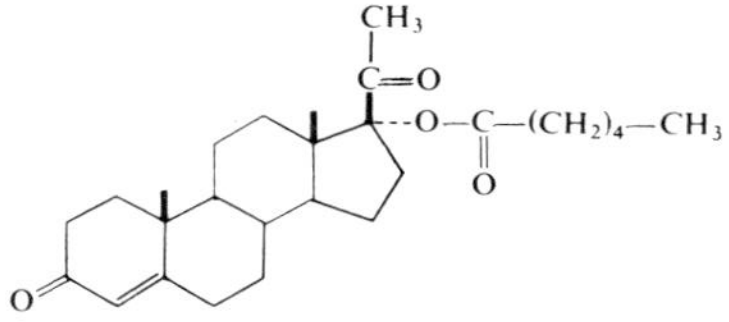

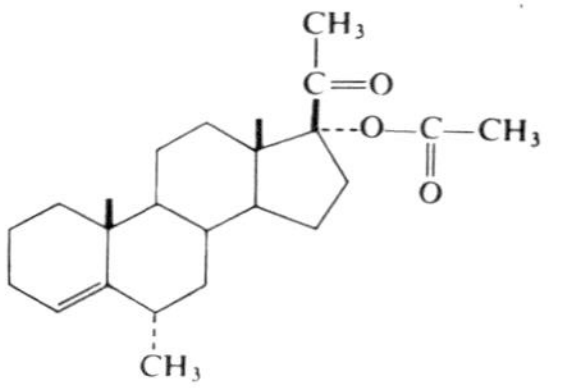

17α-Hydroxyprogesterone caproate
4-Pregnen-17α-ol-3,20 dione caproate

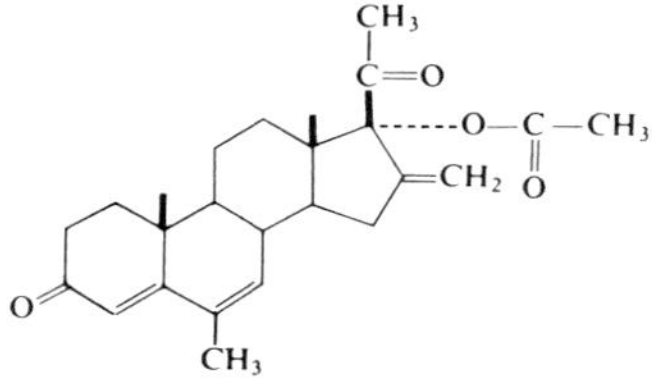

Melengestrol acetate
6-Methyl-16-methylene-4,6-pregnadien-
17α-ol-3,20-dione acetate

9α-Bromo-11-ketoprogesterone
9α-Bromo-4-pregnen-3,11,20-trione

Megestrol acetate
6-Methyl-4,6-pregnadien-17α-ol-3,20-
dione acetate

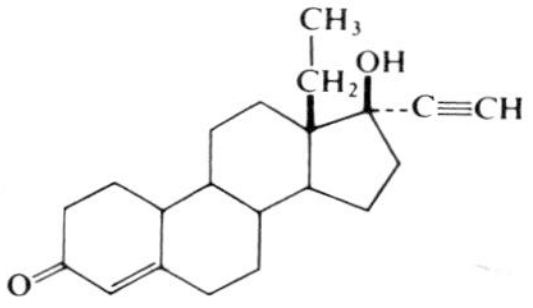

Norgestrel
17α-Ethinyl-18-methyl-4-estren-17β-ol-3-one
17α-Ethinyl-13β-ethyl-4-gonen-17β-ol-3-one

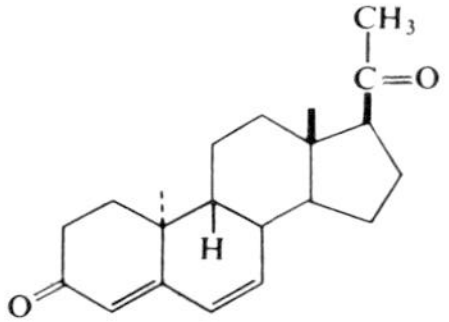

Gestonorone caproate
19-Nor-4-pregnen-17α-ol-3,20-dione caproate

Dydrogesterone
6-Dehydro-retro-progesterone
6-Dehydro-9β,10α-progesterone
4,6,(9β, 10α)-Pregnadien-3,20-dione

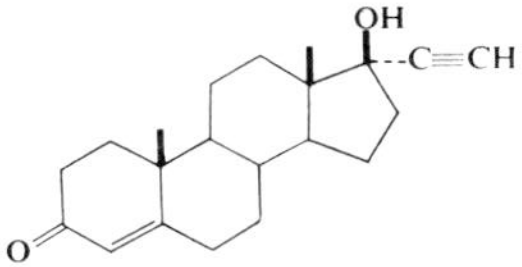

Ethisterone, Ethindrone
Anhydrohydroxyprogesterone
Ethinyltestosterone
17α-Ethinyl-4-androsten-17β-ol-3-one

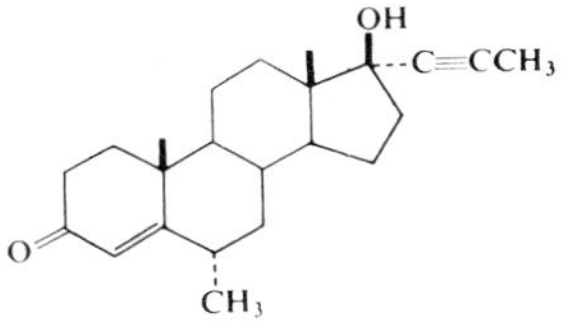

Dimethisterone
Dimethylethisterone
17α-Ethinyl-6α,21-dimethyl-
4-androsten-17β-ol-3-one

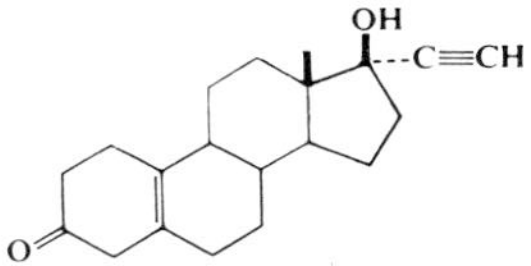

Norethynodrel
17α-Ethinylestranolone
17α-Ethinyl-5(10)-estren-17β-ol-3-one

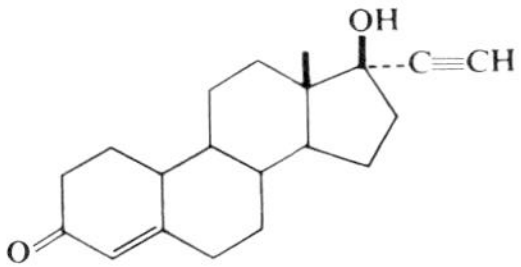

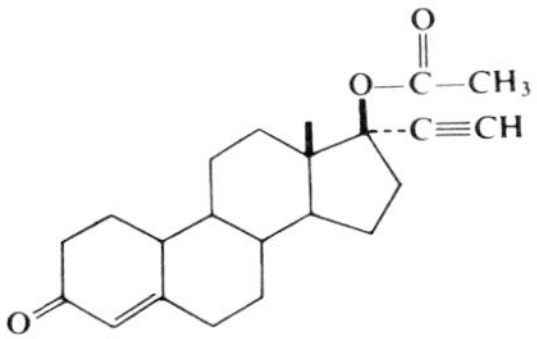

Norethisterone, Norlutin, Norethindrone
Ethinyl-19-nor-testosterone
17α-Ethinyl-4-estren-17β-ol-3-one

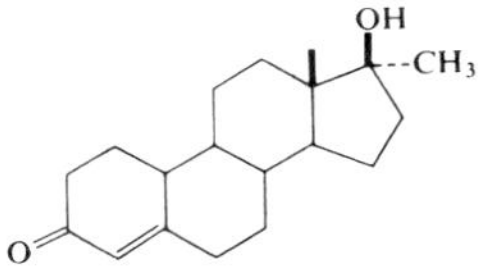

17α-Methyl-19-nor-
testosterone
17α-Methyl-4-estren-
17β-ol-3-one

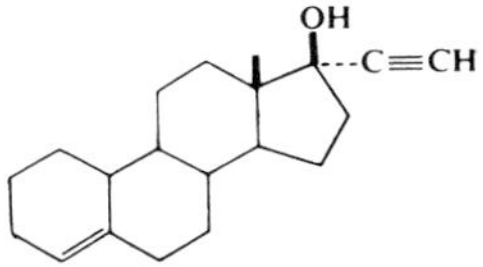

Lynestrenol
17α-Ethinyl-4-estren-17β-ol

Norethisterone acetate
17α-Ethinyl-4-estren-17β-ol-3-one acetate

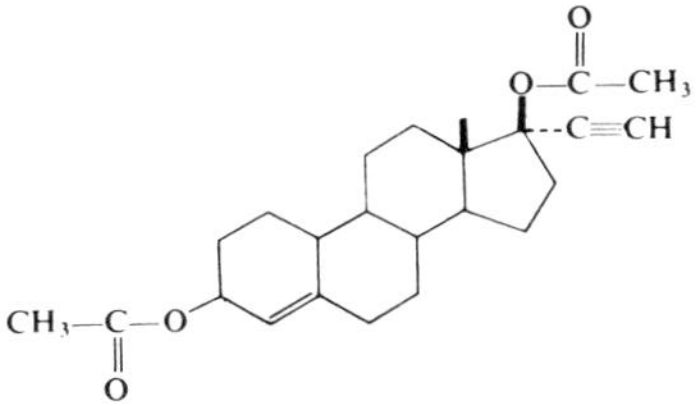

Ethynodiol diacetate
Norethisterone diacetate
17α-Ethinyl-4-estren-3β,17β-
diol diacetate

Fig. 4.8. Synthetic progestogens.

Table 4.6. *Available oral contraceptives of the combined type*

UK	USA	Other	Firm	Estrogen		Progestogen		Total days
Anovlar 21			Schering AG			Norethisterone acetate (= Norethindrone acetate in USA)	4 mg	21
Gynovlar 21		Anovlar mite	Schering AG	0.05 mg Ethinyl-estradiol			3 mg	21
Norlestrin and	Norlestrin	Etalontin	Parke-Davis				2.5 mg	20 and 21
Norlestrin 21		Orelestrin, Orlest						
Norlestrin 1 mg	Norlestrin 1 mg	Prolestrin	Parke-Davis				1 mg	21 and 21[a]
Minovlar			Schering AG				1 mg	21
Minovlar ED			Schering AG				1 mg	21[a]
Volidan and			BDH	0.05 mg Ethinyl-estradiol		Megestrol acetate	4 mg	20 and 21
Volidan 21								
Nuvacon[b]			BDH	0.1 mg Ethinyl-estradiol		Megestrol acetate	2 mg	21
	Provest		Upjohn	0.05 mg Ethinyl-estradiol		Medroxyprogesterone acetate	10 mg	21
Conovid[b]	Enovid-10 (Enovid)	Enavid-10	Searle	0.15 mg	Mestranol	Norethynodrel	10 mg	20
Conovid E[b]	Enovid-5	Enavid-5, Enadrel	Searle	0.075 mg			5 mg	20
Norolen[b]	Enovid-E	Enavid-E	Searle	0.1 mg			2.5 mg	20
Prevision[b]			W. J. Rendell	0.075 mg			3 mg	21
			Roussel	0.1 mg			2.5 mg	20

Preparation	Trade name	Manufacturer	Estrogen	Estrogen	Progestogen	Progestogen	Days
Lyndiol[b]		Organon	0.15 mg	Mestranol	5 mg	Lynestrenol	20
Lyndiol 2.5[b]		Organon	0.075 mg	Mestranol	2.5 mg	Lynestrenol	22
Minilyn[c]		Organon	0.05 mg	Ethinyl-estradiol	2.5 mg	Lynestrenol	22
	Norinyl 1 + 80	Syntex	0.08 mg	Mestranol	1 mg	Norethisterone	21[a]
Norinyl-1	Norinyl-2	Syntex	0.05 mg	Mestranol	2 mg	(= norethindrone in USA)	21
	Norinyl-1	Syntex	0.05 mg	Mestranol	1 mg		21
Ortho-Novin 2 mg[b]	Ortho-Novum 2 mg	Ortho (Cilag-Chemie)	0.11 mg	Mestranol	2 mg		21
Ortho-Novin 1/80[b]	Ortho-Novum 1 mg		0.08 mg	Mestranol	1 mg		21
	Ortho-Novum 10		0.06 mg	Mestranol	10 mg		21
Ortho-Novin 1/50[c]			0.05 mg	Mestranol	1 mg		21
Ovulen 50[c]		Searle	0.05 mg	Ethinyl-estradiol	1 mg	Ethynodiol diacetate	21
Demulen		Searle	0.1 mg	Ethinyl-estradiol	0.5 mg	Ethynodiol diacetate	21
Ovulen 1 mg[b]	Metrulen-M, Ovulen	Searle (Boehringer, Mannheim)	0.1 mg	Mestranol	1 mg	Ethynodiol diacetate	21
Ovral	Stediril	Wyeth	0.05 mg	Ethinyl estradiol	0.5 mg	Norgestrel	21
Eugynon 28[a] and Eugynon		Schering AG	0.05 mg	Ethinyl-estradiol	0.5 mg	Norgestrel	21[a]
Aconcen		Merck AG	0.1 mg	Mestranol	3 mg	Chlormadinone acetate	21
		Searle	0.05 mg	Ethinyl estradiol	0.5 mg	Ethynodiol diacetate	21

[a] Plus seven lactose tablets.
[b] All preparations containing more than 0.05 mg estrogen were withdrawn from the UK market in December 1969.
[c] Preparations introduced in December 1969.

4.7). There is then an interval to bring the cycle to 28 days. Some preparations provide placebo tablets for this interval. This type of sequence is more similar to the natural body sequence of hormone secretion but has a slightly higher failure rate. The incidence of "break-through" bleeding is lowest at 0-5%.

3. Progestogen alone

Intramuscular depot injections are given of a long-acting progestogen. Alternatively, a micro-dose of progestogen is taken orally, daily *continuously*. These preparations have been commercially available in the United Kingdom. Their advantages are that the amounts of drug required are very small and therefore the side-effects much less. The most likely compounds are chlormadinone acetate and norethisterone acetate. Regular cyclical bleeding is established but may be at intervals of as little as 12 days. The pregnancy rate is high.

B. MECHANISMS OF ACTION

The first two types of contraceptive act by feedback inhibition of the steroid cycle, i.e. by suppressing pituitary gonadotrophins and hence inhibiting ovulation. Estrogens inhibit the release of FSH and progestogens inhibit the release of LH. Ovulation can be inhibited by either estrogen or progesterone alone. The combined preparations also act on the uterine endometrium to make it unsuitable for ovum implantation and thicken cervical mucus to make it an effective sperm barrier.

The lone progestogen preparations do not appear to act as ovulation inhibitors, but rely partially on cervical mucus changes as a means of contraception. Estrogens alone are not regarded as satisfactory for the long-term suppression of ovulation because the cycles tend to become irregular owing to delayed bleeding from an estrogen-type endometrium and after a few cycles it is not uncommon to get ovulation.

The possibilities of using steroid prophylaxis in other conditions is under active consideration. For veterinary use, vaginal pessaries containing progestogens have been used successfully to synchronize estrus in sheep, and injectable preparations for the same purpose have been tried in pigs and cattle.

C. METHODS OF ASSESSMENT

In the commercially available preparations the estrogens used are universally either ethinylestradiol or mestranol, i.e. the two most potent. It is exceedingly difficult to accurately assess the potency of progestogens in the human female and correlation with animal tests is poor. Several qualitative tests have been used but it is difficult to obtain quantitative results.

1. Greenblatt test for the postponement of menstruation

As controls, a daily dose of 75-100 mg intramuscular progesterone is required to delay menstruation. Usually bleeding occurs 15-30 days after the expected

Table 4.7. *Available oral contraceptives of the sequential type*

Trade name			Firm	Estrogen phase			Progestogen phase			Total days
UK	USA	Other		Estrogen		Days	Progestogen[b]		Days	
C-Quens 21[c]		C-Quens 14/7	Eli Lilly	0.1 mg	Mestranol	14	1.5 mg	Chlormadinone acetate	7	21
Sequens[c]	C-Quens	Estirona	Eli Lilly	0.08 mg	Mestranol	15	2 mg	Chlormadinone acetate	5	20
		Estirona 21	Eli Lilly	0.1 mg	Mestranol	14	1.5 mg	Chlormadinone acetate	7	21
Feminor Sequential[c]			London Rubber	0.1 mg	Mestranol	15	5 mg	Norethynodrel	5	20
Ortho Novin SQ[c]	Ortho-Novum SQ	Novulon-S	Ortho	0.1 mg	Mestranol	14	2 mg	Norethisterone (Norethindrone)	7	21
		Neonovum	Ortho (Cilag-Chemie)	0.1 mg	Mestranol	14	2 mg	Anagesterone acetate	7	21
Serial 28[c]			BDH	0.1 mg	Ethinyl-estradiol	16	1 mg	Megestrol acetate	5	21[a]
	Oracon	Ovin	Mead-Johnson	0.1 mg	Ethinyl-estradiol	16	25 mg	Dimethisterone	5	21
	Norgnen		Syntex	0.08 mg	Mestranol	14	2 mg	Norethisterone	6	20

[a] Plus seven days of lactose tablets.

[b] Given in addition to the same amount of estrogen in the estrogen phase.

[c] All preparations containing more than 0.05 mg estrogen were withdrawn from the UK market in December 1969.

Table 4.8. *Relative oral progestogen potency measured by delay in menstruation*

	ED_{50} (mg)
Norethynodrel	5.3
Norethisterone (without mestranol)	4.3
Melengestrol acetate	2.5
21-Fluoro-medroxy-progesterone acetate	2.5
Megestrol acetate	1.8
Ethynodiol diacetate	1.5

Compounds were given with 0.1 mg mestranol.

period while progesterone is being given. Orally 0.2 mg mestranol and 1000 mg progesterone are required daily. Other oral progestogens may be tried instead of the standard progesterone. It has been found that 30 mg norethindrone daily causes postponement of menstruation for as long as 6 months. Table 4.8 shows some of the most active compounds tested in this way, with estimates of the doses required to delay menstruation in 50% of the trials.

2. Swyer test

The endometrial response to different progestogens is assessed by biopsy in estrogen-primed women with long-standing secondary amenorrhea. Estrogen is given for 20 days, progestogen for the last ten of these and the biopsy taken on the twenty-first day.

3. Prevention of "break-through" bleeding

When given daily with 0.2 mg mestranol for 20-40 days, the minimum amount of progestogen required to prevent bleeding gives an indication of their relative potencies (Table 4.9).

Table 4.9. *Relative progestogen potencies in preventing "break-through" bleeding*

	mg
Ethynodiol diacetate	1
Chlormadinone	4
Norethisterone acetate	7.5
Norethisterone	10
Norethynodrel	13.8
Medroxyprogesterone acetate	30

D. FUTURE DEVELOPMENTS IN FEMALE CONTRACEPTION

1. Continuous progestogen

A potent progestogen, e.g. chlormadinone acetate, norethisterone acetate, is administered orally in small amounts throughout the cycle. It is believed that ovulation is not regularly inhibited and that the mechanism of contraception is due partially to a change in the cervical mucus, which prevents passage of sperms, and possibly partially to changes in the rate of tubal transport of ova and production of ovarian steroids.

2. Long acting oral contraception

Quinestrol (Fig. 4.9) has a greatly prolonged estrogenic effect probably due to storage in body fat with gradual release. A single oral dose of 5 mg lasts

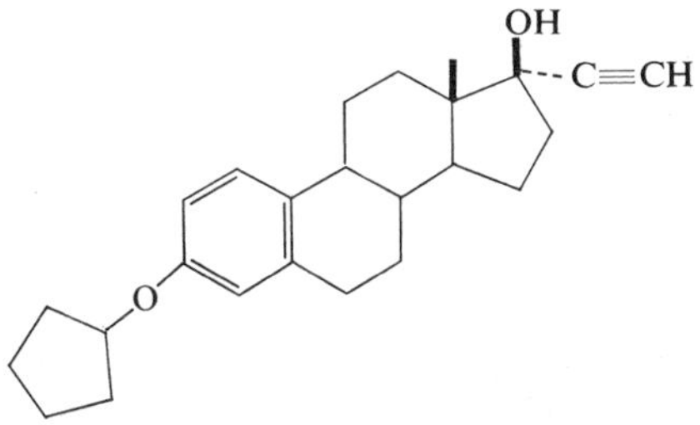

Quinestrol
Ethinylestradiol 3-cyclopentyl ether

Fig. 4.9. A long acting estrogen.

for 6-14 weeks. Efficient contraception involves simultaneous administration of a short acting progestogen, e.g. chlormadinone acetate.

3. Long acting injectable preparations

Estradiol enanthate and 17α-hydroxyprogesterone caproate are suitable components.

4. Implantation

Experiments are in progress in the search for pellet forms of long acting estrogens and progestogens. These would last almost indefinitely.

5. Post-coital and non-steroid contraceptives

Various synthetic estrogens have been shown to be effective post-coital contraceptives (the "morning-after" pill) and seem to act by preventing implantation of the fertilized ovum. Large doses of estrogens, e.g. 5-50 mg diethyl-stilbestrol or 0.5 mg ethinyl-estradiol given for 4-5 days after coitus will prevent

5

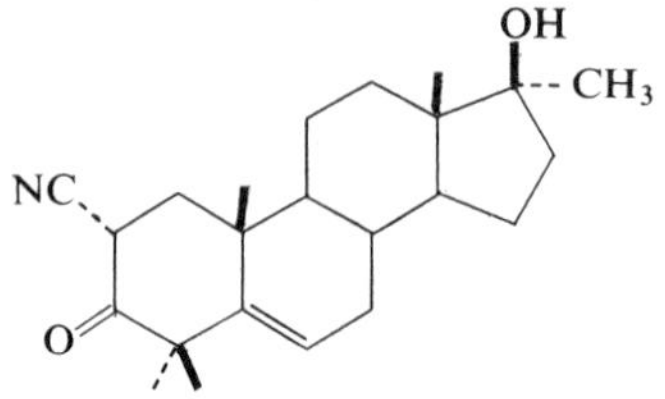

Cyanotrimethylandrostenolone
2α-Cyano-4,4,17α-trimethyl-
5-androsten-17β-ol-3-one

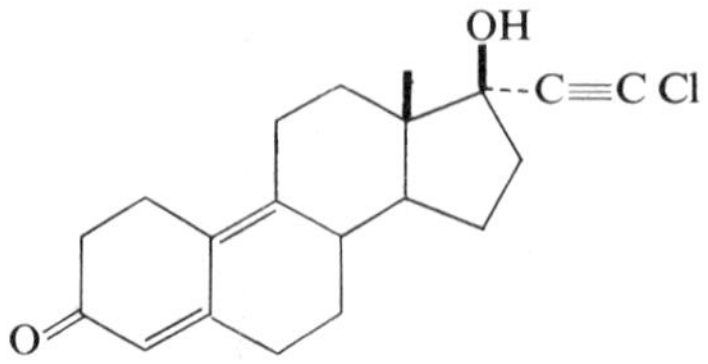

Mk-665, Ethynerone
17α-Chloroethinyl-4,9-estradien-
17β-ol-3-one

Fig. 4.10. Some new inhibitors of steroidogenesis.

pregnancy. The effects may be teratogenic and cause deformation in the infant if implantation is not prevented. There is at present no hormonal pill which will satisfactorily remove an early (2-week) pregnancy (the "abortion pill").

A number of new steroids with unusual ring additions may prove to be effective contraceptives, e.g. a cyanoketone (Fig. 4.10) has been shown to be a potent inhibitor of various 3β-hydroxysteroid dehydrogenases and thus might interfere with progesterone synthesis. Similarly MK-665 is a potent inhibitor of certain steroidogenic steps in human testicles.

Several non-steroidal weak estrogens and anti-estrogens (Fig. 4.11) also inhibit implantation or interfere with corpus luteum function, e.g. ORF-3858

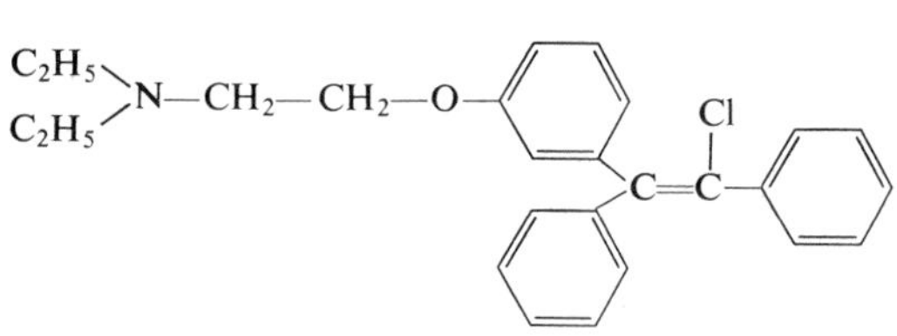

"Clomid"
Clomiphene

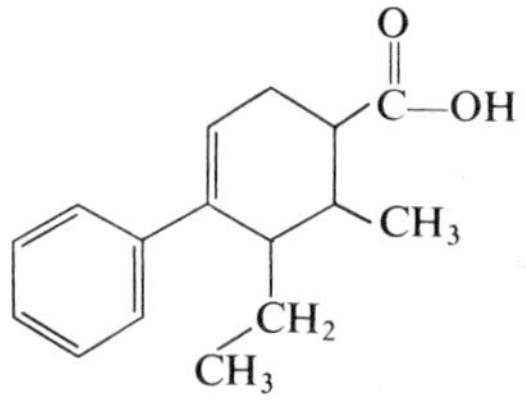

(Ortho) ORF-3858
2-Methyl-3-ethyl-4-phenyl-Δ⁴-cyclo-
hexene carboxylic acid

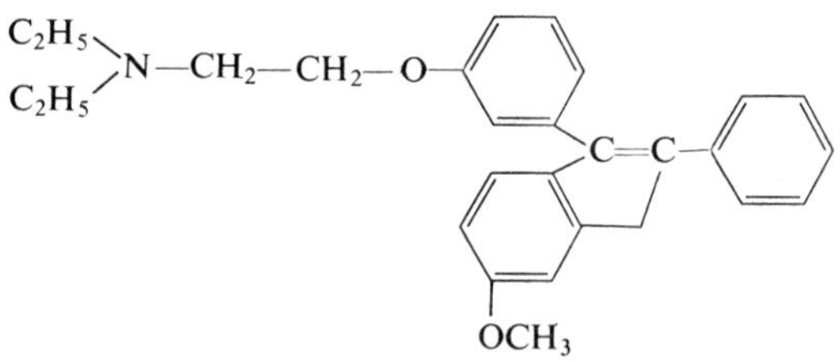

(Upjohn) U-11, 555A

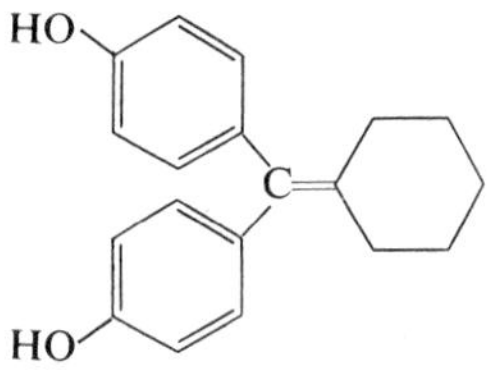

(Ferrosan) F-6060

Fig. 4.11. Some non-steroidal estrogen antagonists.

which is effective post-coitally in rabbits and monkeys and appears to have no teratogenic effects. F-6060 inhibits 3β-hydroxysteroid dehydrogenase of human corpus luteum *in vitro*. Clomiphene is used in the human species for the induction of ovulation, which seems to result from stimulation of FSH secretion. It also alters the structure of the endometrium.

6. Immunological contraception

It has been shown that certain females agglutinate the sperm of certain males and that this effect appears to be acquired by exposure to sperm. It is possible that immunological incompatibility may be adapted to contraception.

E. ESTRUS SYNCHRONIZATION IN DOMESTIC ANIMALS

The development of artificial methods for regulating the estrus cycle in various classes of farm animals has long been a goal of animal physiologists. For beef and dairy cattle it is more productive to have all the calves born on the same day. Control of the onset of estrus in sows by weaning at the appropriate time is widely practised in the intensive production of pigs but no comparable means are available for regulating the time of estrus in gilts (female nulliparous pigs). If estrus could be synchronized in gilts it would make the rearing of the piglets more economical and would enable artificial insemination to be given at the correct and more easily determinable time. By running vasectomized rams with ewes about a month before the time of normal mating at the transition period between the non-breeding and the breeding seasons, it is possible to bring estrus forward and to achieve an earlier lambing. A degree of synchronization can be achieved by this method and it is commonly used by sheep farmers to induce earlier breeding.

The first successful synchronization of estrus in cattle resulting from an oral progestogen was reported in 1960. The compound, 6-methyl-17α-acetoxy-progesterone (MAP), was mixed in soya bean oil meal and about 4 lb of this meal fed to each animal daily for 20 days. Artificial insemination was carried out 3-5 days after the withdrawal of treatment or 10-12 h after the start of estrus. Similar results have been obtained with "Lutinyl" and melengestrol acetate (Fig. 4.12).

Similar effects have been obtained with ewes by the oral and intramuscular administration of progestogens. Vaginal pessaries made of polyurethane impregnated with "Cronolone" (Fig. 4.13) have also been used to synchronize estrus in ewes. Synchronization of estrus in gilts with progestogens is much more difficult than in cattle and sheep, as the dose has to be much more carefully controlled so that luteinized or cystic follicles are not produced. A successful method is to suppress gonadotrophin secretion with "Methallibure" given orally in the follicular phase of the cycle, at 100 mg for 20 days when estrus occurs 4-9 days after withdrawal.

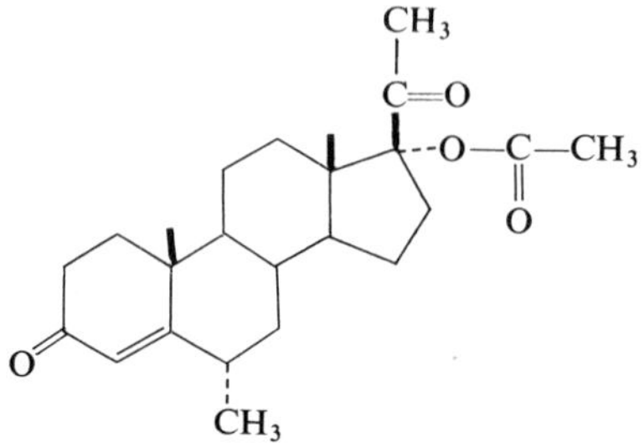

MAP
Depo-Provera
6α-Methyl-17-acetoxyprogesterone
6α-Methyl-4-pregnen-17α-ol-3,20-
dione acetate

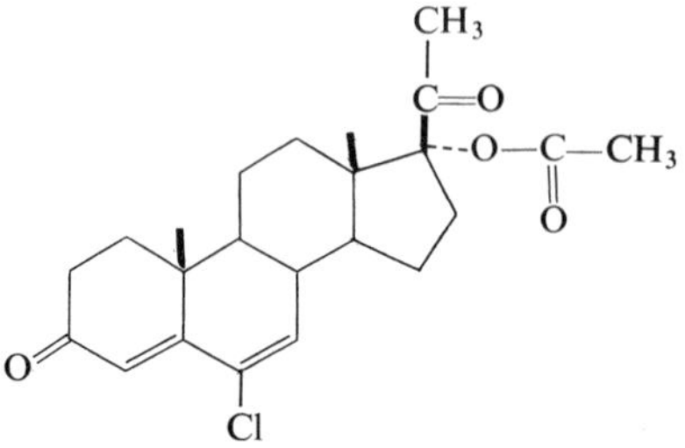

CAP, Chlormadinone acetate
Lutinyl
6-Chloro-Δ⁶-dehydro-17-acetoxy-
progesterone
6-Chloro-4,6-pregnadien-17α-ol-
3,20-dione

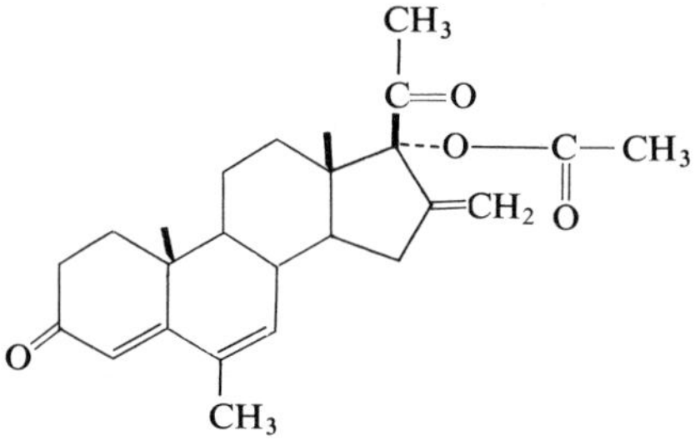

Melengestrol acetate
6-Methyl-16-methylene-4,6-pregnadien-17α-ol-3,20-dione acetate

Fig. 4.12. Compounds used for estrus synchronization.

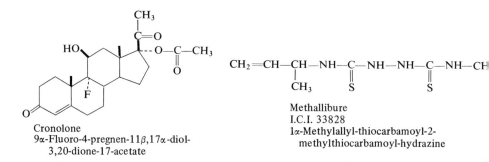

Cronolone
9α-Fluoro-4-pregnen-11β,17α-diol-
3,20-dione-17-acetate

Methallibure
I.C.I. 33828
1α-Methylallyl-thiocarbamoyl-2-
methylthiocarbamoyl-hydrazine

Fig. 4.13. Compounds used for estrus synchronization of pigs.

5

TARGET ORGAN EFFECTS–B. ANDROGENS AND ANABOLICS

I. INTRODUCTION

Androgens are compounds which produce and maintain the secondary characteristics of the adult male or their vestigal remains in the female. These are increased size of the phallus (penis or clitoris); growth and pigmentation of the scrotum (or labia majora); development of the prostate and seminal vesicles; deepening of the voice; stimulation of the sebaceous secretion; and the appearance of sexual hair. Androgens show a generalized anabolic effect, causing increased protein formation, particularly of muscle and bone, which causes an increased rate of linear growth in the immature animal. Administration of androgens results in a retention of nitrogen, phosphorus and potassium together with a lowering of the respiratory quotient, which implies the use of dietary or body fat for protein biosynthesis. Subcutaneous fat is lost and veins become prominent under the skin. Growth of the beard lags well behind the other events of puberty while recession of hair at the temples occurs in those subjects with genes for baldness. In females, androgens have a progestational action. Androgens are also believed to be responsible for linear bone growth in both males and females, probably in conjunction with somatotrophin.

II. GROWTH HORMONE

Somatotrophin causes linear bone growth and increase in body tissue weight in hypophysectomized rats continuously for up to 90 days. The action on body tissues, especially muscle, is probably due to increased protein synthesis rather than decreased protein catabolism, i.e. growth hormone is anabolic. An immediate effect in intact young animals is to lower plasma and liver amino nitrogen. There is body retention of nitrogen, sodium, potassium and phosphorus. Nitrogen retention induced by growth hormone is greater in animals receiving a high fat than a high carbohydrate diet and this may be due to the ability of growth hormone to stimulate insulin secretion. It is now known that elevation of blood sugar suppresses secretion of growth hormone and that administration of human growth hormone results in impaired glucose tolerance in normal subjects. In animals treated with growth hormone the respiratory quotient is lowered suggesting increased fat oxidation and increased blood non-esterified fatty acids. Growth hormone causes muscle glycogen deposition and appears to have a direct effect on the renal tubular transport of phosphorus and calcium. There is an elevation of serum phosphorus and calcium.

Body growth is influenced by somatotrophin, thyrotrophin, gonadotrophin and ACTH. The cessation of growth after puberty is not due to lack of somatotrophin but to the ossification of the epiphysial cartilage discs brought about by the sex hormones. The influence of thyrotrophin on body growth is easily seen in cretins and can be corrected by the administration of thyroid extract or thyroxine. The administration of ACTH or of corticosteroids results in depression of the growth of children and the stimulating influence of somatotrophin on body growth is counteracted by ACTH in hypophysectomized animals. In man, most but not all of the sex difference in adult height arises at puberty. The pubertal spurt in height takes place earlier, is shorter and of less intensity in girls and is generally believed to be due to adrenal androgens. The greater increase in male height at puberty is nearly all attributable to the greater amount of androgen secreted. It is not known how androgens promote skeletal growth but there is evidence that they potentiate the skeletal growth response to somatotrophin.

III. ANDROGENS
A. BIOLOGICAL ASSAY
1. Capon comb growth test

After castration there is a marked involution of the cock's comb and the administration of androgen restores the comb to its normal size. Birds are ready for use 6 months after castration. At the beginning of the assay the length and height of the combs is determined. The androgen is then given, usually by intramuscular injection, for 3-5 days. The combs are then remeasured and the difference in both length and height is determined. An alternative to injection is to inunct an oily solution of the androgen directly onto the comb. This method is much more sensitive than intramuscular injection. Some workers remove the comb at the end of the test, weigh it, and express results in terms of comb weight to body weight. The original capon unit was the amount of androgen to cause a 20% increase in comb area. In the place of capons, young Leghorn chicks, 2-3 days old, may also serve as test animals. Androgens are applied by inunction, the chicks killed 24 h after the last application and the combs weighed. This method is more sensitive, more convenient but less precise than the capon comb.

2. Pfeiffer's test

The bill of the English sparrow (*Passer domesticus*) responds to androgens by a marked blackening. The test animals can be either castrated males, or normal females. The androgens may be given either by intramuscular injection or applied directly to the bill. The test has been little used.

3. Mathieson and Hays test

The administration of androgens to the castrated male rat leads to an increase in the weight of the seminal vesicles. The androgen is usually injected intramuscularly and the weight of the seminal vesicles determined after 72 h and compared with untreated controls. The prostate gland also increases with androgens and can be used as a second assay in the same animals.

4. Hamilton's test

This is a human clinical assay based on the rate and amount of axillary hair growth. It is easy to use, but difficult to interpret and can be used only either on volunteers for short periods, or on patients receiving androgen therapy.

B. POTENCY

The definition of androgenic action of a steroid as being its effect on the secondary male characteristics is very vague, since the secondary male characteristics are localized in many different tissues and vary considerably between species. The extent to which these different tissues are restored after the administration of androgens can differ widely among the various compounds. Arbitrarily it is generally agreed that for the purpose of pharmacological bioassay of steroids in mammals, the term "androgenic activity" is restricted to the effect of such compounds on organs directly involved in the production and transport of semen. However, the ratio of the effects of various steroids on the different parts of the male genital tract is also variable, e.g. androstanedione has a ratio of responses on rat ventral prostate and seminal vesicles of about 3.8 whereas androstanolone has a ratio of 1.1. This implies that a comparison of the androgenic activity of various compounds can be made only on the basis of a comparison of their effects on the same organ in comparable test animals. The weight of the testes appears to be related to the amount of FSH secreted, while the weight of the ventral prostate and of seminal vesicles appears to be related to the amount of ICSH (LH) secreted.

The most potent naturally occurring androgens are testosterone and dihydro-testosterone and either may be the physiologically active androgen although their concentrations in body tissues and fluids is so small that they cannot be detected in many of them. Less active are some of their oxygenated 5α-andro-stane derivatives (i.e. belonging to the allo and not the normal series). Dehydroepiandrosterone and androst-4-ene-3,17-dione are weak androgens. Table 5.1 shows some relative potencies obtained from a consideration of the results obtained by all the methods.

Table 5.1. *Relative potency of the natural androgens (%)*

Testosterone	100
5α-Androstan-17β-ol-3-one (5α-dihydrotestosterone)	90
5α-Androstane-3α,17β-diol (androstanediol)	60
Androstenedione	20
Dehydroepiandrosterone	10
Androsterone	10
Etiocholanolone (5β-androsterone)	0
Epitestosterone	0

C. CLINICAL INDICATIONS

1. Hypopituitarism

Dwarfs with normal body proportions are known as midgets and suffer from ateliosis which is defined as a condition in which neither growth nor develop-ment is arrested, though both are indefinitely retarded. Sexual and asexual forms may be distinguished depending on whether sexual development is or is not normal. The two forms cannot be distinguished with certainty until at least 25 years of age, as puberty occurs spontaneously in the sexual form at a relatively late age. Growth retardation is not normally noticed until 2-3 years of age. Such hypopituitarism is an uncommon cause of dwarfism in children, accounting for less than 10% of the cases, about two-thirds of which have no evidence of pituitary tumour.

The treatment of choice is two units of intramuscular human somatotrophin daily for the first 15 days of 4 months, with a rest of 4 months and so on until a height of at least 5 ft is reached. Growth can be increased by as much as three times, giving up to 3 in. a year. If secondary sexual characteristics do not develop by the age of 12 years, supplements of sex hormones are given. In males this is 200-400 mg intramuscular testosterone enanthate once a month and in females 10-20 mg oral methyltestosterone daily is required to produce axillary and pubic hair. It may also be necessary to give 1-2 mg oral stilbestrol daily for 6-9 months in the females. These doses of androgens will also cause increase in linear growth if human somatotrophin is not available. Younger children of either sex may be given 1.25 mg fluoxymesterone every 12 h.

2. Impotence and male sterility

The administration of androgens in impotence produces mainly psychological benefits. Some improvement in sperm counts can be achieved as a rebound effect after suppression of pituitary gonadotrophin secretion by androgen but fertility in oligospermic males is not usually achieved. Smaller doses, e.g. 50-100 mg testosterone enanthate every 2 weeks, together with serum gonadotrophin, may stimulate spermatogenesis. Secondary sexual characteristics can be improved, e.g. in eunuchs and males castrated in adult life by 250 mg intramuscular testosterone enanthate every 3-6 weeks.

3. Cancer

Androgens have been used in breast cancer when excision or radiotherapy have failed to control the progress of local recurrent disease. They are also used in cases where the primary tumour is inoperable or is unsuited for, or resistant to, radiotherapy. Hormones are also widely used in cases of disseminated carcinoma, which occurs in the majority of breast cancer patients. Many tumours arising in the breast retain the normal estrogen dependence of breast tissue and androgens are given to antagonize the effects of circulating estrogens. The most common treatment is 100 mg intramuscular testosterone propionate three times a week which produces subjective improvement in about 20% of cases. Many other androgens and anabolic steroids have been used.

IV. ANABOLICS

A. BIOLOGICAL ASSAY

1. Levator ani test

The weight of the levator ani muscle (in the perineal muscle complex) is an indication of the myotropic potency of the compound administered to the castrated male rat. There are many variations in technique and length of the test

5*

while its theoretical basis is open to doubt. Nevertheless, this is the only test in general use which enables rapid pharmacological screening and the qualitative parallelism between results and the nitrogen-retaining properties of a compound in general is remarkable.

2. Nitrogen retention

Test animals are force-fed on a fixed diet and need to be stabilized for about a month prior to test. Both rats and monkeys have been used. In man the additional nitrogen retained by maximally effective doses of an anabolic steroid amounts to about 20% of the urine nitrogen value found in the control period. Hydroxystenazole and methylnorandrostenolone have no nitrogen-retaining potency in rats but hydroxystenazole produces substantial nitrogen retention in primates as well as man. Norethandrolone produces only a small nitrogen retention in monkeys but is a useful compound in man.

B. POTENCY

Animal experiments have given conflicting results and it is not possible to arrange the anabolic steroids in order of potency. All androgenic compounds have an anabolic effect and the synthetic compounds have been designed to reduce the androgenic effect without reducing the anabolic effect. Testosterone is considered to have an anabolic : androgenic ratio (i.e. therapeutic index) of one. The best of the anabolic steroids have a therapeutic index of two to three and the least effective are nearer one. Their structures are shown in Fig. 5.1. It appears that all anabolic steroids given in maximally effective doses have the same quantitative effect on protein metabolism. Anabolic steroids may be given as an intramuscular injection in an oil, e.g. nandrolone phenylpropionate, nandrolone decanoate and methenalone enanthate. Orally-active compounds usually have a 17α-alkyl substituent which is believed to protect the 17β-hydroxyl group from oxidation by the liver. Some relative potencies are given in Table 5.2 for intramuscular administration and in Table 5.3 for oral administration.

C. CLINICAL INDICATIONS

1. Debility

The body of a normal adult male weighing 70 kg has a total protein content of about 8-12 kg, of which about 50% is in the supporting structures (bones, connective tissue, skin), 40% in muscle and about 10% in the viscera. The turnover of connective tissue collagen, which constitutes about 30% of total body protein, is some years. The overall turnover rate is about 5-10 g/kg per day (i.e. about five times the daily protein intake). In normal individuals the balance between catabolism and anabolism is so fine that the external nitrogen balance is

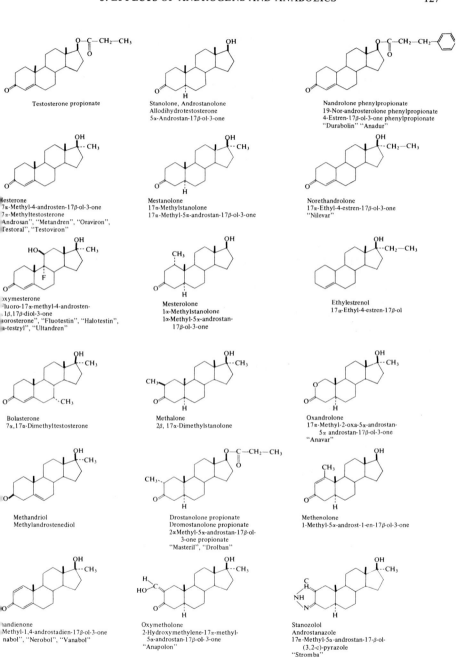

Fig. 5.1. Synthetic androgenic and anabolic steroids.

zero. Almost all disease states are catabolic and lead to negative nitrogen balance. Both testosterone and anabolic steroids have proved disappointing as therapeutic substances in acute illness or trauma which is in the catabolic phase. The period

Table 5.2. *Some comparative intramuscular androgenic and anabolic potencies*

	Androgenic activity	Myotropic activity	Approximate androgenic: myotropic ratio
Testosterone	100	100	1
Testosterone propionate	93-115	96-147	0.9
Testosterone enanthate	6	7	0.9
7α-Methyltestosterone propionate	161-222	352-452	0.5
5α-Dihydrotestosterone (stanolone)	146-168	138-156	0.7
7α-Methyl-19-nortestosterone acetate	126-143	299-328	0.4
Fluoxymesterone, "Fluosterone", etc.	72-122	84-235	0.6
Norandrolone phenpropionate, "Durobolin," "Anadur"	80-97	286-488	0.2
Methenolone enanthate, "Primobolan Depot"	52-56	78-108	0.6
Drostanolone, "Masteril", "Drolban"	44-59	77-144	0.5
D-Homo-testosterone propionate	40-61	28-112	0.6
17α-Methyl-19-nortestosterone	19-24	48-68	0.4
Norethandrolone, "Nilevar"	24-25	60-69	0.4
Androstane-3, 17-dione	5-30	5-23	1.4
5α-Androstane-3α, 17β-diol dipropionate	18-31	10-31	1.2
5α-Androstane-3β, 17β-diol diacetate	12-17	7-9	1.5
4-Androsten-3α, 17β-diol diacetate	49-92	36-96	1.2
4-Androsten-3β, 17β-diol diacetate	105-183	66-127	1.6
Androsterone	6-8	4-7	1.4
17α-Methyl-5-androstene-3β, 17β-diol	17-28	16-17	1.4
17β-Hydroxy-17α-vinyl-4-androsten-3-one (vinyltestosterone)	11	6	1.8

of recovery is characterized by anabolism with a positive external nitrogen balance when the nitrogen retained may be as much as 23% of that absorbed. During this phase the administration of anabolic steroids may have some value. There is an increase in appetite and in the feeling of well-being in children, women and hypogonadal adults of both sexes. In normal adult males this effect is either transient or non-existent. All these steroids have some virilizing effect and chronic administration to normal males may cause feedback inhibition of gonadotrophin secretion and hence testicular atrophy.

2. Osteoporosis

Osteoporosis has been defined as a reduction in bone mass per unit volume with no known change in chemical composition. It is found in Cushing's syndrome, hypogonadism, rheumatoid arthritis, malnutrition and many other conditions. It is most commonly seen in post-menopausal women and in the

Table 5.3. *Some comparative oral androgenic and anabolic potencies*

	Andro-genic activity	Myotro-pic activity	Approximate androgenic: myotropic ratio
Fluoxymesterone	100	100	1
1-Dehydro-11β-hydroxy-17α-methyl-testosterone	18	18	1
4, 5α-Dihydro-2(hydroxymethylene)-testosterone	< 5-11	4	2.8
7α, 17-Dimethyltestosterone	54-65	108-112	0.5
9α-Fluoro-11-keto-17α-methyl-testosterone	80-86	85-92	0.8
4-Hydroxy-17-methyltestosterone	5-12	22-36	0.3
11β-Hydroxy-17α-methyltestosterone	31	39	0.8
17β-Hydroxy-17α-methyl-5α-androstane-3, 11-dione	41-55	46-98	0.7
Methenolone acetate	72-84	148-320	0.3
17-Methyl-5α-androstane-11β, 17β-diol	17-32	18-20	1.3
17α-Methyl-5α-androstane-3β, 11β, 17β-triol	40-62	14-70	1.2
Methyltestosterone	9	5	1.8

aged of both sexes. Anabolic steroids have been used extensively in the treatment of this condition together with a high-protein, high-calcium diet. Subjective improvement, e.g. the relief of pain, is often apparent but radiological improvement is rare.

3. During treatment with corticosteroids

Glucocorticosteroid treatment in man has a catabolic effect on the skeletal muscles, bone and skin and leads to protein depletion and osteoporosis, while there is an anabolic effect on the liver. It is believed that the resulting iatrogenic

Cushing's syndrome is caused by suppression of the adrenal-pituitary axis. Growth is arrested in the young. In short-term balance studies, anabolic steroids have been shown to effect an amelioration and sometimes a reversal of the negative nitrogen and calcium balance induced by glucocorticoids. Long-term studies are not so favourable and there may be an increase in glucocorticoid side effects, e.g. acne, hirsutism.

V. ANTI-ANDROGENS

Anti-hormones are defined on the basis of their effects on target organs in preventing the effects of the positive hormone. Thus, anti-androgens are defined as substances which decrease the effectiveness of exogenously-administered androgens when the target organ effect that is being measured is one of the biological assays described previously, e.g. weight of the seminal vesicles in the castrated rat or mouse, or weight of the comb of the chick. In the former type of methods androgens are removed by castration and replaced in one group of test animals by subcutaneous injection. This has the effect of allowing the growth of the seminal vesicles. In another group of animals, androgens and anti-androgens are given at the same time and the degree of prevention of growth of seminal vesicles is a measure of the anti-androgenic potency. A variety of anti-androgenic compounds of different structures have been described, e.g. estrogens and carcinogenic hydrocarbons such as benzpyrene and methylcholanthrene. The most potent anti-androgens are structurally related to progesterone and are often potent progestogens, e.g. chlormadinone acetate, cyproterone acetate (Fig. 5.2).

Progesterone itself has anti-androgenic properties in animals, including antagonism of testosterone-induced growth of seminal vesicles in the rat. Its derivatives, cyproterone acetate and chlormadinone acetate, antagonize testosterone-induced capon comb growth and growth of the seminal vesicles, ventral prostate and levator ani in rats. They also antagonize the effect of testosterone on the hypothalamus and block direct effects of androgens on the testes. When given to pregnant rats, cyproterone acetate antagonizes the foetal testicular androgens leading to feminization of male offspring. Such compounds may provide effective treatment for acne, hirsutism, virilization, precocious puberty and prostate disease. They may also have a use as male contraceptives if side effects, such as impotency, can be eliminated.

Estrogens may directly antagonize selected androgenic actions, e.g. chick comb growth, but other anti-androgenic effects, e.g. decreased size of secondary sexual organs, are due to suppression of pituitary gonadotrophin secretion which in turn results in decreased androgen secretion by the testes. Estrogens do not antagonize most of the actions of androgens on secondary sexual structures when both are administered to castrate animals.

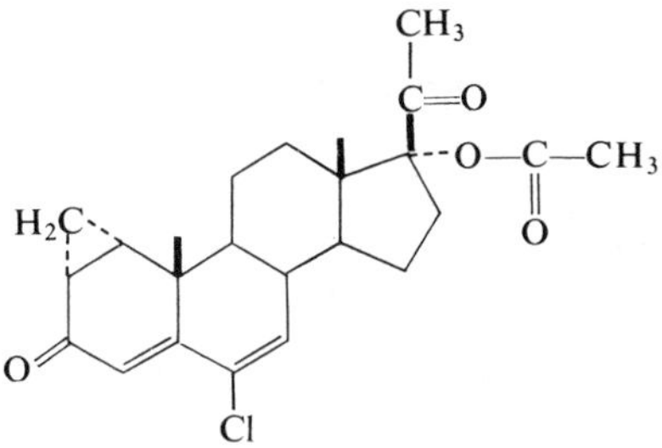

Cyproterone acetate
6-Chloro-1α,2α-methylene-4,6-pregnadien-
17α-ol-3,20-dione acetate

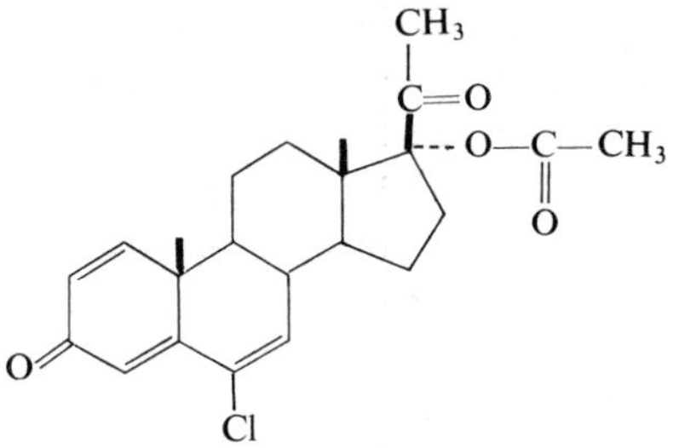

Δ¹-Chlormadinone acetate
6-Chloro-1,4,6-pregnatrien-
17α-ol-3,20 dione acetate

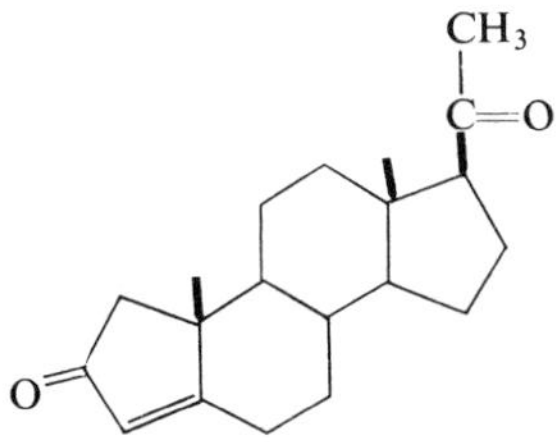

A-Nor-progesterone

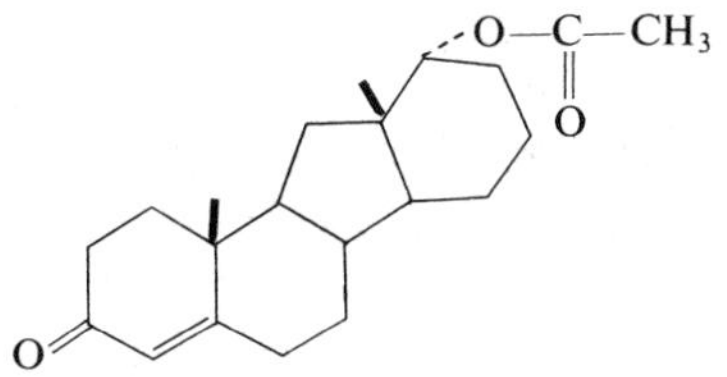

C-Nor-D-homo-17α-epitestosterone acetate
C-Nor-D-homo-4-androsten-17α-ol acetate

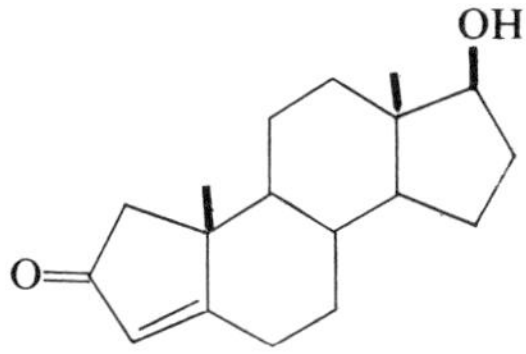

A-Nor-testosterone

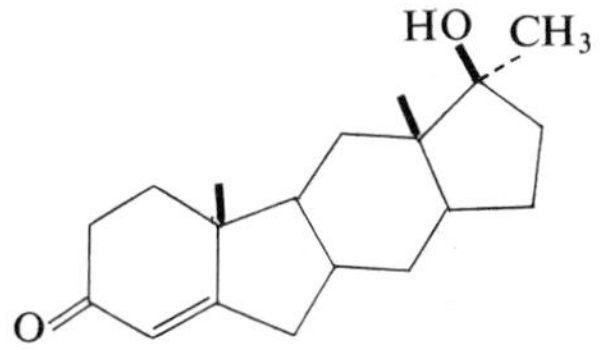

17α-Methyl-B-nor-testosterone
17α-Methyl-B-nor-4-androsten-
17β-ol-3-one

Fig. 5.2. Some anti-androgens related to testosterone and progesterone.

VI. EFFECTS OF STEROIDS ON SKIN, HAIR FOLLICLES AND SEBACEOUS GLANDS

A. SKIN

The skin is an important target organ for both estrogens and androgens. There is a general proliferative effect on the epidermal cells with a stimulation of mitosis and turnover rate of the skin. In man the turnover rate is about 30 days from cell division in the basal layer to loss of the cell from the horny layer. Estrogens are believed to be responsible for the softness and suppleness of female skin and the decline in estrogen production at the menopause is believed to cause thinning, tightening and drying of the skin. Similarly in males decrease in androgen production with age is believed to be responsible for some of the ageing effects in skin. Aged skin is much thinner, having fewer layers of cells in the spinous layer and the rete pegs at the base of the undulating epidermis tend to become flat. Estrogens have been used in cosmetics for the postmenopausal woman from some 35 years and the US Food and Drug Administration (FDA) has set an upper limit of 10,000 IU per oz. Progesterone or pregnenolone acetate are often also present. It is now recognized that topical estrogens exert their effects by water retention producing a non-pitting edema of the skin. In this way the skin becomes firmer, plumper and smoother. Wrinkles are stretched out and seem to disappear. One of the best compounds producing this effect is pregnenolone which has no hormonal properties. Such hormone creams are of use in the treatment of mucous membranes and vulvo-vaginal tissues. Systemic effects are prevented by omitting cholesterol from the formulation so that the active constituents are retained in the epithelial tissue.

B. SEBACEOUS GLANDS

Androgens and estrogens exert a profound effect on the sebaceous glands, whose activity is usually measured by the amount of sebum produced. Sebum can be blotted or eluted from a particular area of skin, weighed and analysed into its constituent fatty acids, esters, alcohols, hydrocarbons and steroids. Administration of androgens causes enlargement of the sebaceous glands and increased sebum production in animals. In man, increased circulating androgens at puberty exert the same effect and in some cases are responsible for acne. The average age of onset of acne is 14 years and the age of maximum incidence is 16 years when about 60% of boys have acne on the face, 20% on the chest and 25% on the back. Acne is less severe and less frequent in girls. There is a decreased incidence after the age of 20. Sebaceous secretion of adult males, in contrast to prepubertal males, cannot be further increased by the administration of androgens and it is believed that the binding sites in the target organ are already saturated with endogenous androgens. The administration of androgens to adult females can cause a slight increase in sebum production. Ovarian and adrenal androgens play a key role in sebaceous gland activity in the female and the latter appear to be the sole source of stimulation before the menarche and after the menopause.

Progesterone, or more probably its metabolites, also exerts a stimulatory effect on the sebaceous glands in the female and is believed to be responsible for the premenstrual flare of acne. Very large endogenous doses of progesterone are required to cause an increase in sebum production and it is possible that the effect is really androgenic. Many progestogens have significant androgenic properties and it is possible that the compound responsible for the acne of the progestational phase of the menstrual cycle is some other compound produced in minor amounts.

It is commonly accepted that estrogens suppress human sebaceous gland secretion. In the human female sebaceous secretion decreases with the decrease in circulating estrogen with age. Estrogens have been used in the treatment of acne but very large doses are required in the male, e.g. 2.5 mg ethinylestradiol per day. It is believed that the effect is not a direct suppression of the sebaceous glands but that feedback inhibition occurs and less androgen is produced. Estrogen treatment of males with acne is not recommended because of other anti-androgenic effects, e.g. on the testes. Recently, females with acne have been successfully treated with estrogens in the form of the contraceptive pill and again the effect is probably by feedback inhibition. Topical anti-androgens which confine their activities to the skin have not yet succeeded in suppressing male sebum secretion.

C. HAIR GROWTH

The individual hair has a definite life span varying from a few weeks to several years, which always terminates with the death of the hair and its replacement by a new one. This is due to a gradual lessening of mitotic activity in the hair matrix at the bottom of the follicle. The lower end of the hair degenerates and partly detaches itself from the now quiescent, resting follicle. This is the telogen or resting stage. When the hair cycle restarts with active proliferation in the follicle, this is the anagen phase. The catagen phase is characterized by cessation of active proliferation. On the general body surface about equal numbers of follicles are resting and active at any one time so that the numbers remain constant. The minimum length of the hair cycle on the scalp is about 16 months for males and 20 months for females. On the bearded area the cycle lasts 7-11 months. Sex hormones promote the final development and maintenance of the secondary sexual hair, most of which are lost in women after the menopause. The effect seems to be due to androgens in both males and females as estrogens suppress hair growth in the rat and dog. Male pattern baldness also appears to be due to androgens, when each successive generation of hair lessens in diameter until the follicle no longer produces hair and progressive immaturity ends in atrophy of the follicle. Thus, androgens stimulate the growth of hair in some parts of the skin and inhibit it in others. It is possible that different androgens are taken up by slightly different receptor sites in these target areas. The skin can be considered not as a single target organ but as containing a number of different target receptor sites for a variety of hormones.

Baldness is a dominant *sex-limited* genetic trait. That baldness is not due to a *sex-linked* gene is clear from the fact that bald fathers, depending on whether they carry two or only one baldness gene, transmit their baldness to all or half of their sons. The genes for baldness derived from father and mother are identical so that a male can be bald when neither of his parents is so, in which case his baldness gene will have come from his mother. The action of the baldness gene differs very markedly in the two sexes due to the action of the male sex hormones on the genotype. No amount of androgens will produce baldness in males who have not inherited the necessary genes. Administration of androgens to eunuchs will produce baldness in only those with baldness genes. Women inheriting a baldness gene from each parent, becoming homozygous for baldness, experience thinning of the hair or partial baldness but complete hereditary baldness of the masculine type in the female is extremely rare. Although some men (and women) manifest their baldness genes while comparatively young, e.g. in their twenties and thirties, it cannot be considered that all people who have baldness genes have exhibited them until they are at least fifty. The frequency of bald men over fifty is about 75% which represents the frequency of the genotypes *BB* and *Bb* in the population where *B* is the (dominant) gene for baldness and *b* the (recessive) gene for non-baldness. The gene frequencies of *B* and *b* are 0.500 and the frequency of *BB* is 25%. The figure agrees very well with the figure of 20% of adult women who complain of diffuse thinning of the hair and who are homozygous for baldness.

VII. ANTI-SPERMATOGENIC COMPOUNDS

A. SPERMATOGENESIS

A good deal is now known about spermatogenesis in rats and mice. Mammalian spermatogenesis is divisible into two main phases, i.e. the formation of morphologically-mature spermatozoa in the seminiferous epithelium lining of the testis tubules, followed by their liberation, collection into and transport through the epididymus via the vas deferens into the urethra. Here the prostrate and seminal vesicles contribute their secretions. The rat testis is largely composed of an intricate arrangement of minute convoluted tubules, lined throughout by seminiferous epithelium in which spermatogenesis commences with spermatogonia, which lie at the periphery of the tubule. The earliest recognizable cell is called spermatogonia type-A and it undergoes five mitotic and one meiotic division, resulting in young spermatozoa in the lumen of the testis (Fig. 5.3). The cells produced by mitotic division of spermatogonia type-A gradually change morphologically and are known as intermediate and type-B spermatogonia. Some type-A cells remain to function as stem cells. Type-B spermatogonia divide into resting spermatocytes which undergo a long meiotic prophase before undergoing meiosis to form secondary spermatocytes. A final division of these cells rapidly follows and spermatids are formed, the process from type-A spermatogonia taking 12 days. The transformation of spermatids into morphologically-mature spermatozoa is then a long, complex metamorphosis lasting a further 36 days. While this is taking place, three other generations of type-A spermatogonia commence development at intervals of 12 days so that successive waves of sperm liberation follow each other. One complete cycle thus

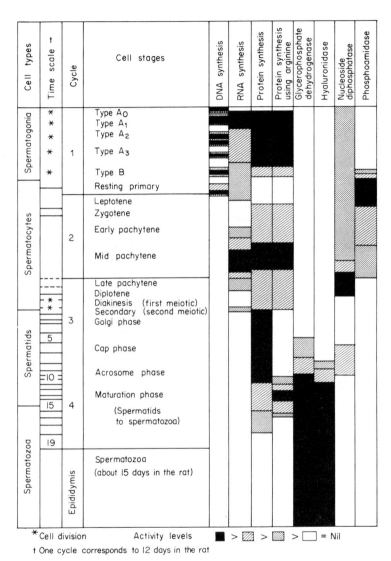

Fig. 5.3. Stages of spermatogenesis and spermiogenesis in the rat. (After B. W. Fox and M. Fox, *Pharmac. Rev.,* 1967, **19**, 21.)

takes 48 days during which three other cycles are started. In the mouse the same situation occurs except each cycle takes 8.2 days. Mature sperm, from the seminiferous tubules, are collected by a number of ducts which discharge their contents into the epididymus where they are believed to undergo a further maturation process and are non-mobile. The duration of the epididymal phase in the rat is about 15 days. Sertoli cells act as "nurse" or sustaining cells for spermatids and spermatozoa, and appear to assist in the transfer of important nutrient material from the basal membrane to the developing germinal cells.

In contrast to other mammalian species, the arrangement of germ cells in the human seminiferous tubule is completely irregular, although generations of spermatogonia, spermatocytes and spermatids are grouped in a few well-defined cellular associations. One cycle of the seminiferous epithelium lasts 16 days and the whole process of spermatogenesis takes about 64 days (9 weeks).

B. HORMONAL CONTROL

It is now believed that both the interstitial cells (Leydig cells) and the cells of the seminiferous tubule can synthesize testosterone, although the former contribute some 90% of the testicular secretion of androgen. Circulating testosterone inhibits the secretion of gonadotrophin by the pituitary gland by feedback inhibition. Treatment of male rats with testosterone propionate (0.1 mg per day) inhibits this pituitary secretion and hence the function of the testis. Spermatogenesis is arrested at the level of the secondary spermatocyte and early spermatid. The same effect can be produced by estrogens and by feedback inhibition of gonadotrophin secretion. Larger doses overshadow the inhibition of gonadotrophin secretion and maintain the testis directly.

In man, injections of 50 mg testosterone propionate three times weekly cause a progressive fall in sperm count to very low levels which can be maintained. There is no loss of libido and of potency. Suppression of gonadotrophin secretion with the same oral estrogens and progestogens used in female contraception also arrests spermatogenesis but with loss of libido and potency. An orally-active testosterone derivative has not yet been developed which will not inhibit potency. A number of steroidal "anti-androgens" have been found to arrest spermatogenesis with the simultaneous suppression of libido, e.g. cyproterone acetate. These compounds have strong progestational activity.

C. CYTOTOXIC DRUGS

A number of cytotoxic drugs have been used in the inhibition of spermatogenesis and fall into certain well-defined groups (Table 5.4).

Most of these groups of compounds were discovered while the effects of cytotoxic drugs on cancer cells were being investigated. The main problem is to find drugs capable of acting on spermatogenesis specifically without a simul-

Table 5.4. *Cytotoxic anti-spermatogenic drugs*

Chemical group	Examples
Purine and pyrimidine antimetabolites	6-Azauracil
Alkylating agents	
Nitrogen mustards	Tretamine
Alkylesters of alkane sulphonic acids	Busulphan
Bis (dichloroacetyl) diamines	WIN 18,446
Dinitropyrrole derivatives	ORF 1616

taneous depression of cell division and maturation throughout the body. The effect of these drugs tends to be differential, in that rapidly dividing tissues such as cancers and seminiferous epithelia are inhibited while the other tissues are not affected.

Purine and pyrimidine metabolites seem to be the least specific of the cytotoxic drugs, there being a general depression of fertility throughout the major part of the spermatogenic cycle. Alkylating agents have been extensively investigated in cancer chemotherapy and mainly combine with DNA. Tretamine (Fig. 5.4) has been found to produce infertility in rats and mice by action on the type-A spermatogonia and on spermatids. Several derivatives of ethyleneimine

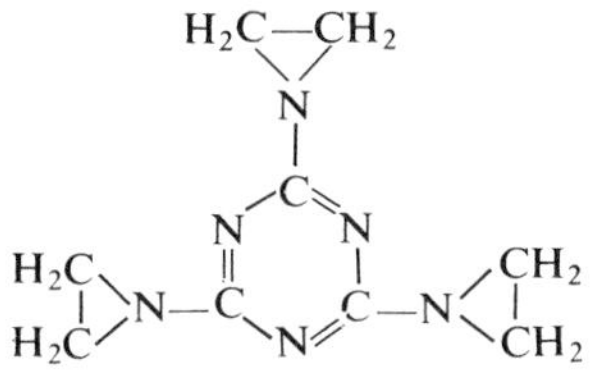

TEM
Tretamine
Triethylene melamine
2,4,6-Triaziridin-1'-yl-1,3,5-triazine

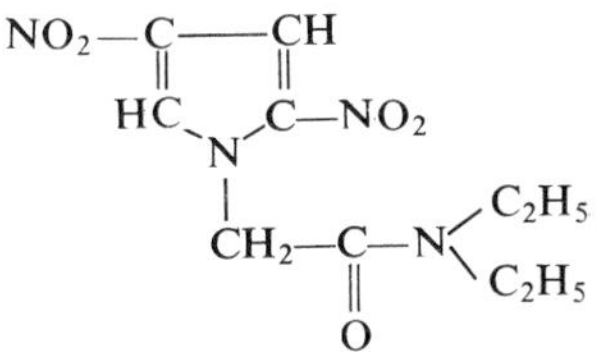

ORF 1616
1-(*N,N*-Diethylcarbamylmethyl)-
2,4-dinitropyrrole

$$CH_3-SO_2-O-CH_2-CH_2-CH_2-CH_2-O-SO_2-CH_3$$

Busulphan
Myleran
1,4-Di-(methanesulphonoxy) butane
Tetramethylenedimethane sulphonate

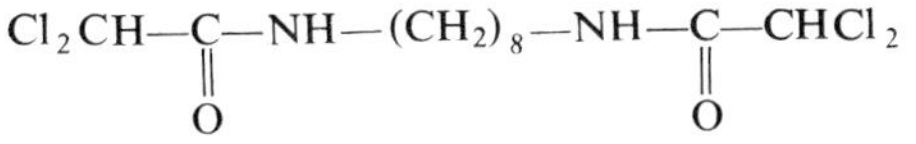

$$Cl_2CH-\underset{O}{\overset{}{C}}-NH-(CH_2)_8-NH-\underset{O}{\overset{}{C}}-CHCl_2$$

WIN 18,446
N,N'-bis(dichloroacetyl)-1,8-octanediamine

Fig. 5.4. Some cytotoxic anti-spermatogenic drugs.

have been tested on spermatogenesis in the rat. Alkyl esters of alkane sulphonic acids deliver an alkyl group to an active nucleophilic centre within biological material and the nature of the biochemical lesion produced depends on the structure of the alkyl group. "Busulphan" ("Myleran"), used in the treatment of chronic myeloid leukemia, has been shown to interfere with early developmental processes in the myeloid, intestinal and spermatogenic systems. It causes sterility in male rats about 9 weeks after a single dose due to the arrest of the first division of the spermatogonia.

Other important groups of compounds are derivatives of dinitropyrrole, e.g. ORF 1616, of nitrofuran and of methylhydrazine. An important group of compounds are the bis(dichloroacetyl)diamines, e.g. WIN 18,446. These suppress spermatogenesis in the monkey, rat, dog, mouse and guinea pig without affecting gonadotrophin secretion. These studies led to trials in male prison inmates and aspermia was found without loss of libido with doses of WIN 18,446 of 0.5-1.5 g daily for 9-54 weeks. There was a gradual drop in sperm count in the first 9 weeks. Histology showed the Sertoli cells were undamaged. On cessation of treatment, sperm counts began to recover after 8-9 weeks and were fully recovered by 12-14 weeks. This compound was put out on a trial in the general population and great disappointment occurred when it was discovered that the consumption of minute amounts of alcohol caused severe vasomotor disturbances similar to drunkenness in persons receiving the drug.

6

TARGET ORGAN EFFECTS–C. CORTICOIDS

I. INTRODUCTION

Adrenocorticosteroids are divided into two groups depending on their biological activity. The mineralocorticoids affect the excretion of fluid and electrolytes and are principally characterized by causing sodium retention. Some compounds which stimulate sodium excretion may also be placed in this group. The glucocorticoids affect intermediary metabolism and suppress inflammatory processes. A large number of compounds exist which possess both glucocorticoid activity and either sodium-retaining or sodium-excreting action and may be classified as both glucocorticoid and mineralocorticoid.

The steroids produced by the adrenal cortex are essential for life and replacement therapy is necessary after adrenalectomy. Survival tests have been used in adrenalectomized animals to assay the potency of these steroids. The time of survival is noted together with changes in body weight. Drakes, rats, mice, hamsters and dogs have been used and Table 6.1 shows that the mineralocorticoids (aldosterone and 9α-fluoroprednisolone) appear the most potent. In clinical practice, most adrenalectomized patients can be maintained fairly well without mineralosteroids provided they have a liberal salt intake and glucocorticoid therapy.

Table 6.1. *Life maintenance potencies in the dog.*

Aldosterone	20-40
Cortisone	1.0
Cortisol	0.05
Prednisolone	0.0125
9α-Fluoro-prednisolone	20-40

Deoxycorticosterone = 1.

II. MINERALOCORTICOIDS

A. WATER BALANCE

The hormones that are of the greatest importance in regulating water and electrolyte metabolism exert their principal effects on renal function, the kidney nephron being the target organ. By far the most important of these hormones are the anti-diuretic hormone (ADH) of the posterior pituitary, which has been identified as arginine vasopressin, and to a lesser extent aldosterone, the sodium-retaining hormone of the adrenal cortex. Other hormones have relatively minor significance under ordinary conditions but many assume importance under pathologic conditions.

The kidney contains about one million nephrons, each being a tube 20-50 μ wide and about 50 mm long (Fig. 6.1). The glomerulus is composed of a cluster of capillaries which lie in a space whose peripheral wall is known as the glomerular (or Bowman's) capsule. These capillaries share a central stalk of mesenchymal cells, the cytoplasm of which forms one continuous cytoplasm while the outer part of the stalk is hollowed out to form the capillary loop. The composition and volume of the extracellular fluid is controlled by glomerular filtration and tubular reabsorption or secretion. In one day about 180 litres of almost protein-free fluid is filtered through the glomerular capillaries into the glomerular space and thence into the tubule. Eventually about 1 litre emerges as urine. About 120 ml of filtrate are separated from the 600 ml of plasma which pass through the kidneys each minute and the glomerular filtrate contains all the diffusable, ultrafiltrable substances present in plasma. It contains about 30 mg protein per 100 ml which represents about 50 g of protein per 24 h.

The tubule reabsorbs or prevents the reabsorption of the contents of the tubular fluid and secretes into the tubular lumen substances which are either circulating in the peritubular venous capillaries or which are formed by the tubule cell. These processes are under the control of a wide variety of hormones, plasma electrolyte concentrations and gas pressures. The proximal tubule reabsorbs about 80% of the total solids and water, e.g. protein and glucose are almost completely reabsorbed but there is little or no reabsorption of urea and creatinine. Sodium chloride is partly reabsorbed and the fluid in the proximal tube always remains isotonic with arterial blood although its pH may change.

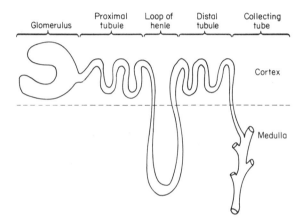

Fig. 6.1. Diagram of a kidney nephron.

The loop of Henle makes the interstitial fluid in the medulla hypertonic and the tubular fluid hypotonic by reabsorbing sodium and chloride against a concentration gradient. The distal and collection tubes adjust the pH, osmolarity and electrolyte content of the urine. Sodium is reabsorbed by a cation exchange process for hydrogen and potassium, and ammonia is synthesized by the tubular epithelium and diffuses into the tubular lumen where it forms ammonium ions with hydrogen ions. All these processes are stimulated by aldosterone-like steroids and are inhibited by aldosterone antagonists (spironolactones). The distal tubule receives the hypotonic fluid from the loop of Henle and in the presence of ADH it is permeable to water so that isotonic fluid in comparatively low volume is delivered into the collecting duct. The collecting duct passively reabsorbs water in the presence of ADH so that a small volume of hypertonic urine is excreted.

The anti-diuretic hormone of the posterior pituitary (arginine vasopressin) promotes the conservation of water by increasing the water-permeability of the cells lining the distal portions of the nephron. It is secreted in response to dehydration and is very sensitive to slight increases in extracellular osmolarity. The water that is reabsorbed dilutes the extracellular fluids and corrects the hyperosmolarity. A decrease in the osmolarity of extracellular fluid below about 280 milliosmols per kg of water normally leads to the cessation of ADH secretion. Growth hormone (GH) promotes the retention of extracellular fluid.

B. ALDOSTERONE

Aldosterone secretion is controlled by the secretion of renin from the juxtaglomerular apparatus. The blood supply to the medulla passes through those glomeruli which are nearest to the medulla and their blood supply is different from the other glomeruli. In each nephron, the first part of the distal tubule rises from the medulla and comes to lie near the glomerulus of that nephron. At this point the afferent arteriole to the glomerulus touches the distal tube and this area of contact is known as the juxtoglomerular apparatus. The cells of the afferent arteriole contain cytoplasmic secretory granules of renin which are secreted into the general circulation in response to a reduction in the extracellular fluid volume, i.e. a higher osmolarity. Renin reacts with plasma angiotensinogen to produce the vasoconstrictor peptide angiotensin which stimulates the adrenal cortex to produce aldosterone. In normal subjects there is a diurnal rhythm in plasma renin activity, the lowest levels occurring in the afternoon and this is probably the major factor in the diurnal rhythm of aldosterone secretion. Aldosterone secretion is also influenced by the concentration of potassium in body fluids, potassium depletion diminishing aldosterone secretion.

Since normally in man 97-100% of the filtered sodium undergoes tubular reabsorption, a change of only 3% will account for the most extreme variations in sodium excretion. Only a relatively small fraction of filtered sodium is under the control of adrenal steroids as about 98% of the filtered sodium is reabsorbed in the absence of the adrenals. Aldosterone causes the increased reabsorption of sodium and chloride in the distal tubule and the increased secretion of potassium and hydrogen ions. The reabsorption of sodium and chloride increases the osmolarity of the extracellular fluid which stimulates the production of ADH. A very delicate balance of the two hormones occurs. Within 40 min after the intravenous injection of adrenal cortical extract, sodium reabsorption is increased to 98.8% and reaches a maximum of 99.8% in 60-120 min, an increase of only 2%. This effect can also be brought about by the administration of 11-deoxycorticosterone (DOC) which is thus a "pure" mineralocorticoid although it only has about 1% of the activity of aldosterone. Potassium excretion is brought about in exchange for sodium retention. When normal subjects are given a prolonged course of DOC or aldosterone, sodium retention is maintained for only approximately 7-10 days when sodium balance is regained, usually after delivering part of the retained sodium. The sodium retention produced by mineralocorticoids can be blocked by the associated administration of adequate amounts of glucocorticoids. Increased production of aldosterone is a most important homeostatic mechanism in situations demanding conservation of sodium by the body.

It is now believed that mineralocorticoids do not act directly on the molecular machinery of sodium transport systems as there is a delay of 30-120 min between administration and effect, and the plasma half-life of aldosterone is only about 35 min. Tissue uptake of aldosterone reaches a steady state maximal level in 30 min but there is a latent period of 60-90 min in the response. Mineralocorticoids have a trigger-like action and there is evidence that they regulate sodium transport by induction of protein synthesis at the level of DNA-directed RNA synthesis. Autoradiography has shown that the physiologically-specific mineralocorticoid receptors are intranuclear and are proteins. The protein whose synthesis is induced by aldosterone is believed to act as a "permease" to admit more sodium into the transport pathways of the tissue.

Mineralocorticoid activity is usually assayed by salt retention tests in the adrenalectomized dog or rat. Sodium and potassium are estimated in the urine 4-6 h after the administration of steroid. Some relative potencies are shown in Table 6.2. In the rat several classes of steroid can be recognized:

(a) no effect;
(b) primary sodium retainers, e.g. aldosterone, deoxycorticosterone. Glucocorticoid activity is minimal or absent relative to sodium-retaining potential;
(c) glucocorticoids showing sodium-retaining action, e.g. 9α-fluoro-2α-methylcortisol;
(d) glucocorticoids showing sodium-excreting action, e.g. triamcinolone;
(e) primary sodium excretors.

Table 6.2. *Comparative sodium-retaining potencies in the dog.*

Cortisol	0.04
Prednisolone	0.03
6α-Methylprednisolone	0.02
9α-Fluoro-cortisol acetate	5.0
9α-Fluoro-6α-methyl-cortisol	4.4
9α-Fluoroprednisolone	9.0

In man the oral mineralocorticoid of choice is now 9α-fluorohydrocortisone which has the same salt-retaining potency as aldosterone. Even more potent is 2-methyl-9α-fluorohydrocortisone.

C. ALDOSTERONE ANTAGONISTS

The aldosterone antagonists are a group of steroidal compounds structurally related to the natural hormone and characterized by a spirolactone configuration at C-17. They competitively inhibit the peripheral actions of aldosterone at its target site in the nephron. When administered alone, these antagonists produce little change in renal excretion of water and electrolyte in man provided that a diet of high sodium content is being consumed. In the presence of low sodium intake, there is increased urinary excretion of sodium and water with a decrease in potassium excretion. The full effect of these drugs becomes apparent when they are given together with a diuretic acting more proximally in the nephron, which ensures that a substantial amount of sodium is presented to the distal tube where in the presence of an aldosterone antagonist it cannot be reabsorbed. The aldosterone antagonist most often used is spironolactone ("Aldactone") (Fig. 6.2) which is remarkably free from toxic and side effects.

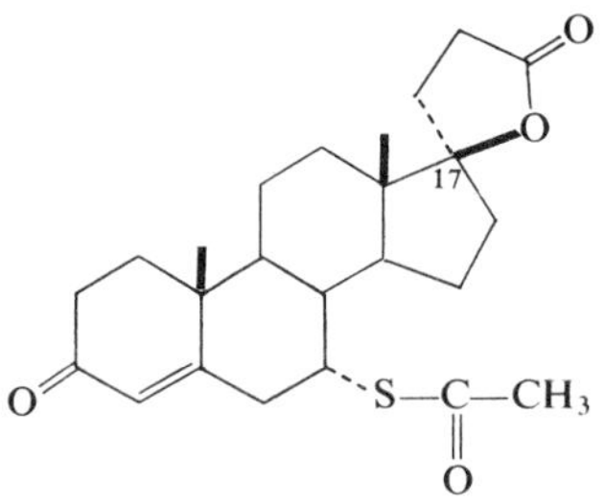

"Aldactone"
Spironolactone
3-(3-Oxo-7α-acetylthio-17β-hydroxy-4-
androsten-17α-yl) propionic acid γ-lactone

Fig. 6.2. "Aldactone".

III. GLUCOCORTICOIDS

A. GENERAL EFFECTS

The corticosteroids of the adrenal cortex are essential for life. The glucocorticoids play an important role in the regulation of protein, carbo-hydrate, lipid and nucleic acid metabolism. They are primarily catabolic, causing increased breakdown of extrahepatic proteins to amino acids.

In the liver, glucocorticoids produce increased glycogen deposition, increased gluconeogenesis, increased uptake of amino acids and increased synthesis of RNA and protein, i.e. anabolic effects. These are believed to be primary effects whereas the production of urea and ketone bodies are believed to be secondary. It seems likely that increased urea production occurs as a consequence of increased mobilization of amino acids to the liver and ketone body production is related to the mobilization of fat to the liver. In adipose tissue, muscle, skin and lymphatic and connective tissue, glucocorticoids inhibit glucose utilization, but these effects are not demonstrable in the presence of insulin. One of the major metabolic effects of glucocorticoids is on lipid mobilization. A decrease in fat utilization and an increase in body lipid are seen in adrenalectomized animals. The production of urea causes an increased excretion of urinary nitrogen.

Administration of glucocorticoids to animals results in increases in the activity of a number of enzymes, e.g. most of the enzymes of the glycolysis cycle, the urea cycle and amino acid-metabolizing enzymes of the liver. It is believed that these increases, in most cases, represent an increase in the synthesis of enzyme protein. One of the first enzymatic activities observed to increase following glucocorticoid treatment of animals is the amino acid-metabolizing enzyme, tryptophan pyrrolase.

The metabolic effects of the glucocorticoids are opposed by insulin. In the regulation of carbohydrate, protein and lipid metabolism these two hormones play key roles. Both the amelioration of diabetes by adrenalectomy and the production of steroid diabetes are well-known. Insulin increases glucose utilization, corticoids inhibit it, but the action of insulin predominates. The corticoids promote lipid mobilization and insulin prevents it. Insulin stimulates extrahepatic protein synthesis and the glucocorticoids have the opposite effect, but these actions are reversed in the liver. Corticoid induction of various hepatic enzymes is blocked by insulin.

Glucocorticoids have a hypocalcaemic effect which results primarily from inhibition of calcium absorption by the gastrointestinal tract, which is normally induced by vitamin D. There is a general antagonism to the action of vitamin D by glucocorticoids. Reduced calcium absorption may cause a decrease in serum calcium, hypersecretion of the parathyroid glands and hence increased bone resorption. There is a dimineralization of bone following excess glucocorticoids.

B. ASSAY OF CATABOLISM

1. Nitrogen loss

The magnitude of the urinary nitrogen loss can be used as an assay of glucocorticoid potency. In man, cortisol produces a nitrogen deficiency of 70 mg/24 h whereas prednisolone causes a loss of 150 mg/24 h. The effects on nitrogen balance are decreased by insertion of an α-hydroxy group at C-16.

2. Liver glycogen deposition

Bioassay techniques using both the adrenalectomized rat and adrenalectomized mouse have been extensively used. Male rats are adrenalectomized and fed a 55% protein diet and tap water containing 1% NaCl. On the fourth postoperative day, the food is removed and the following day water is also withheld. Subcutaneous injections of steroid in a suitable oil are given at four intervals of 2 h and the liver removed for glycogen determination after a further

3 h. Liver glycogen levels do not begin to increase for at least 2-4 h after a single dose; maximum levels are attained in 8-12 h, decreasing to control values within 24-32 h. Plasma glucose levels also increase significantly within 30-60 min and reach a maximum in about 4 h. Table 6.4 (p. 158) shows some relative potencies. Intact animals yield results at least as good as adrenalectomized animals when tests are limited to pure steroids and no toxic solvents are used.

C. STRESS AND ULCEROGENESIS

The simplest definition of stress is "the rate of wear and tear on the body". The accumulated results of such wear and tear are what we call ageing but the rate at which the wear and tear progresses at any one time is stress. The body has a built-in defence mechanism that tends to repair the damage caused by stress. This is accomplished largely through nervous and hormonal reactions. Among the latter, increased production during stress of hormones such as ACTH and corticoids is especially important. There appear to be two mechanisms by which stress brings about an increase in ACTH secretion. ACTH release following haemorrhage and endotoxin stresses cannot be suppressed by dexamethasone whereas that caused by trauma can. Amongst the most common agents causing stress in man are psychic and nervous stimuli, infections, trauma, hypersensitivity reactions, muscular work, haemorrhage, intoxication with various drugs and nutritional deficiencies. The production of sex hormones is diminished at times when the body must produce an excessive amount of ACTH and corticoids. This results in diminishing sexual desire and may induce temporary impotence or frigidity. In the male, sperm production may be severely impeded and in the female there may be a cessation of menstruation (amenorrhea). Milk secretion in the lactating female may also be diminished by stress. Maladjustment to stress can produce a variety of diseases, e.g. nervous and mental diseases, high blood pressure, cardiac diseases, various types of arthritis and duodenal ulcers. In most of these diseases, hereditary predisposition and previous personal experiences are principally responsible for determining which organ system will break down as a result of stress. Characteristically, the glucocorticoid-induced ulcer is gastric in location, is associated with little pain and is featured pathologically by a modest inflammatory reaction and lack of scar formation on

Table 6.3. *Relative ulcerogenic properties of corticoids.*

Hydrocortisone	1.0
Prednisolone	2.5
6α-Methylprednisolone	8.0
Triamcinolone	30
Dexamethasone	87

healing. Possible causative mechanisms may be increased hydrochloric acid and pepsin production or decreased formation of protective mucus. The relative potency of glucocorticoids can be assessed by ulcerogenesis tests, e.g. female rats are fasted for 4 days and steroids injected daily subcutaneously. After 4 days the gastric mucosa is examined. The percentage of animals with pyloric ulcers, the severity and number of ulcers is calculated and an "ulcer index" calculated (Table 6.3).

IV. ANTI-INFLAMMATORY STEROIDS

A. INTRODUCTION

Glucocorticoids exert a suppressive effect on the response of tissue to injury. This effect is variable, depending on the mechanism by which the injury was produced. It may be a specific anti-allergic suppression or a non-specific anti-inflammatory suppression. The principle types of injury are trauma, infection and allergy. There is considerable evidence that injuries may also be due to auto-immune processes, e.g. in rheumatoid arthritis. Injuries of all types are followed by inflammation.

B. THE INFLAMMATORY RESPONSE

The four cardinal signs of inflammation are redness, swelling, heat and pain. Inflammation can be defined as the local response to injury of a tissue and manifests as a tissue exudate and the infiltration of cells into the injured tissue.

1. Inflammatory exudates

The first response to tissue injury appears to be vasodilation. A transient arteriolar constriction is followed by a prolonged dilation of arterioles, capillaries and venules. During this period of vasodilation, blood flow at first quickens and then becomes sluggish. The stasis of blood which may develop is probably due to loss of water from the venules, leaving behind clumped masses of erythrocytes. The loss of fluid is due mainly to increased permeability of the walls of the blood vessels to plasma proteins. At the same time leukocytes leave the centre of the blood stream and lie up against the vascular epithelium. Plasma protein escapes from both venules of 8-100 μ diameter and also from capillaries. Increased vascular permeability is due to the transient formation of gaps between endothelial cells of the blood vessels through which the plasma proteins infiltrate. It seems likely that molecular sieving occurs during the subsequent passage through the basement membrane, as inflammatory exudates usually have more albumin and less of the larger globulins than plasma. Once outside the vessels the protein exudate is slowly reabsorbed by the lymphatics with the exception of fibrinogen which will become partly polymerized to form fibrin, deposits of which form a major feature of inflammatory exudates.

In addition to water, salts and plasma proteins, the inflammatory exudate contains large numbers of cells. In acute inflammations large numbers of cells migrate from the blood to the site of injury but if the stimulus persists or is of a low intensity, the inflammation becomes chronic. The exudate resolves, or may never have formed, there is a proliferation of tissue cells of the reticulo-endothelial system and granulomas are formed. In chronic infections due to micro-organisms the typical response is a granuloma. Foreign-body granulomas are also a typical inflammatory response, e.g. to paraffin.

2. Cellular infiltration

(a) Neutrophils

Normally the blood contains 5000-8000 leukocytes per mm^3 of which 48% are monocytes and 21-35% are lymphocytes (Fig. 6.3). The predominant cells accounting for 56-78% of the total leukocytes are the polymorphonuclear leukocytes or granulocytes, so called because of their lobed nuclei and the presence of granules in the cytoplasm. The polymorphs are formed in the bone marrow and initially have a round nucleus. The proportion of immature granulocytes in the blood, with the round nucleus, is usually about 3-6% but can increase to 20% in acute infections. Most of the polymorphs are neutrophils, i.e. their cytoplasm granules do not stain with either acidic or basic dyes. These cells account for about 54-73% of the total blood leukocytes and are the first line of defence in acute infections. During the period of most intense reaction, the neutrophils pass through the walls of the blood vessels into the tissues and make up the major component of the cellular infiltrate, being the chief component of pus. They move at a rate of 20 μ/min and take about 2-13 min to pass through the vessel wall by inserting pseudopodia between the endothelial cells until their whole body lies between the endothelium and the endothelial basement membrane, through which they then pass. Their main function is phagocytosis and they are often called microphages. They are only able to engulf smaller objects such as bacteria and can digest fibrin and inflamed tissue. In acute bacterial infections, burns and severe injuries the proportion of neutrophils in the blood can rise to 80-95% of the total leukocytes.

(b) Eosinophils and basophils

Some 2-4% of the blood polymorphs are eosinophils, i.e. their cytoplasmic granules stain with eosin. They are found invading the tissues in the later stages of many inflammations especially in hypersensitivity of the atopic type, e.g. asthma, hay fever. There is also usually an eosinophilia of the blood when the proportion of eosinophils may reach 20% of the total leukocytes. About 0-1% of blood polymorphs are basophils or mast leukocytes which are different morpho-logically from the tissue mast cells in that they are smaller, more rounded and have a polymorphorus nucleus. They do not increase in the blood during acute

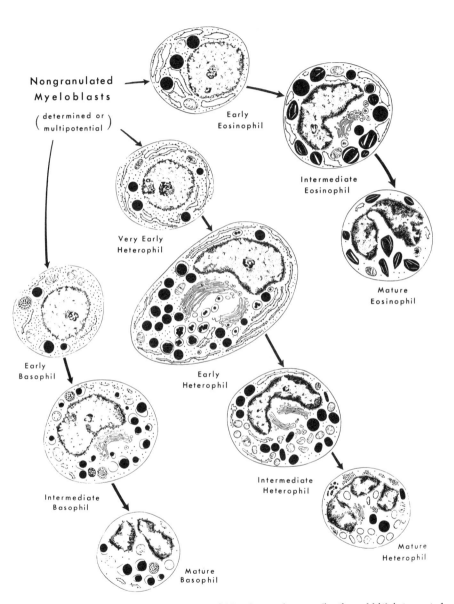

Nongranulated
Myeloblasts

(determined or multipotential)

Early
Eosinophil

Intermediate
Eosinophil

Very Early
Heterophil

Mature
Eosinophil

Early
Basophil

Early
Heterophil

Intermediate
Basophil

Intermediate
Heterophil

Mature
Heterophil

Mature
Basophil

Fig. 6.3. Stages in the development of blood granuloctyes (in the rabbit) interpreted from electron microscope pictures. (From B. K. Wetzel, R. G. Horn and S. S. Spencer, 1967.)

6

infections but they do infiltrate tissues in chronic inflammations, i.e. when fresh connective tissue is being laid down.

(c) Monocytes

In the later stages of an acute inflammation mononuclear cells dominate the cellular infiltrate as the polymorphs move away or disintegrate. Most of these cells come from the blood monocytes but move about four times more slowly than the neutrophils and therefore arrive later. In fixed, stained tissue they appear round with cytoplasm better defined than the polymorphs although lacking granules. The nucleus is unlobed but often appears indented. Once in the' tissue, the monocytes undergo transformations into macrophages, giant cells, epithelial cells or histiocytes. There is also a resident population of these types of cells of the reticulo-endothelial system in the tissues of all organs of the body, especially in skin. Histiocytes normally occur in very small numbers around some of the blood vessels. They induce the formation of abundant reticulin fibres (precollagen) and possess the ability to phagotize bacteria and particulate matter with their lysosomal enzymes. They are much increased in many inflammatory conditions especially the granulomas. Macrophages are the large phagocytic cells which are believed to be formed from the blood monocytes and tissue histiocytes by fusion or nuclear division without cellular division to form giant cells. They usually contain large amounts of ingested matter. Great numbers of giant cells are present in certain foreign body granulomas. Acquired immunity to bacterial infections depends in part on the presence of numerous macrophages. When macrophages ingest tubercle bacilli they become transformed into epitheloid cells which possess abundant, slightly eosinophilic cytoplasma and often pseudopodia. They tend to become organized into groups, "tubercles", of interlocking cells with large pale staining nuclei in which the cytoplasm of neighbouring cells often appears coalesced. They are found in a variety of granulomas as a result of a hypersensitivity or immunologic reaction. They are capable of forming reticulin fibres and as the granuloma heals they may condense into collagen. Subcutaneous "rheumatoid" nodules may occur in rheumatoid arthritis which show several foci of fibroid degeneration each of which is surrounded by histiocytes. In the intermediary stroma of the nodule, there is a chronic inflammatory filtrate with some proliferation of the blood vessels and fibrosis.

(d) Lymphocytes and plasma cells

Lymphocytes also migrate from the blood vessels and from lymphoid tissue and there is a striking infiltration in chronic infections. They are the predominant cells in chronic inflammation and do not divide and carry out phagocytosis. Among their functions is the formation of antibodies. Plasma cells occur in small numbers in most chronic inflammatory infiltrates and granulomas although they rarely enter the blood stream. They have abundant cytoplasm which is deeply basophilic, homogeneous and sharply defined. Their functions are the synthesis of γ-globulin and antibodies.

(e) Tissue mast cells

Mast cells occur in the loose connective tissues of mammals, especially around the blood vessels, between the fat cells and in the peritoneum. They are characterized mainly by their globular cytoplasmic granules which stain metachromatically with various basic dyes, e.g. toluidine blue, due to the presence of acid mucopolysaceliasides. Mast cells were named by Paul Ehrlich and "mast" means food supplying. The mast cell granules contain histamine and heparin. The latter is believed to be the precursor of the hyaluronic acid of the tissue ground substance. The mast cells of certain animals, but not man, also contain serotonin (5-hydroxytryptamine). In injuries of the antibody-antigen type, histamine is released from the mast cell granules which causes increased permeability of blood vessels. It is believed that the primary function of infiltrated eosinophils is to neutralize released histamine.

3. Mediators of inflammation

Histamine is a mediator of inflammation, which may be defined as an endogenous chemical agent which takes an active part in the development of the inflammatory response. It can be isolated from the inflammatory site, the inflammatory response can be repressed by specific antagonists, the antihistamines, and when histamine liberators are used to deplete the tissue histamine it is not possible to provoke the usual inflammatory response. It causes marked vasodilation and increased permeability of the small vessels to fluid and proteins. Other known mediators of inflammation are serotonin, the polypeptides bradykinin and kallidin and macromolecular kinins.

C. ANTIBODY FORMATION

An antigen is a substance which, when introduced parenterally into animal tissue, stimulates the production of an antibody, and which, when in contact with that antibody, reacts specifically with it. An antibody is a globulin present in blood or body fluids which reacts specifically with an antigen. An antibody which causes lysis is called a lysin, haemolysin or bacteriolysin; one which causes agglutination is called an agglutinin; and one which causes precipitation is called a precipitin. Antibodies are γ- or immuno-globulins and occur in immune-sera. Complement is the heat-labile factor occurring in normal (non-immune)-sera which is essential, in addition to antibody, for the immune lysis of red blood cells and certain bacteria. Several proteins occurring in the euglobulin and pseudoglobulin fractions have been shown to be constituents of complement. In an immune reaction, first the foreign macromolecule (antigen) is detected and marked by combination with antibody and then the antigen-antibody complex is disposed of by reaction with complement, i.e. complement fixation. Adjuvants are substances which when mixed with antigens improve antibody production or other immune responses.

1. Plasma cells

It is now believed that plasma cells are the principal site of synthesis of antibodies. These cells have abundant cytoplasm which is deeply basophilic, homogenous and sharply defined, possessing large numbers of microsomes and ribosomes for protein synthesis. The ultrastructure of the plasma cell is unique and its origin is still unknown. Immunological and morphological evidence exists that there are at least two types of plasma cells involved in antibody formation, one apparently producing 7S γ-globulin and one producing 19S γ-globulin.

The site of antibody formation depends to a considerable extent upon the site of injection of the antigen and occurs in surrounding tissue and in the regional lymph nodes. If antigen is injected intravenously, the antibodies are produced in the spleen and lymphoid tissue. In response to antigen, immature plasmablasts divide rapidly and greatly increase their RNA and ribosomal content. Mature plasma cells produce large amounts of antibody protein.

2. Lymphocytes

Other types of cell have been found to contain γ-globulin, e.g. about 1% of the small lymphocytes in thoracic duct lymph and in the spleen. It is not known whether antibodies are synthesized in these cells or are acquired from the circulation.

There is a good deal of evidence to suggest functionally that there are two distinct varieties of lymphocytes, one in the bone marrow involved primarily in haemopoiesis and one in other parts of the lympho-myeloid complex and serving immunological needs. They are believed to originate from primitive reticular cells, via lymphoblasts, and large and medium lymphocytes to the small lymphocyte. The nucleus is rounded with a slight indentation and is characterized by dense, coarse aggregates of chromatin and a relatively thick nuclear membrane. The cytoplasm is relatively sparse and lightly basophilic with few mitochondria. There is no rough endoplasmic reticulum but there are some ribosomes and polysomes indicating some protein synthesis. Embryologically, lymphocytes appear to arise from undifferentiated epithelial cells of the primordial thymus and from the reticular cells of lymph nodes, spleen and appendix. After exposure to antigen, the small lymphocyte is "activated" with a higher RNA and protein turnover, and they may proliferate. It is thought that these cells have become immunologically competent and are capable of antibody synthesis. They are involved in the recognition, effector and memory aspects of immunological phenomena. They have a very long life in the body (greater than

10 years) and are continually and quickly circulating through blood and lymph via the tissues and lymph nodes.

4. The thymus

The thymus is a lymphoid organ which differs considerably from other lymphoid organs both structurally and functionally. It is composed of a medulla and a cortex, and contains two main types of cells. The lymphocytes are densely packed in the cortex where they outnumber the epithelial reticular cells which predominate in the medulla. The epithelial reticular cells are characterized under electron microscopy by their desmosomes, tonofibrils and long cytoplasmic processes. They are a permanent thymus-specific population of cells whose function appears to be to modify the lymphocytes circulating through the thymus so that they become immunologically competent and can react with antigens.

D. THE ALLERGIC OR IMMUNE RESPONSE

There are four main modes of response by which an individual, who has been "sensitized" by a previous experience of the antigen (allergen), may react, and if the reaction is intense enough suffer tissue damage due to the allergic state (Fig. 6.4).

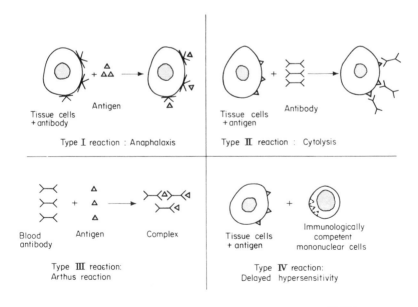

Fig. 6.4. Types of allergic response. (From Gell and Coombs, 1968.)

1. Type I reaction, anaphalaxis, immediate hypersensitivity

This is initiated by antigen (or allergen) reacting with tissue cells passively sensitized by antibody production elsewhere and leads to the release of pharmacologically-active substances. Reactions may be local, e.g. in skin urticaria, in hay fever and asthma and in certain forms of food allergy. The antibodies are passively absorbed onto the membranes of all the tissue cells. Among the pharmacologically-active substances liberated is histamine which produces dilation of the capillaries and contraction of smooth muscle. Other mediators of inflammation are also released. Atopic individuals produce a type of non-precipitating heat-labile antibody (reagin) which passively sensitizes tissue cells after ordinary exposure to otherwise innocuous substances in the environment. The skin reaction is immediate, being maximal in 10-20 min and resolving in 1-1½ h. The urticarial weal and erythematous flare are frequently accompanied by itching. The peripheral arteriole is a focal point for the production of tissue edema and eosinophil cells predominate.

2. Type II reaction, cytolysis

This is initiated by antibody reacting with either an antigenic component of a tissue cell or an antigen (or hapten, i.e. drug) which has become intimately associated with the tissue cells. Complement is usually but not always necessary to effect the cellular damage. Thus, this type of reaction is almost the opposite of type I reaction in that it is the antigens that are absorbed onto the surface of the cells and the antibodies that attack. Examples of when the antigen is a component of the tissue cells are transfusion reactions and haemolytic disease of the new-born. Typical reactions where antigens are acquired by cells are in bacterial infections and drug reactions. In many of these conditions the principle effect is lysis of the erythrocytes.

3. Type III reaction, Arthus reaction

This is initiated when excess antigen is injected into the individual and reacts in the tissue spaces with potentially precipitating antibody from the blood, forming microprecipitates in and around the small vessels and causing secondary damage to cells. Complex formation is sometimes aided by complement.

A variation of the Arthus reaction is serum sickness where the excess injected antigen circulates in the blood and reacts with the produced antibody as it enters the circulation from the lymphoid tissue. A soluble circulating complex is formed which is deposited in the blood vessels and walls and causes local inflammation.

Once the complexes are formed and deposited they produce a local histamine release and possibly the release of cytotoxic compounds. Circulating leukocytes are effected and become aggregated. Local vascular endothelium is activated and promotes the deposition of the aggregated leukocytes, platelets and thrombin with resultant thrombosis and haemorrhage. According to the amount of complex formed, anything from transient polymorph infiltration and edema to extensive vascular thrombosis and local nercrosis may develop. Examples of the Arthus reaction are no longer common but can sometimes be seen after several injections of horse tetanus antitoxin. Sensitivity to penicillin is an Arthus reaction where metabolic products of penicillin combine with protein to form an antigen.

4. Type IV reaction, delayed hypersensitivity

This is initiated by the reaction of specifically modified mononuclear cells containing a substance of mechanism capable of responding specifically to allergen deposited at a local site. It is manifested by the infiltration of cells, mainly of reticulo-endothelial origin and takes 24-48 h to become fully developed. There is no circulating antibody. Examples are delayed skin reactions of the tuberculin type and contact dermatitis. It is assumed that the initial sensitization alters cells, probably in the lymphoid system to contain something like an antibody, sometimes called "fixed-cell antibody".

5. Homografts and transplants

A homograft is a piece of tissue or a whole organ which is transplanted from one individual to another of the same species. Initially the homograft "takes", i.e. becomes established and survives in the host, but sooner or later lympho-cytes and plasma cells begin to accumulate in the graft, any circulation which has been established in the graft slows and stops, the cells of the graft die and the graft is either cast off or gradually replaced by tissue derived from the recipient, i.e. the graft is rejected. This local reaction is typically accompanied by enlargement of the regional lymph nodes with the associated appearance of large cells with pale staining nuclei and sometimes by systemic manifestations, e.g. enlargement of the spleen. Rejection of homografts does not occur between identical twins.

Homograft rejection is an immunological phenomenon stimulated by antigens liberated from the graft and circulating recipient cells play an important part in the reaction. The reaction is most similar to the type IV immune reaction.

E. EFFECT OF GLUCOCORTICOIDS ON THE INFLAMMATORY AND IMMUNE RESPONSES

Glucocorticoids exert a suppressive effect on the inflammatory reaction. They are important in maintaining vascular integrity, increase capillary resistance and potentiate the vasoconstrictive action of noradrenalin. The mast cells, which liberate the histamine which acts as a powerful vasodilator, show morphological changes and suppression of activity under the influence of glucocorticoids.

Steroids do not suppress the potent globulin permeability factor, which also causes vasodilation, or the immediate wheal and flare produced by histamine. Nevertheless it is believed that glucocorticoids support the integrity of the micro-circulation by suppressing excessive local formation of histamine, by suppressing the action of histidine decarboxylase on histamine, and therefore maintaining a balance between vasodilator and vasoconstrictor influences. Symptoms of asthma and other atopic type I reactions can be dramatically relieved by the administration of corticoids, but the mechanism of action remains unknown.

Glucocorticoids suppress the endothelial sticking of leukocytes with subsequent retardation of leukocyte accumulation at the site of injury. There is also inhibition of diapedesis and impaired migration of lymphocytes and phagocytes. The composition and polymerization of essential components of mesenchymal connective tissue are influenced by these steroids, e.g. acid mucopolysaccharide formation is reduced in granulation tissue and hyaluronic acid formation is inhibited. There is also an inhibition of collagen production by fibroblasts.

There is a decreased resistance to infection following glucocorticoid administration probably due to the inhibition of phagocytosis of the cells of the reticulo-endothelial system. Glucocorticoids impair humoral antibody production and inhibit proliferation of germinal centres of the spleen and lymph nodes in the primary response to antigen. This effect is maximal if the steroid is given before the introduction of the antigen. In this way it is similar to radiation-induced immunosuppression and different from anti-metabolite suppression of antibody formation which occurs in the induction period. Once immunity has been established, the secondary (anamnestic) response is suppressed only partially or not at all by steroids. In "cortisone-sensitive" species (rats, mice, rabbits), administration of glucocorticoids causes reduced synthesis of γ-globulin and suppression of circulating antibody but this effect cannot be readily demonstrated in "cortisone-resistant" species (man, guinea pigs). Passively induced Arthus reactions are not altered by glucocorticoids, but the active Arthus reaction which requires large amounts of endogenous antibody is diminished owing to steroid suppression of antibody production. Glucocorticosteroids do not influence the rate of disappearance of passively administered antibody.

Steroids may influence production and transport of the mediator of delayed hypersensitivity reactions, as they cause a marked decrease in the weight of lymphoid tissue and a prompt fall in circulating lymphocytes. Glucocorticoid regression of thymus tissue is very striking. An intact thymus is necessary for the establishment of lymphoid tissue that is responsible for recognition of antigenicity and effective antibody production. Involution of lymphoid tissue occurs by lymphocyto-karyorrhexis, inhibition of mitosis and suppression of DNA synthesis. Suppression of mitosis may be due to steroid-induced inhibition of DNA synthesis. Small lymphocytes and thymus cells are more susceptible to the effects of corticosteroids than are reticular and large immature lymphoid cells. The corticosteroid effect on lymphoid tissue is manifested by lymphopenia in hyperadrenalcorticism and by hyperplasia of lymphoid tissue in adrenal insufficiency.

The prompt fall in peripheral blood lymphocytes and eosinophils following glucocorticoid administration is accompanied by a marked increase in circulating neutrophils but this does not appear to be due to increased production of these cells but rather to their redistribution. It is believed that their egress from the blood is prevented.

Glucocorticoids do not block the union of antigen and antibody as manifested by the precipitin reaction nor do they appear to affect the binding of complement by antigen-antibody reaction. It is believed that the tissue reaction which mediates the antigen-antibody union is suppressed.

The capacity to reject homografts may be reduced by exposing the recipient shortly before or after the graft is made to whole body irradiation, cytotoxic drugs and anti-inflammatory steroids, all of which prevent the formation of antibodies. Modern practice is to give a mixture of cytotoxic drugs, e.g. 6-mercaptopurine, and of immuno-suppressive (anti-inflammatory) steroids.

F. BIOLOGICAL ASSAY OF ANTI-INFLAMMATORY STEROIDS

1. Thymus involution tests

The effects of glucocorticoids on the lymphoid tissues are very dramatic. Decrease in thymus size and weight following the administration of corticoids to adrenalectomized immature rats or mice is one of the most widely used assays. The animals receive the corticoids immediately following adrenalectomy. The thymus tissues are removed 1-3 days later and accurately weighed. They are then compared with untreated controls. As handling and injection may by themselves induce thymus atrophy, it is important that the controls be similarly treated.

2. Granuloma pouch tests

A pouch is formed by injecting a given amount of air, say 25 ml, into the loose subcutaneous connective tissue of the dorsal skin of the rat. If an irritant is introduced into the cavity, its lining is rapidly transformed into a granulomatous membrane and the air is gradually displaced by a more or less haemorrhagic inflammatory exudate. Many types of granuloma tissues can be obtained with different irritants, e.g. formalin induces a predominant fibroblastic reaction, croton oil causes an intensely fibrous capsule containing a haemorrhagic exudate, mustard powder results in the production of innumerable foreign-body giant cells, turpentine predominantly causes pus formation and carrageenan or carboxymethylcellulose transforms the connective tissue lining almost entirely

6*

into metachromatically-staining "pseudomastocytes". A common technique is to implant non-sterile cotton pellets subcutaneously in the adrenalectomized rat when the end-point of the assay is the weight of the granuloma produced after 4 days, the weight of the pellet being subtracted. With irritants which produce inflammatory exudates, the volume of the exudate is the end-point of the assay. Corticoids suppress the formation of these granulomata and may be given systematically or directly to the pouch. Tables 6.4 and 6.5 show some relative anti-inflammatory potencies obtained by granuloma pouch methods, compared with other methods.

Table 6.4. *Relative potencies of glucocorticoids in adrenalectomized male rats*

	Liver glycogen deposition	Thymus involution	Anti-granuloma
Hydrocortisone acetate	1.0	1.0	1.0
Cortisone acetate	0.5	0.5	0.5
Prednisone acetate	2.6	0.9	1.0
Prednisolone acetate	5.0	4.0	2.7
6α-Methylprednisolone	13.0	3.0	6.0
Paramethasone	23.1	45.1	63.6
9α-Fluoroprednisolone	27.0	4.4	17.7
Fluocinolone	44.0	8.5	19.7
Betamethasone	59.0	11.7	35.8
Dexamethasone	90.4	47.0	104.0
Triamcinolone acetonide	108.0	37.7	48.5
Fluocinolone acetonide	138.0	263.0	446.0

3. Experimental arthritis tests

An experimental arthritis may be induced in rats by the subcutaneous injection of irritants, e.g. formalin, dextran, carrageenan, just beneath the

Table 6.5 *Relative potencies of oral glucocorticoids in intact male rats*

	Body weight depression	Thymus involution	Adrenal weight depression[a]	Granuloma inhibition
Hydrocortisone	1.0	1.0	1.0	1.0
Prednisolone	3.9	3.3	3.2	3.7
6α-Methylprednisolone	0.4	5.2	4.4	5.4
Triamcinolone	3.6	2.7	3.5	3.2
Dexamethasone	144	113	121	154

[a] Due to suppression of pituitary secretion.

plantar skin of the hind paws. A few minutes after injection, there is intense congestion and diffuse edema of the whole paw but particularly in the metatarsal region. Two days later, the acute reaction tends to localize at the joint level and the mobility of the paw is limited. During the following ten days, the articular inflammatory process enters a chronic phase. Most of the edema has subsided but the surrounding skin remains intensely hyperaemic and the peri-articular tissue begins to proliferate especially in the ankle-joint region. The end-point of the assay is usually the volume of the swollen paw. Steroids may be given orally (Table 6.6) or injected directly into the joint. These tests are more commonly used for assessing non-steroidal anti-inflammatory agents of potential use in rheumatoid arthritis rather than for assessing the potency of anti-inflammatory steroids.

Table 6.6 *Doses (mg/kg) of anti-in-flammatory agents, given by mouth once daily, required to produce at least 50% inhibition of increase in thickness of the injected rat hind paw*

Paramethasone Dexamethasone Betamethasone	1
Triamcinolone Prednisolone	10-20
Cortisone	50-100
Acetylsalicylic acid Sodium salicylate	100-200

4. Eosinopenia tests

Male mice are adrenalectomized and maintained with 1% NaCl instead of drinking water and on replacement corticosteroid therapy (15 mg pellets of deoxycorticosterone acetate, DOCA, implanted at time of operation). Three days after operation, 5 µg adrenalin is given subcutaneously and 4 h later the steroid in a suitable oil. Blood samples are taken from the tail before and 3 h after steroid injection. The reduction in the number of blood eosinophils is counted. Eosinopenia tests have also been carried out in man after intravenous, intramuscular and intra-articular applications of steroids. Table 6.7 shows that the results were not always in agreement for the same species.

G. FIBROBLASTS AND WOUND HEALING

Loose connective tissue, e.g. the dermis of the skin, consists of a collagenous protein matrix interspersed with ground substance and with cells of different types. The protein matrix consists mainly of collagen fibrils 650-1000 Å in diameter which are aggregated into bundles and interspersed with fibroblasts. Elastin fibres about 70 Å in diameter lie entwined among the collagen bundles and are characterized by having no cross striations. Reticulin fibrils are

Table 6.7. *Relative corticosteroid potencies by the eosinopenia test*

	Mouse	Man
Corticosterone	0.4	0.06
Aldosterone	0.3	25-50
Prednisolone	3.3	4
6α-Methylprednisolone	1.7	5
9α-Fluoroprednisolone	7.2	20
Triamcinolone	3.2	5
Dexamethasone	9.3	28

also present in the dermis especially just beneath the basal layer of the epidermis where they form a meshwork. They are about one-half or one-third as wide as collagen fibrils but have the same periodicity, 640 Å long. The ground substance consists of polysaccharides and glycoproteins.

In normal tissue the only cells present belong to the reticulo-histiocytic-fibroblast group and the most common are the fibroblasts. These have oval or spindle-shaped nuclei, a distinct membrane, and PAS positive, diastase-resistant granules in their cytoplasm. The resident fibroblasts are divided into active fibroblasts which are associated with the production of the dermal fibre system and inactive fibrocytes which may act as reserve cells when a need for replacement and proliferation arises. Replacement of lost cells and tissues is accomplished by cell migration and cell proliferation. In wounds of the skin, the cells chiefly concerned are the fibroblasts, vascular endothelium and epithelium. Fibroblasts enlarge and migrate from surviving tissue into the blood clot at a later time than the polymorphs and monocytes. At the same time the endothelial cells of the capillaries at the edge of the wound swell, divide and begin to migrate. These form loops of cells and eventually more capillaries. Gradually a new tissue is built up under the clot—"granulation tissue" which appears to the naked eye to be composed of pink granules. These granules consist of newly formed capillary loops, fibroblasts and leukocytes. A new mesenchymal tissue is built up and epithelial cells migrate across its surface in sheets. The fibroblasts are responsible for the synthesis of collagen. Only the smallest collagen fibrils are manufactured inside the fibroblasts, i.e. about 100 Å diameter, while mature collagen fibres aggregate together extracellularly. Fibroblasts also form some of the mucopolysaccharides of the ground substance.

An early observation concerning the influence of cortisone in the treatment of patients with various types of diseases was that there was an inhibition of wound healing following surgical operations and it was assumed that this was due to inhibition of collagen formation. Prolonged daily local applications of various corticosteroids produce a thinning of the skin with a diminution in both epidermal cells and in the connective tissue components. The effect on the dermis becomes maximal after a period of time and then ceases. Keloids are prominent scars in which there has been excessive formation of new collagen. If they are treated with corticosteroids up to a year following their formation, a considerable reversal or diminution in the collagen of the ketoid may occur. It appears that corticosteroids can both prevent the formation of new collagen and also promote the removal of already formed collagen.

Corticosteroids also inhibit the production of ground substance as shown by the incorporation of S^{35}-sulphate into chondroitin sulphate. Ground substance seems to be produced by both the fibroblasts and the mast cells. Fibroblasts will take up and store in granular form not only heparin but a wide variety of naturally occurring and synthetic polysaccharides, when they appear to be a type of mast cell (mastocytoid). These polysaccharides are eventually released and added to the ground substance. Corticosteroids also effect the viscosity of ground substance.

Fibroblasts have been used *in vitro* to investigate the effects of corticoids on collagen and polysaccharide synthesis and also to assay the potency of anti-inflammatory steroids. Several established cell lines are available, e.g. L-929 clone of mouse skin fibroblasts, 3T3 mouse fibroblasts and WI-38 human foetal lung fibroblasts. These cell lines were originally isolated from tissue explants by the outgrowth of cells. When mesenchymal tissues are grown, many eventually yield what appears to be uniform populations of fibroblasts and it is possible to achieve clones from these cells. Although the cells become altered in tissue culture, e.g. the number of their chromosomes becomes variable with a model number usually greater than that of the parent animal, fibroblast cell lines behave very similarly to their behaviour *in vivo*, e.g. in the manufacture of collagen and ground substance. Small amounts of corticoids in the physiological range inhibit the growth of fibroblasts *in vitro* and Table 6.8 shows some relative anti-inflammatory potencies obtained by biological assay with L cells.

H. STRUCTURE OF ANTI-INFLAMMATORY STEROIDS

The formulae of the most commonly used anti-inflammatory steroids are shown in Figure 6.5. Cortisone and prednisone derivatives are entirely inactive as anti-inflammatory agents unless they are given orally or by intramuscular injection, when their activity depends entirely on their conversion to the corresponding hydrocortisone and prednisolone derivatives by the action of an

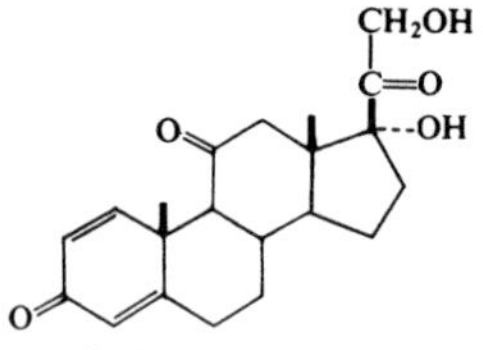

CH₂OH structure — Prednisone
1,2-Dehydrocortisone
Deltacortisone

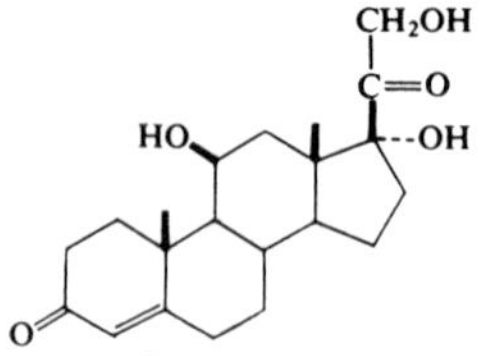

Cortisol
Hydrocortisone

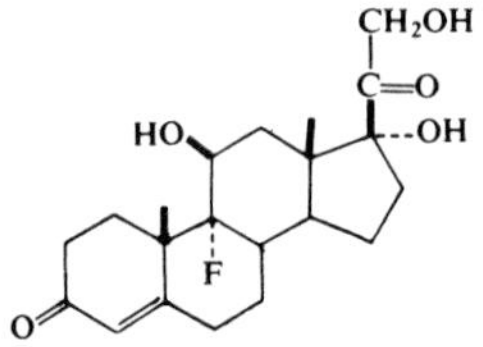

Fludrocortisone
9α-Fluorohydrocortisone

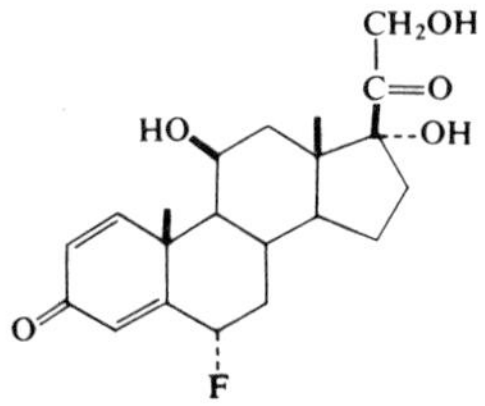

Fluprednisolone
6α-Fluoroprednisolone

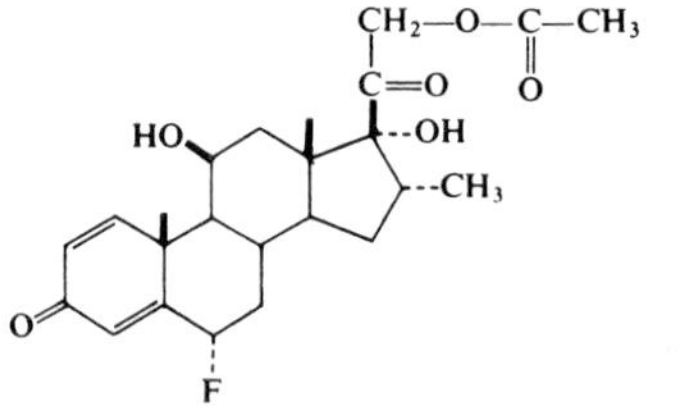

Paramethasone acetate
6α-Fluoro-16α-methylprednisolone
21-acetate

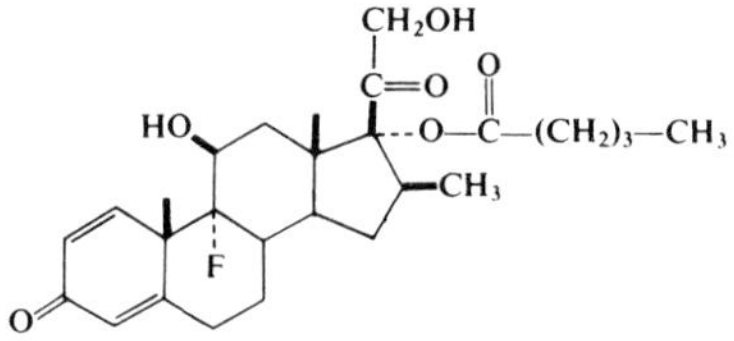

Betamethasone valerate
9α-Fluoro-16β-methyl-prednisolone-
17-n-valerate

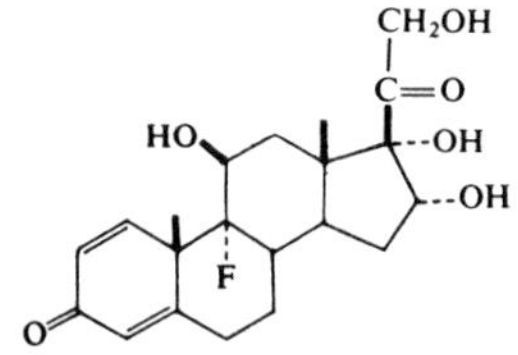

Triamcinolone
9α-Fluoro-16α-hydroxyprednisolone

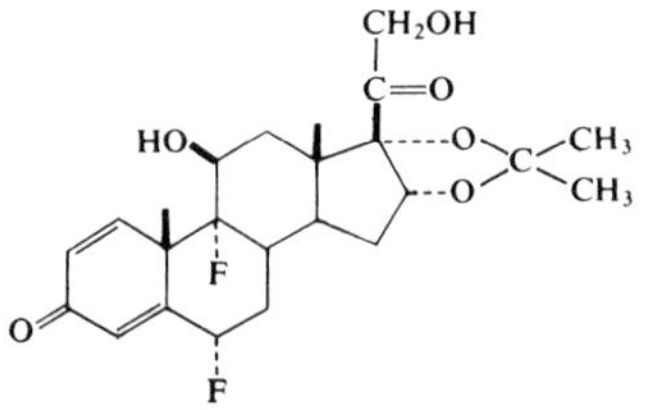

Fluocinolone acetonide
6α,9α-Difluoro-16α-hydroxyprednisolone
16,17-acetonide

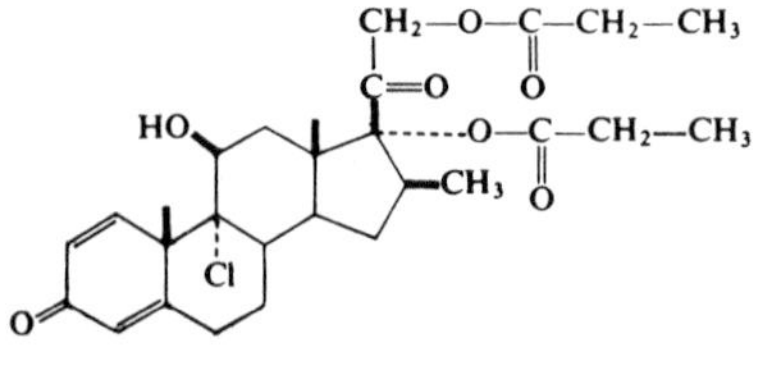

Beclomethasone dipropionate
9α-Chloro-16β-methylprednisolone 17,21-
dipropionate

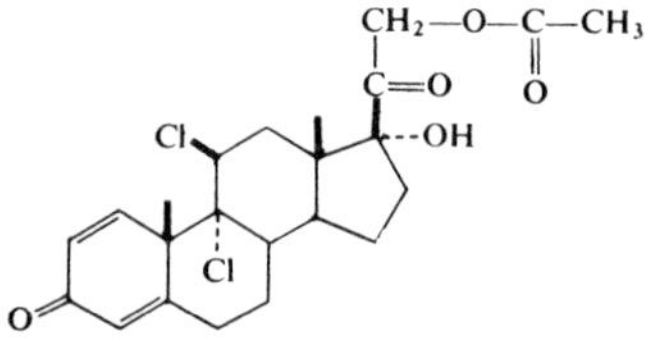

Dichlorisone acetate

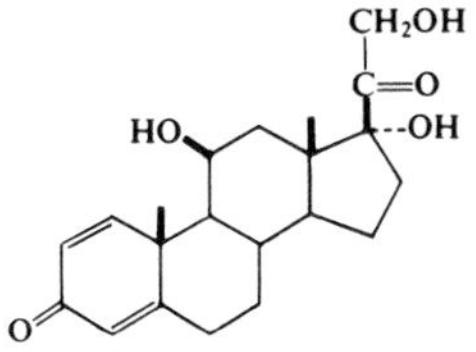

Prednisolone
1,2-Dehydrocortisol
Deltacortisol

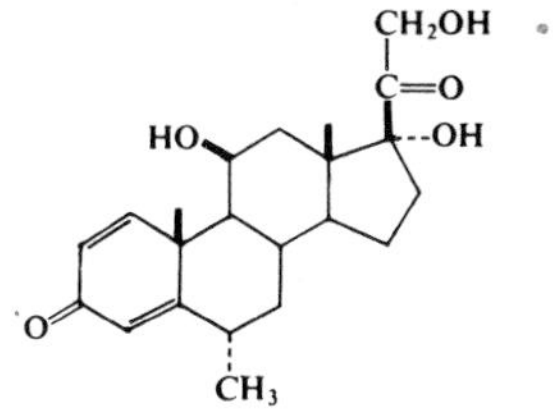

6α-Methylprednisolone

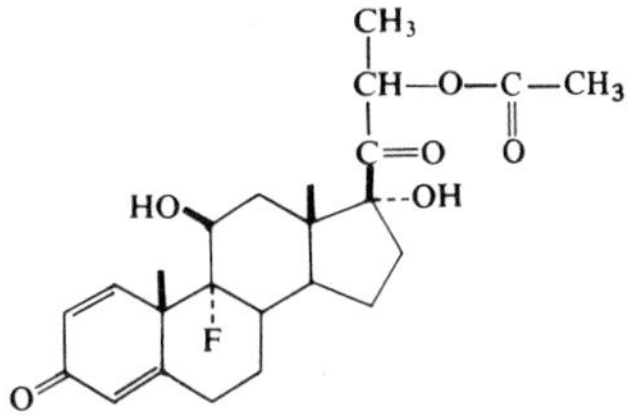

Fluperolone acetate
9α-Fluoro-21-methylprednisolone
acetate

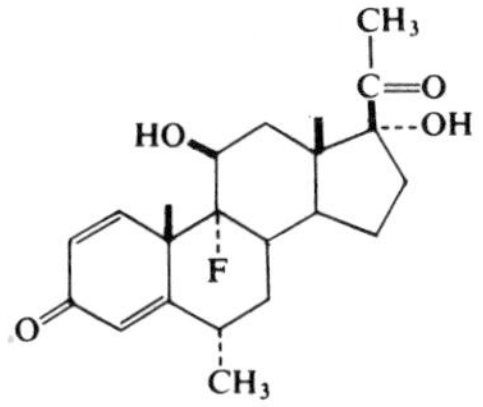

Fluorometholone
9α-Fluoro-6α-methyl-21-deoxy-
prednisolone

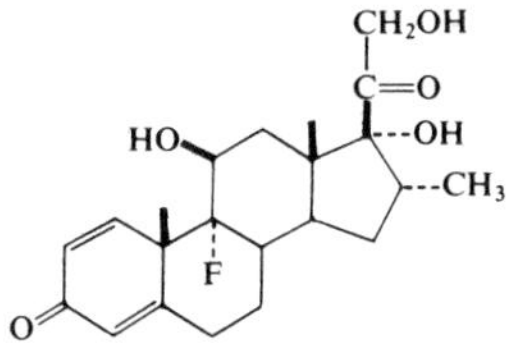

Dexamethasone
9α-Fluoro-16α-methylprednisolone

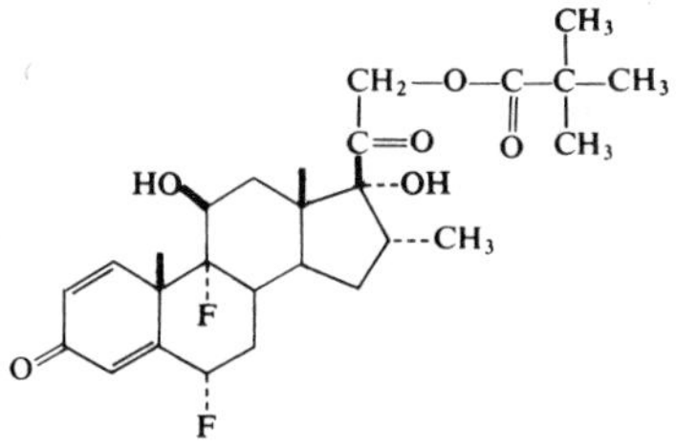

Fluomethasone pivalate (or trimethylacetate)
6α,9α-Difluoro-16α-methylprednisolone
21-pivalate

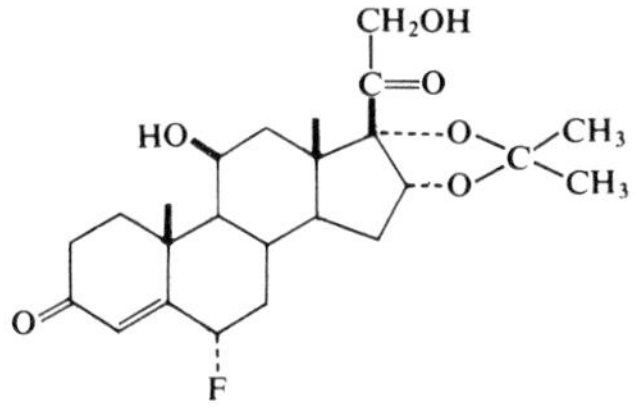

Flurandrenolone
6α-Fluoro-16α-hydroxyhydrocortisone
16,17-acetonide

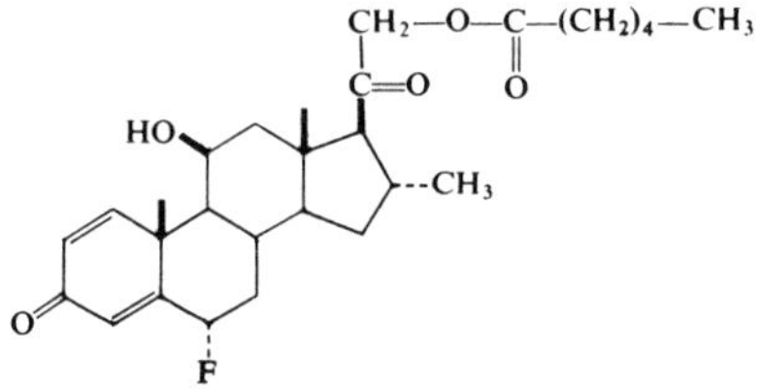

Fluocortolone caproate
6α-Fluoro-16α-methyl-1-dehydro-
corticosterone 21-caproate

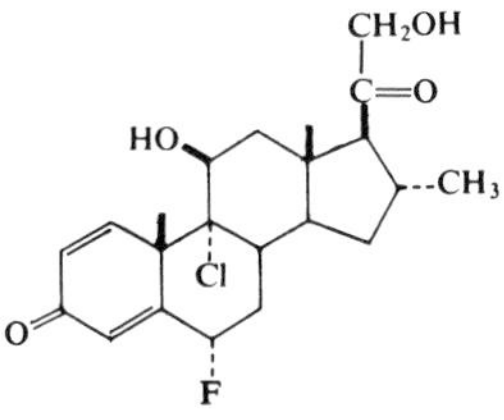

Chlocortolone
6α-Fluoro-9α-chloro-16α-methyl-
1-dehydrocorticosterone

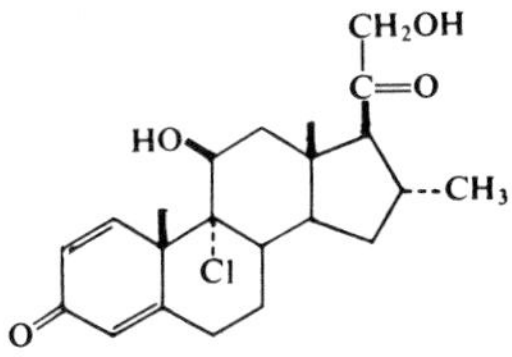

Desfluoclocortolone
9α-Chloro-16α-methyl-1-dehydro-
corticosterone

Fig. 6.5. Some anti-inflamatory steroids.

Table 6.8. *Relative potencies of anti-inflammatory steroids by fibroblast assay*

Cortisol	1
Prednisolone	1.7
Dexamethasone	7.5
Paramethasone	11.3
Triamcinolone acetonide	156
Fluocinolone acetonide	440

11β-dehydrogenase. The skin is unable to bring about this conversion and topical cortisone and prednisone are totally inactive. Only about 70% of cortisone and prednisone are converted by the body to hydrocortisone and prednisolone respectively and this agrees well with their estimated relative potencies, e.g. that oral cortisone is 70% as potent as oral hydrocortisone. All the active anti-inflammatory steroids have an 11β-hydroxy group with the exception of dichlorisone which has an 11β-chloro group and has some topical anti-inflammatory activity. Most of the commonly used compounds are derivatives of hydrocortisone in that they have a 17α-hydroxyl group but there is a small group of compounds, e.g. fluocortolone, which are derivatives of corticosterone. Insertion of a double bond at C-1, methyl groups at C-16 and C-6, fluoride or chloride groups at C-6 and C-9 all serve to enhance the potency of these steroids. The most potent compound appears to be fluocinolone. One of the objects of the structural modifications is to separate the mineralocorticoid, glucocorticoid, catabolic and anti-inflammatory effects of these compounds. The only properties that vary independently with structure are the anti-inflammatory effect and the sodium retention. Otherwise equivalent doses of synthetic steroids have the same effect on glycogen and protein metabolism.

1. Oral anti-inflammatory steroids

Prednisone (as prednisolone) has five times the anti-inflammatory action of cortisone (as hydrocortisone) and has less tendency to produce sodium retention. It has therefore tended to replace cortisone for oral therapy. A large dose of 6 mg per day, equivalent to 300 mg of cortisone, is essential in the acute phase of many illnesses and this quantity may be continued for 2-3 weeks without producing serious side-effects or permanent inhibition of adrenal or pituitary function. However, carefully controlled maintenance therapy is necessary to avoid these complications as side-effects may occur on as little as 5-10 mg per day. When prednisone causes edema, 4-8 mg 6α-methylprednisolone or 1-2 mg dexamethasone per day may be used. Both these compounds have no sodium-retaining properties (Table 6.9). Triamcinolone is not usually recommended because of its higher proportion of side-effects, e.g. erythema, bloating, abdominal cramps. The anti-inflammatory effect of ACTH is attributable to a stimulation of hydrocortisone production by the adrenal cortex.

Table 6.9. *Relative oral anti-inflammatory and mineralocorticoid effects*

	Dose (mg/day)	Anti-inflammatory effect	Mineralocorticoid (salt-retaining) effect
Hydrocortisone	25	1	1
Cortisone	30	0.8	0.8
Prednisone	5	5	0.6
Prednisolone	5	5	0.6
6α-Methylprednisolone	4	6	0
Triamcinolone	4	6	0
Dexamethasone	1	25	0
Betamethasone	1	25	0
Paramethasone	2	12	0
Aldosterone	—	0.1	100
9α-Fluorocortisol	0.1	12	100

2. Topical steroids

There are several possible routes for the penetrance of compounds into the epidermis of the skin, namely through the cells of the stratum corneum, between the cells of the stratum corneum, through the walls of the hair follicles or through the walls of the sweat glands. The hair follicles were formally thought to be the main route of percanteneous absorption and are certainly very important in the penetration of some substances, e.g. surface active agents. Such compounds easily reach the dermis and the systemic circulation. It is now thought that the major route of penetration is the epidermis itself, although it is not known conclusively whether the pathway is through or between the cells of the stratum corneum. It is believed that the main barrier to skin penetration is the fully formed keratin layer of the stratum corneum, the lowest layers of which offer the most resistance to penetration. Compounds which penetrate through the stratum corneum readily reach the epidermis but there appears to be another barrier between the epidermis and the dermis and hence the systemic circulation, which only some of the compounds can penetrate.

The keratin of the stratum corneum can be readily hydrated and when this is accomplished with an occlusive dressing, water loss from the skin surface is decreased and the skin temperature increases. Under these circumstances, the penetration of some anti-inflammatory steroids can be increased 100-fold.

Patients treated with a topical steroid and total occlusion, i.e. from neck to wrists and ankles, usually receive about 30 g of ointment or cream per treatment per 24 h. This results in a variety of amounts of steroids being received according to the concentration in the ointment. Under these conditions all the commercially available preparations, which are also clinically effective, produce some adreno-cortico-suppression due to penetration into the systemic circulation. This is usually measured as a decrease in 17-hydroxy-steroids in 24 h urine specimens from about 10-15 mg to about 5-8 mg. To obtain accurate measurements of this suppression, it is usual to give the base for 3 days, the active steroid for 3 days and then the base for 3 days. It is very unusual to get a drop in urinary 17-hydroxy-steroids to about 1 mg/24 h and slight Cushing's signs have only been seen occasionally in a few cases of gross over-treatment. Whole body occlusion is now rarely used as when such large doses of steroids are necessary, it is now considered better to administer them orally, when a better control of dose is obtained.

The most important factor in skin absorption is the nature of the substance itself and the vehicle in which it is presented to the skin surface is only of subsidiary importance. An evenly balanced solubility between water and lipid, i.e. a partition coefficient of one, favours skin penetration. This can be achieved with corticoids by the preparation of a variety of esters, e.g. triamcinolone has five times the systemic activity of hydrocortisone but only one-tenth its topical activity, but conversion to the acetonide enhances its penetration 1000-fold. Similarly, betamethasone has thirty times the systemic activity of hydrocortisone but only ten times its topical activity, while conversion to the 17-*n*-valerate produces the highest topical activity. It is necessary to dissolve the steroids before incorporation into a cream or ointment as even microfine particles in suspension are almost ineffective. Lipid solvents such as benzene and ethanol, facilitate the absorption of both water-soluble and lipid-soluble substances. Hydrophilic solvents, e.g. propylene glycol, dimethyl sulphoxide (DMSO), have also been shown to enhance the penetration of some steroids.

Formulation plays a less important part in the penetrance of topical corticoids into the skin and hence their clinical efficacy. Most steroids are offered either as a cream or an ointment although very little work has been done on relative penetrance from the two forms. Creams are oil-in-water emulsions, and are hydrophilic or "washable" ointments. They are stable over a wide range of pH and are suitable for the incorporation of anionic or non-ionic medicaments. The oil phase which constitutes some 30% of the cream is usually a mixture of oils, soft and hard waxes and the emulsifying agent is anionic, e.g. sodium lauryl sulphate. For the incorporation of cationic medicaments, a more suitable emulsifying agent is cetrimide emulsifying wax. Ointments are water-in-oil emulsions. The oil phase represents about 50% of the ointment and is composed of a mixture of oils and waxes. Cholesterol or mixed wool alcohols may be added as an emulsifying agent. This appreciably diminishes the penetration of water-soluble substances and hence may prevent them reaching the dermis and causing systemic effects, but increasing the penetration of lipid soluble substances. Pastes are recommended for exudative acute and subacute dermatoses and ointments for markedly dry, chronic inflammatory dermatoses. Creams are intermediate in use between pastes or ointments and have a broad range of indications.

Assessment of topical anti-inflammatory steroids presents special problems as animal tests do not mimic the human skin. Experimental inflammations have been induced in human volunteers, e.g. with ultra-violet light or tape stripping or by the application of irritants such as croton oil. None of these techniques are

Table 6.10. *Topical potency of steroids*

	THFA assay	Clinical assessment
Hydrocortisone	1	1
Triamcinolone	0.1	
Prednisolone	1.8	2
6α-Methylprednisolone	4.7	5
9α-Fluorohydrocortisone	9.0	10
Dexamethasone	19.0	10
Fluorometholone	42.0	40
Triamcinolone-16,17-acetonide	33.0	40

satisfactory and most screening tests for topical steroids now rely on the vasoconstriction assay. Topical steroids produce a pallor in normal skin and there is a rough correlation between vasoconstrictor potency and clinical usefulness. The results reflect the ability of the steroid to penetrate the normal human stratum corneum and to a lesser extent, the rate of clearance of the absorbed drug. Steroids are usually applied to the arm in ethanol or acetone solution, the solvent allowed to evaporate off, an occlusive dressing applied for 16 h and the degree of pallor assessed either visually or by relectance measurements or the examination of coloured photographs. When the percentages of test sites are plotted against the reciprocal of the log dose, a sigmoid curve is produced and the relative potencies of compounds can be ranked.

Table 6.10 shows some relative potencies obtained using the erythema produced by tetrahydrofurfurylalcohol (THFA) under an occlusive dressing. When steroids were added simultaneously, the erythema was prevented. Results agree well with potency assessed clinically.

Table 6.11 shows the trade names and concentrations of some of the more important topical fluorinated steroids available. Most of these are very powerful and this is reflected in the small concentrations present. These steroids can all be obtained plain or admixed with a variety of fungicides and bactericides (Table 6.12). There are also a large number of topical preparations containing hydrocortisone, hydrocortisone acetate, prednisolone, prednisolone acetate and 6α-methylprednisolone together with a variety of bactericides and fungicides.

Table 6.11. *Topical plain fluorinated anti-inflammatory steroids*

Trade name	Manufacturer		Steroid
Adcortyl-A	Squibb	0.1%	Triamcinolone acetonide
Betnesol	Glaxo	0.1%	Betamethasone disodium phosphate
Betnovate	Glaxo	0.1%	Betamethasone 17-valerate
Drenison (Cordran)	Eli Lilly	0.5 mg/ml	Flurandrenolone
Fluoderm plain	BDH	0.025%	Fluomethologne
Haelan	Dista	0.0125%	Flurandrenolone
Haelan-X	Dista	0.05%	Flurandrenolone
Ledercort	Lederle	0.1%	Triamcinolone acetonide
Ledercort D	Lederle	0.01%	Triamcinolone acetonide
Locorten	Ciba	0.02%	Flumethasone pivalate
Methral	Harvey Pharm.	0.1%	Fluperolone acetate
Propaderm	Allen & Hanbury	0.025%	Beclomethasone dipropionate
Synalar	I.C.I.	0.025%	Fluocinolone acetonide
Synalar Forte	I.C.I.	0.2%	Fluocinolone acetonide
Synandone	I.C.I.	0.01%	Fluocinolone acetonide
Ultralanum Plain	Schering Chem.	⎰0.25%	Fluocortolone
		⎱0.25%	Fluocortolone caproate

These substances are not so powerful and are therefore present in higher concentrations for effective use. In general, the use of plain topical steroids is not recommended if infection is present as they inhibit the body's natural defence mechanisms and the infection may get much worse, although the inflammation may appear to heal at first.

V. STEROID ANAESTHETICS

In the course of experimental studies on the pharmacology of steroids, it was discovered that sudden, intense overdosage with deoxycorticosterone acetate (DOCA) produced an initial state of excitation, followed by complete surgical anaesthesia in the rat, mouse, dog and in many other mammals. Similar results were obtained with progesterone which also produced the same action in man. Anaesthesia in man has also been produced by hydroxydione (Fig. 6.6).

Table 6.12. *Topical fluorinated steroids with germicides*

Trade name	Manufacturer	Steroid		Additions
Adcortyl-A with Graneodin	Squibb	Triamcinolone acetonide	0.1%	2.5 mg/g Neomycin
Aureocort (ointment)	Lederle	Triamcinolone	0.1%	0.25 mg/g Gramicidin
Betnovate-N	Glaxo	Betamethasone 17-*n*-valerate	0.1%	0.5% Neomycin sulphate
Betnovate-C	Glaxo	Betamethasone 17-*n*-valerate	0.1%	3% Chinoform (vioform)
Decaspray	Merck, Sharp & Dohme	Dexamethasone	10 mg/90 g aerosol	50 mg/90 g Neomycin sulphate
Drenison with Neomycin	Eli Lilly	Flurandrenolone	0.5 mg/ml	5 mg/ml Neomycin
Fluoderm	BDH	Fluorometholone	0.025%	0.50% Chlorphenesin
				3% Chioquinol
Ledercort acetonide cream with Neomycin	Lederle	Triamcinolone acetonide	0.1%	0.35% Neomycin sulphate
Locorten N	Ciba	Flumethasone pivalate	0.02%	0.5% Neomycin sulphate
Locorten Vioform	Ciba	Flumethasone pivalate	0.02%	3% Iodochlorhydroxyquinolone (chinoform)
Propaderm-C	Allen & Hanbury's	Beclomethasone dipropionate	0.025%	3% Chinoform
Propaderm-A	Allen & Hanbury's	Beclomethasone dipropionate	0.025%	3% Aureomycin
Remiderm	Squibb	Triamcinolone acetonide	0.025%	0.75% Halquinol
Synalar with Chinoform	I.C.I.	Fluocinolone acetonide	0.025%	3% Chinoform
Synalar-N	I.C.I.	Fluocinolone acetonide	0.025%	5% Neomycin sulphate
Synandone-N	I.C.I.	Fluocinolone acetonide	0.01%	0.5% Neomycin sulphate
Tri-adcortyl	Squibb	Triamcinolone acetonide	1 mg/g	2.5 mg/g Neomycin
				0.25 mg/g Gramicidin
				100,000 units/g Nystatin
Ultralan (um)	Schering	Fluocortolone	0.025%	2.5% Clemizole hexachlorophenate
		Fluocortolone caproate	0.025%	

Intravenous injections with hydroxydione sodium succinate produces uncon-
ciousness in about 4 min but venous spasm and thrombophlebitis are not
uncommon. Steroid anaesthetics are very little used.

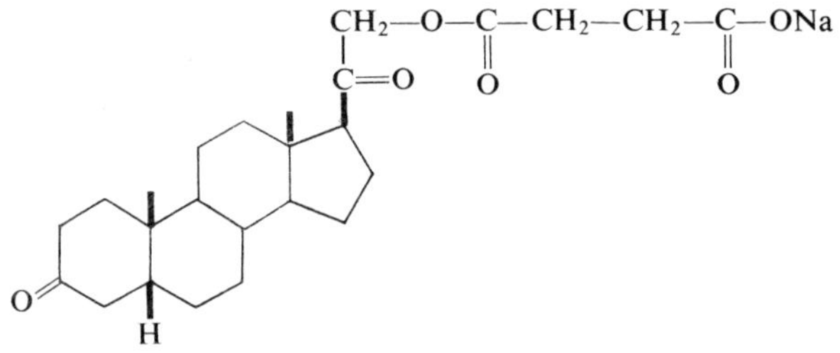

Hydroxydione sodium succinate
Sodium 21-(3-carboxypropionoyloxy)-5β-pregnane-
    3,20-dione
5β-Pregnan-21-ol-3,20-dione sodium
    succinate

Fig. 6.6. Hydroxydione.

7

EFFECTS OF NON-HORMONAL STEROIDS

I. CHOLESTEROL

A. MEMBRANE STRUCTURE

1. Bimolecular leaflet models

The cell membrane, or plasma membrane, forms the outer boundary of animal cells. It varies in thickness between 75 and 105 Å and is probably composed principally of protein and phospholipid arranged in a highly organized manner. In the Danielli model there are two protein monolayers on the outer and inner surfaces of the membrane and lipid molecules form a double internal layer. Each lipid molecule has a hydrophobic, non-polar end extending towards the centre of the membrane, where there is a narrow gap between the opposed non-polar ends of the two layers of lipid molecules. The membrane is not

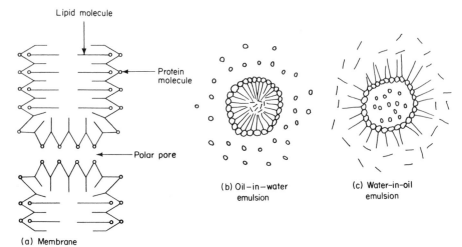

Fig. 7.1. Structure of bimolecular leaflet biological membranes and of emulsions. (Diagram (a) from Stein and Danielli, 1956.)

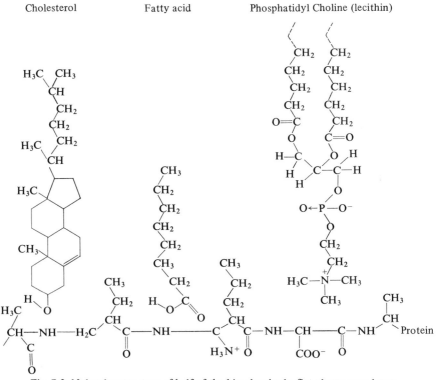

Fig. 7.2. Molecular structure of half of the bimolecular leaflet plasma membrane.

continuous, but is interrupted by lipid pits, protein pits and by pores of about 10 Å diameter. Cells in contact with similar cells often have specialized structures on the contact surfaces, e.g. desmosomes (Figs. 7.1a and 7.2).

Membranes also exist inside cells. The nuclear envelope is composed of two separate membranes each of which shows the typical structure. There is a gap between these two membranes and nuclear pores 500-200 Å in diameter pass through both. In the cytoplasm the rough and smooth endoplasmic reticulums appear as complex systems composed of pairs of membranes enclosing interconnecting cavities. Rough endoplasmic reticulum has ribosomes attached and synthesizes protein. The membranes of mitochondria are thinner than cell membranes, but show the same laminated structure. Lysosomes are cytoplasmic bags containing hydrolytic enzymes and are bounded by a membrane.

Analysis of cell membranes shows that they consist of lipid and protein in the ratio of 1.7 to 1.0. The lipids are mainly cholesterol and phospholipids, of which cholesterol accounts for 15-30% of the total lipids. The phospholipids account for 55-75% of the total lipids and are mainly lecithin and cephalin. On average, the membrane has 75-90 molecules of lipid for every molecule of protein. Cholesterol and the phospholipids are the chief emulsifying agents of the body for the formation of water-in-oil emulsions.

Most lipids of animal cell membranes occur in five organelles: plasmolemma (cell surface), endoplasmic reticulum, Golgi complex, mitochondria, and nuclei. The types of membranes found in, or around, particular cells are highly variable. Animal cells generally contain three types of lipids: phospholipids, glycolipids and sterols, usually cholesterol. Sterols are absent from most bacterial cell membranes and in plant membranes the glycolipids are glycerol esters whereas in animal cells they are sphingolipids. Sterol esters and triglycerides do not occur as membrane components. Cholesterol is only a minor component of the membranes of mammalian mitochondria.

Cholesterol has a condensing effect on phospholipids. It has been suggested that the presence of a *cis* double bond in the 9:10 position of the hydrocarbon chain of a phospholipid is ideally suited for combination with a cholesterol molecule. Cholesterol enters the cavities between phospholipid molecules and does not increase the overall size of a membrane. A possible role for cholesterol in membranes is to control the fluidity of the hydrocarbon chains of the phospholipids, providing a coherent structure stable over a wide temperature range and permitting some latitude in the fatty acid content of the component lipids.

There is also an important carbohydrate component of cell membranes and this may occur as an outside coat. The chemical composition and structure of glycoproteins associated with cell surfaces and those excreted by cells are quite different, e.g. a higher galactosamine: glucosamine ratio and lack of mannose. The protein mostly shows a predominance of serine and threonine linked to carbohydrate rather than to asparagine. Neuraminic acid (a sialic acid) appears to be an important component of many diverse membrane systems.

2. Micellar models

On the basis of observations made with the electron microscope on macromolecular lipid complexes, apparently composed of globular micelles, it has been suggested that it is not necessary to consider structures containing a high proportion of phospholipids solely in terms of bimolecular leaflets. It is suggested that globular micelles of lipid are in dynamic equilibrium with the bimolecular leaflet structure within membranes. Such globular micelles would have lipophilic cores of about 40 Å in diameter and the overall diameters of the micelles would be about 50 Å, provided that the polar groups of the phospholipid molecules are arranged tangentially to the surface of the globular units. Adjacent micelles might be held together by hydrogen bonds. The stability of such a flat sheet of micelles may be dependent upon interaction with protein (or perhaps glycoprotein) molecules on the surface of the lipid layer. In this model the polar groups of the phospholipids, and their associated counter ions, line the pores, each of which has an effective radius of about 4 Å at its narrowest point.

B. MEMBRANE PERMEABILITY

1. Types of permeability

Substances may enter cells either by free diffusion, diffusion through pores, pinocytosis, or active transport. Both types of diffusion are in response to a concentration gradient, do not require energy and are passive phenomena. The ability to pass through a membrane by diffusion largely depends on the lipid: water partition coefficient of the compound, which should be about one for maximum permeability. Smaller molecules penetrate faster than expected on the basis of their partition coefficient and this is believed to be due to the pores. The rate of diffusion is much increased by temperature. Only non-electrolytes can penetrate by diffusion and ions are largely taken up by active transport. This appears to be the result of the plasma membrane being charged. Cell membranes in different parts of the body have different amounts of cholesterol. The more cholesterol present, the more water can diffuse into the cell.

Active transport through a membrane is indicated when a substance is taken up against a concentration gradient, or when the uptake is dependent on respiration energy (ATP), e.g. uptake of potassium, amino acids and glucose. It is believed that a carrier molecule is involved. At the outer surface of the plasma membrane the substance to be transported forms, in the presence of an enzyme, a complex with an organic carrier molecule containing an energy rich bond. The membrane is permeable to the complex, which moves through the membrane to its inner surface. Here the substance is split off from the complex by another enzyme. Metabolic energy is believed to be required for the synthesis of the carrier and possibly for splitting of the complex.

Very large molecules, e.g. protein and DNA, are taken up by pinocytosis. This is a process whereby a certain area of the surface membrane of the cell encloses a droplet of the surrounding medium, separates from the surface and migrates into the cell. Pinocytosis and phagocytosis are two different types of a basically similar process.

2. Effect of steroid hormones on membrane permeability

It has been suggested that there may be a correlation between the type of physiological action caused by any given steroid hormone and the substituents of the molecule, particularly at C-3 and C-17, as a result of the packing of the steroid into lipoprotein membranes. Steroids could pack with their long axis parallel to the hydrocarbon chain of the phospholipids in a bimolecular leaflet. Physiological action would then be determined mainly by the polar groups thus exposed at the hydrophilic surface of the membrane. On this hypothesis, the ability of a steroid molecule to act on any particular cell will depend on the capacity of the steroid to enter and remain within the plasma membrane. This, in turn, will be governed chiefly by the molecular shape of the steroid, its affinity for particular phospholipids already in the membrane, and on the action which any proteins associated with the hydrophilic surface of the lipid might have upon it. This also applies to the membranes inside the cells. Since all active steroids are much shorter than cholesterol, it has been suggested that four molecules of steroid may be packed end-to-end across the width of a bimolecular leaflet membrane when as many as three hydrophilic pools could develop at different levels within the membrane.

An alternative hypothesis is that steroid hormones form local areas of micellar configuration with a membrane by becoming orientated parallel to the interface. Cholesterol, which has only one polar group, is still believed to pack vertically into monolayers, but steroid hormones have two or more polar groups and may pack horizontally. In such a situation the polar groups of the steroid could interact with ions and polar molecules passing through the pores between the phospholipid micelles. The lengths of steroid hormone molecules are such that it seems possible that the polar groups at each end may project into two adjacent pores. The molecular specificity of estrogens, androgens, progestogens and corticoids, does seem to be associated with the number of polar groups in the molecule. This also affects the degree of serum protein binding.

The effects of steroid hormones on a number of membrane systems have been investigated. The effects of cortisone on liver mitochondria are profound. Multiple defects are caused in the mitochondrial respiratory chain and oxidative phosphorylation is uncoupled. There is a striking decrease in the number of mitochondria per liver cell and an increase in the average mitochondrial volume. A decrease in succinate oxidase activity in isolated liver mitochondria has also been demonstrated. Treatment of rats with cortisone and other glucocorticoids has been observed to diminish both the substrate and ATP-dependent accumulation of calcium by isolated liver mitochondria. This is probably a result of interference with the utilization of either ATP or the respiratory substrate necessary to support the uptake process.

Glucocorticoids, and especially anti-inflammatory steroids, also have a profound effect on lysosomal membranes. Lysosomes contain a variety of powerful hydrolytic enzymes and are involved in the uptake and degradation of antigenic molecules. Glucocorticoids are believed to stabilize lysosomal membranes and hence prevent the release of the tissue-damaging enzymes. Vitamins A, D, E and K, sterols, endotoxins, streptolipin and UV-radiation all release lysosomal enzymes. Steroid sulphates are not easily transported across membranes whereas the glucuronosides move across easily.

Membrane stabilization can be brought about by hormonal steroids, bile acids, non-ionic detergents, vitamin A, the phenothiazine group of tranquilizing drugs and some alcohols and anaesthetic drugs. The different types of compounds appear to act preferentially upon different types of membranes, e.g. when the membranes of nerve cells are stabilized anaesthesia results. Membrane stabilization, i.e. the protection of membranes against disruption by mechanical or osmotic means, is a biphasic phenomenon as higher concentrations of the same compounds produce cell lysis, e.g. vitamin A causes lysis of lysosomes and swelling of rat liver mitochondria at 3.5×10^{-5} M but at 3.5×10^{-6} M it causes the protection of erythrocytes against osmotic haemolysis. Membrane lysis by corticosteroids is well known, e.g. on rabbit liver lysosomes at 5×10^{-4} M, while at 10^{-5} M release of lysosomal enzymes is inhibited. A wide variety of steroids at low concentrations, e.g. pregnanolone, androsterone, testosterone, cortisone but not their water soluble derivatives, cause the stabilization of erythrocytes to hypotonic solutions, while at high concentrations they cause lysis or precipitation. The bile steroids, lithocholic acid and sodium taurocholate also exert a biphasic stabilization-lysis effect on erythrocytes. Certain steroids also inhibit the lysis of erythrocytes caused by sulphydryl inhibitors. The degree of erythrocyte stabilization correlates with the potency of steroids as anaesthetics.

C. ANTIGENIC CELL SURFACES

Most substances of large molecular weight are antigenic (under appropriate conditions) and it appears that many species-specific antigens are membrane components of all cells of the body. These membrane antigens may be protein or lipopolysaccharide in nature.

Complement fixation is also a membrane phenomenon. The sequential activation of nine complement components is necessary at the cell membrane before lysis ensues. The reaction is initiated by the binding and activation by the fixed antibody of the first component of complement ($C'1$), which then acts on $C'4$ (which is a well-characterized serum protein) whose binding-site becomes activated and for a short period can bind to the cell membrane or to the antibody molecules. The binding is believed to be hydrophobic in nature and it is not necessary to postulate specific binding sites on the cell membrane. Later $C'3$, another well-characterized serum protein, which occurs in concentrations in excess of 1 mg/ml, is activated and a large amount is bound to the cell membrane.

In man and most animal species, a distinct type of immunoglobulin is adsorbed passively onto the membrane of basophils and mast cells, and possibly also onto other cells. This is the reagin or anaphalactic antibody and combination with specific antigen activates a pathway which leads to degranulation of mast cells and basophils, and to liberation of histamine and other mediators of inflammation.

D. BLOOD CHOLESTEROL

1. Occurrence

Blood plasma collected from a fasting normal human adult contains between 300 and 800 mg of lipid per 100 ml. This lipid is a mixture of free and esterified cholesterol, together with glycerides, phospholipids and non-esterified fatty acids. Figure 7.3 shows how total blood cholesterol in normal men and women

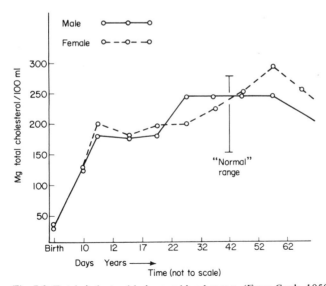

Fig. 7.3. Total cholesterol in human blood serum. (From Cook, 1958.)

rises from about 50 mg/100 ml at birth, to about 180 mg/ml at puberty, with a further gradual rise throughout life.

In normal adult men the mean concentration of cholesterol in blood plasma is 200 mg/100 ml (i.e. about one-third of the total lipids). Of this cholesterol, 70% is present as esters with various fatty acids, and 30% as the free sterol. The fatty acids esterified to plasma cholesterol are (for healthy adult male Europeans) shown in Fig. 7.4.

Both cholesterol and its esters are insoluble in water and are present in plasma in loose chemical association with specific globulin proteins, forming the plasma lipoproteins. These share many of the chemical and physical properties of ordinary globulins, and differ primarily in their lower density. This property can be used to separate them from other plasma proteins, for in high centrifugal fields (100,000 g) lipoproteins float while almost all other proteins sediment.

By the use of an analytical ultracentrifuge it is possible to separate and distinguish a range of specific lipoproteins of differing densities. The cholesterol content of these fractions varies widely. Table 7.1 lists the major properties of

Table 7.1. *Some properties of plasma lipoproteins*

Fraction	Flotation rate sf	Density	Starch electro- phoresis	Composition		
				Protein %	Lipid %	Cholesterol (% of lipid)
Low-density (LDL)						
(i)	10^3-10^5	0.96	α^2	1	99	1
(ii)	20-400	0.96-1.006	α^2	7	93	8
(iii)	12-20	1.006-1.019	β	11	89	9
(iv)	0-12	1.019-1.063	β	21	79	10
High-density (HDL)		1.05-1.21	α^1	45	55	8

these various fractions. The amounts and proportions of the various lipoproteins vary with a wide range of factors. Men have higher levels of all low density fractions than women up to the fifth decade. About this age the two sexes become equal and in the 60's women tend to have higher levels than men. Changes in diet affect low density lipoproteins (LDL) primarily. Low fat diets increase LDL (ii) and (iii) but decrease LDL (iv). High fat diets tend to increase all LDL fractions, but the major increase is in (iv). Unsaturated dietary fats tend to decrease all fractions, especially LDL (iv). The level of dietary cholesterol or other sterols is without effect on the lipoproteins of blood.

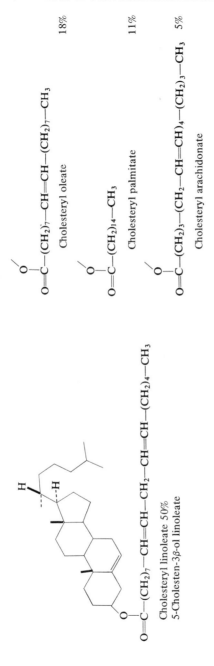

$O=C-(CH_2)_7-CH=CH-(CH_2)_7-CH_3$ 18%

Cholesteryl oleate

$O=C-(CH_2)_{14}-CH_3$ 11%

Cholesteryl palmitate

$O=C-(CH_2)_3-(CH_2-CH=CH)_4-(CH_2)_3-CH_3$ 5%

Cholesteryl arachidonate

$O=C-(CH_2)_7-CH=CH-CH_2-CH=CH-(CH_2)_4-CH_3$

Cholesteryl linoleate 50%
5-Cholesten-3β-ol linoleate

Fig. 7.4. Some cholesterol esters occurring in blood.

2. Determination

(a) Liebermann-Burchard reaction

When concentrated sulphuric acid is added to a solution of cholesterol in acetic anhydride, a series of colour changes occur, going from red through violet to blue-green. At room temperature, cholesterol esters give 10-30% more colour than free cholesterol, but at 0-2°C, only the esters give any colour. A very large number of assay techniques based on this colour reaction have been described. Some use intact, others deproteinized, serum. While there are numerous modifications to choose from, the techniques of Schoenheimer and Sperry seem the most reliable and accurate. Here cholesterol esters are saponified before the colour reaction.

(b) Other colour reactions

Cholesterol will give coloured complexes with any of the following reagents, all of which have been used as the basis of assay methods:

(i) p-toluenesulphonic acid;
(ii) acetyl chloride + zinc chloride in glacial acetic acid;
(iii) ferric chloride + sulphuric acid.

(c) Separation of cholesterol and its esters

The following methods have been employed to separate cholesterol from its esters in serum:

(i) precipitation of free cholesterol as pyridinium cholesteryl sulphate;
(ii) precipitation of free cholesterol by the glycoside tomatin;
(iii) molecular distillation at 10^{-5} mm Hg (free cholesterol distills at 88°C, esters at 155°C);
(iv) countercurrent distribution;
(v) paper or thin-layer chromatography;
(vi) chromatography on columns of alumina or Celite.

(d) Serum low density lipoproteins

These can be estimated turbidimetrically by specific precipitation by dextran sulphate in the presence of calcium ions at pH 9. Normal values in the male aged 20-60 are 500-520 mg/100 ml and in the female 280-470 mg/100 ml.

3. Clinical abnormalities of cholesterol metabolism

Marked increases in plasma cholesterol occur in a variety of pathological conditions (Table 7.2). Some hypercholesteraemic conditions are associated with xanthomas containing cholesterol (abnormal fatty deposits). Rare inherited defects have been reported in which the affected individuals lack either LDL or HDL fractions.

Table 7.2. *Varieties of hypercholesteraemia*

Condition	Lipoprotein fractions increased
1. Essential hypercholesteraemia	LDL (iii) and (iv)
2. Biliary obstruction	LDL (ii), (iii) and (iv)
3. Hyperlipoproteinaemia	LDL (ii)
4. Essential hyperlipaemia	LDL (ii) and (i)
5. Diabetic ketosis	LDL (ii) and (i)
6. Nephrosis	LDL (ii) and (i)

E. ATHEROSCLEROSIS (ARTERIOSCLEROSIS)

The most common site of arteriosclerosis is the aorta. The initial reaction is the formation of fatty streaks or spots on the intimal layer. There is fragmentation of the internal elastic lamina, deposition of increased amounts of acid mucopolysaccharides and proliferation of cellular elements. Increased lipid content can be demonstrated by chemical estimation and histologically. This initial damage is considered to arise from the lumen of the vessel and proceed inwards. Among the many suggested causative agents in blood have been plasma lipoproteins containing cholesterol and its esters; a local increase in macrophages; an increased clotting tendency; platelet sticking; and factors increasing permeability. In syphilitic aortitis the initial lesion is believed to arise from the inward tissue. The second stage is the maturation of the scar with regeneration of the internal elastic lamina and production of collagen fibres. The lipid may disappear if there is healing, but if healing does not occur, the connective tissue degenerates and lipids and calcium salts (mainly phosphate) are deposited.

Atherosclerosis is a recognized pathological entity, but its relationship with myocardial infarction and other forms of heart disease is still uncertain. It is the association of the condition with the coronary arteries supplying the heart which results in morbility or death. Atherosclerosis plaques cause an occlusion of the arteries which may be the cause of blood clots and strain on the heart resulting in ischaemic heart disease, myocardial infarction and death.

Because cholesterol and its esters are found in the plaques of atherosclerotic arteries, and because the feeding of cholesterol to certain animals induces atherosclerosis ("experimental atherosclerosis"), a "cause and effect" relationship between atherosclerosis and/or myocardial infarction and the circulating blood cholesterol has been postulated. Table 7.3 gives a summary of the composition of the normal adult human aorta. Values refer to the medial and intimal layers of the tissue dissected from the aortic valves to the bifurcation of the iliac vessels, after the removal of the adventitial layer which contains a large amount of adipose tissue. In the young adult this tissue weighs 10-15 g, but may

Table 7.3. *Composition of normal human aorta*

	(g/100 g fresh tissue)
Water	70
Total protein, including myosin	20-25
Collagen	7
Elastin	8-9
Mucopolysaccharide ground substance	10
Mineral matter, mainly calcium phosphate	0.3
Lipid	1

increase to over 30 g with increasing age. In old age, the mineral matter increases to 2.5%, of which about 1.3% is calcium phosphate and the rest Na^+, K^+, Mg^{2+} and Cl^-, while the sulphate, which is mainly bound in the mucopolysaccharides, decreases to about 0.2%. Table 7.4 shows the composition of the lipid fraction in normal aorta and in aortic atherosclerotic plaques.

Of the sterol fraction, some 50-65% is esterified mainly with palmitic, oleic and linoleic acids, while palmitic and oleic acids are the principal fatty acids in the triglycerides and phospholipids. Cholesterol is the main sterol present, but cholestanol and cholestane-3β, 5α, 6β-triol may form 5-12% of the fraction. Hydroxy-sterols, e.g. 7α, 7β, 24, 25, 26-dihydroxy-cholesterols, and oxo-sterols, e.g. cholesta-4,6-dien-3-one and cholesta-3,5-dien-7-one, are also present and gas liquid chromatography has shown numerous other compounds present in small amounts. In atherosclerosis the lipid fraction increases to 3-4% and if the weights for *whole* aorta (intimal and medial coats) are taken, the relative increases are five times for phospholipid and forty times for esterified sterols.

Patients with atherosclerosis have a raised blood cholesterol level and routine "check-ups" are now carried out in a number of centres. It is considered that a simple estimation of blood cholesterol, free and esterified, is sufficiently good as a diagnostic index and the more complicated determinations of plasma lipoproteins are not usually required. A plasma level of over 300 mg cholesterol/100

Table 7.4. *Lipid composition of the human aorta*

	Normal (% of total extract)	Atherosclerotic plaques (% of total extract)
Triglycerides	15	9-15
Phospholipid	50-60	33
Total sterols	15	30-60
Free fatty acids	5	1

ml is considered potentially dangerous and merits treatment to prevent myocardial infarction. In some diseases, e.g. essential hypercholestaerolaemia and diabetes mellitus, there is a good correlation between high plasma cholesterol and myocardial infarction. In other diseases, e.g. hypothyroidism, there is not a good correlation.

F. BLOOD CHOLESTEROL LOWERING AGENTS

Various compounds will reduce the total level of plasma cholesterol. The following are some examples:

(a) 10 g or more daily of β-sitosterol lowers pathologically high cholesterol levels. This compound is non-toxic and poorly absorbed in man. It is believed to depress the intestinal absorption of cholesterol;

(b) Large doses of nicotinic acid (5 g) also depress plasma cholesterol. Unfortunately, at this level liver damage is possible;

(c) Certain antibiotics, e.g. neomycin, will lower plasma cholesterol. The mechanism is unknown;

(d) Hypercholesteraemia, due mainly to increases in LDL (iii) and (iv), occurs in myxoedema. Thyroid hormone restores the levels to normal. Large doses of thyroid hormones given to normal people lowers LDL (iv). It is thought that the thyroid hormone increases the rate of conversion of cholesterol to bile acids;

(e) Estrogens increase HDL and decrease LDL. Androgens have the opposite actions. Androsterone has a quite pronounced effect, while etiocholanolone is virtually inert;

(f) A variety of drugs lower plasma cholesterol. Triparanol (Fig. 7.5) is of considerable interest as it completely halts the synthesis of cholesterol at the stage of conversion of desmosterol to 24-dehydrocholesterol in *all* tissues. It dramatically lowers plasma cholesterol, but there is an accumulation of desmosterol so that total plasma sterols are almost unaffected. A number of severe side effects were produced by its use, e.g. cataracts, ichthyosis and alopecia, and it has been withdrawn from the market. A more useful drug is Clofibrate which in doses of 1.5-2.5 g per day causes a significant lowering of plasma cholesterol. This compound blocks the conversion of β-hydroxy-β-methyl-glutaryl-CoA to mevalonic acid.

II. BILE SALTS

A. INTESTINAL ABSORPTION

A large part of the calorie intake of man consists of fat which is water insoluble and is made up of triglycerides possessing long-chain fatty acids. By the coordinated action of the digestive juices and the bile, the dietary lipids are brought into a form that can be absorbed by the intestinal mucosa. In the cells of the mucosa, the absorbed lipids are transformed into discrete particles 0.5 μ in diameter (called chylomicrons) which enter the lymph, and then the general

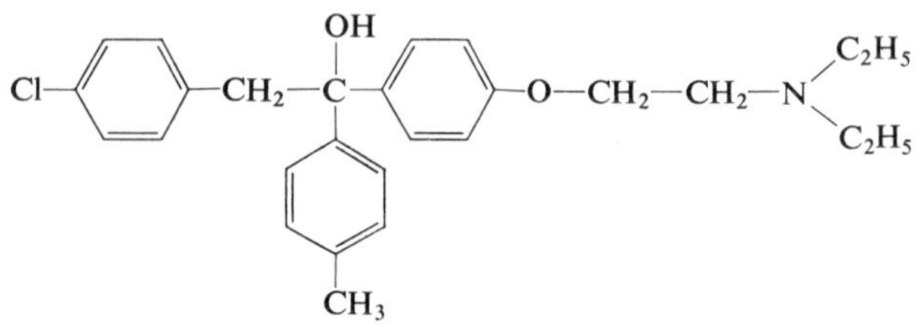

Triparanol
1-[4-(Diethylaminoethoxy)phenyl]-1,1-
(p-ptolyl)-2-(p-chlorophenyl)ethanol

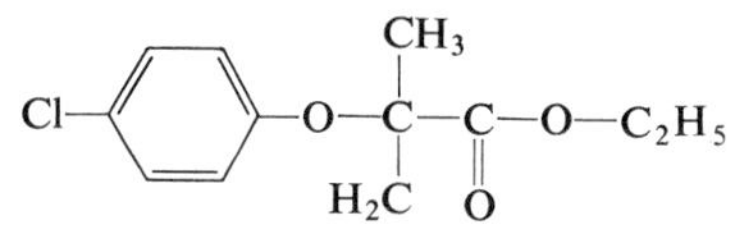

Clofibrate
Atromid-S
Ethyl α-p-chlorophenyl-α-methylpropionate
Ethyl chlorophenoxyisobutyrate

Fig. 7.5. Some plasma cholesterol lowering agents.

circulation via the thoracic duct. Chylomicrons contain about 86% neutral lipids, 3% cholesterol and its esters, 8.5% phospholipids and 2% protein.

The pH of the intestinal contents during digestion is very constant at 6.0-6.5 in the duodenum and upper jejunum. The non-polar triglycerides of the diet are mixed with the bile and partly transformed into more polar substances, the result being a highly complex mixture of non-polar substances (triglycerides, fatty acid, cholesterol) and substances possessing both polar and non-polar structures (bile salts, lecithin). The latter are emulsifying agents and form oil-in-water emulsions. (Figs. 7.1 and 7.6). In higher concentrations, i.e. above the critical micelle concentration, they tend to aggregate and form association-colloids or micelles.

Micellar solutions solubilize non-polar substances which are believed to be taken up into the centre of the micelle. Most of the cholesterol in the intestine is esterified, i.e. non-polar, and is taken up in this way. Amphiphilic or polar solutes are taken up by the mechanism of polar solubilization and are believed to

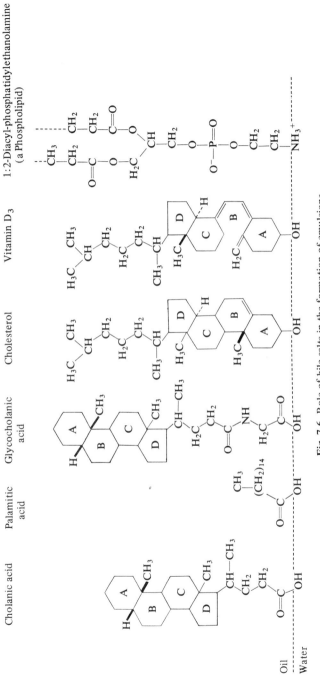

Fig. 7.6. Role of bile salts in the formation of emulsions.

be orientated with and between the polar groups at the micelle surface. When they are present in excess, liquid crystals are formed. An ordinary detergent micelle is considered to be spherical with a radius slightly less than the length of the fully extended paraffin chain. Short-chain monoglycerides, below C-10, are remarkably soluble in bile salt micelles, being solubilized as amphiphiles. Longer chain monoglycerides are solubilized as non-polar solutes and have much lower solubilities.

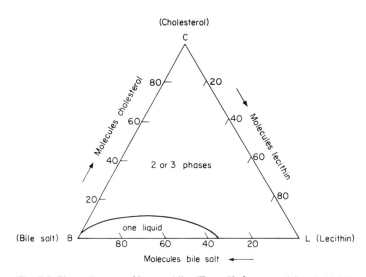

Fig. 7.7. Phase diagram of human bile. (From Hofmann and Small, 1967.)

Lipases only hydrolyse water-insoluble substrates in a heterogeneous system. They are adsorbed at the oil-water interface of emulsions and their action depends on the surface area of the emulsion. Some emulsifying agents increase while others inhibit lipase activity. The bile salts are particularly powerful stimulants of lipase action in the order cholate > taurocholate > deoxycholate and they decrease surface tension in the order deoxycholate > taurocholate > cholate. Bile salts are anionic detergents, but non-biological anionic detergents do not activate lipases. The bile salts are believed to act by exactly aligning the enzyme at the interface.

Bile is a solution of mixed micelles and is a bile salt-water-lecithin-cholesterol system. Over a fairly wide range of bile salts and lecithin concentrations, a maximum amount of 4% cholesterol by weight can be solubilized in a mixed micellar phase. Excess cholesterol is present in crystalline form. Figure 7.7 shows a plot of the area of the micellar phase for 90% water content at 37°C. The addition of cholesterol molecules above the line causes the separation of cholesterol at low lecithin/bile salt ratios and a liquid crystalline phase containing cholesterol at high lecithin/bile salt ratios. The micelles probably consist of bimolecular discs of lecithin molecules stabilized on the sides or ends by bile salt molecules bonded through van der Waals forces to the hydrocarbon chains of the lecithin. Cholesterol would be interdigitated between the lecithin molecules.

The phase diagram predicts the formation of cholesterol crystals but not gallstones. Gallstone formation requires not only nucleation but also continued growth. Cholesterol gallstones appear to have a nucleus of calcium bilirubinate which can arise from hydrolysis of bilirubin glucuronoside. The necessary glucuronidase is present in bile.

B. PHARMACOLOGY

Bile salts are necessary for the intestinal absorption of the fat-soluble vitamins and of carotene, but are of minor importance in the absorption of steroid hormones. They have a mild bacteriostatic effect, inhibiting excessive growth of coliform organisms in the intestinal tract. When given orally or intravenously, bile salts stimulate the liver to increase its output of bile, i.e. they have a choleretic action. The most active compound is dehydrocholic acid which increases the total volume of bile to a much greater extent than it does the total solids and is therefore termed "hydrocholeretic". Glycocholate and taurocholate enhance the flow of bile to a much lesser extent, but both volume and total solids are proportionally increased. Intravenous injection of bile salts causes a marked fall in blood pressure accompanied by bradycardia, probably due to stimulation of the vagal centres as these effects can be reversed by atropine. Dehydrocholic acid is the least potent in producing these side effects and has been used in the treatment of a variety of liver disorders, e.g. in prolonged surgical drainage of biliary fistulas, in biliary obstruction in order to provide bile acids for the absorption of the fat-soluble vitamins, and for the removal of small calculi partially obstructing the flow of bile. Cholestasis may be defined as stagnation of bile formed by the hepatocytes within the intrahepatic and extrahepatic biliary passages, with retention of all biliary substances in the blood. Bile salts have recently been used in the treatment of obesity.

C. GALLSTONES

A variety of solid stones can form in the gall bladder and bile ducts and such stones can attain diameters of up to 5 cm. The commonest stones are composed primarily of cholesterol, the other constituents being bile salts and calcium bilirubinate. Any condition leading to over-concentration of the bile favours stone formation, as even normal bile is supersaturated with cholesterol. Many patients with hypercholesteraemia develop gallstones. Biliary stasis also tends to initiate stone formation.

Examinations have been conducted of bile taken from patients with cholesterol stones. In all cases there are significant increases in total bile solids, but, surprisingly, no increases in either cholesterol or total bile acids. However, most patients do show marked changes in the amounts of individual bile acids present. There is often a decrease in the ratio of trihydroxy to dihydroxy bile acids. Gall bladder bile may show more marked changes than hepatic bile (Table 7.5). It

Table 7.5. *Composition of human bile*

	In liver	In gall bladder
Water, %	97-98	84
Conjugated bile acids, %	0.96-1.2	1.8-6.2
Free bile acids, %	0.28-0.52	20
Bilirubin, mg/100 ml	17-71	50-1000
Cholesterol (non-esterified) mg/100 ml	86-176	100-900
Choline, mg/100 ml	22-92	550
Protein, mg/100 ml	180	450
Fatty acids, mg/100 ml	100-450	80-2400
Lecithins, mg/100 ml	250	350
Carbohydrates, mg/100 ml	60	240
Calcium, mg/100 ml	8-11	25-28
Phosphorus, mg/100 ml	6-24	140

seems likely that gallstones arise from some biochemical lesion of the liver cells. The nature of this lesion is still unknown. At the present time there is no method of treating gallstones other than by surgical removal. Theoretically, a medical treatment could be developed if an agent could be found to stimulate the formation of a dilute bile that would lead to the re-dissolving of the cholesterol stones.

III. VITAMIN D

A. INTESTINAL ABSORPTION

Dietary vitamin D is absorbed in the jejunum and the lower third of the small intestine with the aid of bile salts and enters blood through the lymphatic system where 80% of it appears in the chylomicron fraction. Vitamin D is transported in the blood in the chylomicrons and the lipoproteins, especially with the α_2-globulins to which it is tightly bound. Most oral vitamin D in man accumulates in the liver about 4 h after administration. Within 1-4 h after an intravenous injection of vitamin D_3 or D_4 in rats, maximal incorporation occurs in virtually all the organs, except the liver, and especially in the target organs of bone and intestine. Vitamin D or its products arrive at the target sites long before there is an observable physiological response. In the liver, maximum concentration occurs within a few minutes after administration and is followed by a rapid decline for up to 24 h and then a very gradual decline. Most vitamin D and/or its metabolites are excreted into the small intestine via the bile and appear in the faeces, e.g. 17% of an intravenous dose in the rat appears in the faeces in 24 h. The chemical structures of the excreted products of vitamin D are not yet known.

Most tissues contain at least four metabolites of vitamin D, one of which is an ester of vitamin D and the common long-chain fatty acids. It has been suggested that vitamin D is esterified during absorption in the same way as cholesterol. Vitamin D sulphate has been identified in liver. Most of the vitamin D in cells is believed to be in the heavy microsomal fraction with some in the nuclear debris and mitochondrial fraction, all associated with membranes.

B. CALCIUM METABOLISM

Vitamin D does not have a direct action on the mineralization of bone. Rickets, which is due to a deficiency of vitamin D, is characterized by a failure of the mineralization process to keep pace with the formation of organic matrix of new bone. There is a widening of the epiphyseal plate, with eventual weakening of the bone so that it is unable to support the weight of the animal and becomes bowed and twisted. Osteomalacia is a disease found in adult women, brought about by vitamin D deficiency and characterized by a failure of calcification of matrix which has been decalcified during pregnancy. These bone defects are the result of a deficient supply of calcium and phosphorus to the bone.

Excessive doses of vitamin D cause hypercalcaemia and deposition of bone in the soft tissues, e.g. the kidney, together with a generalized osteoporosis. Intoxication symptoms are weakness, lassitude, headache, nausea, vomiting and diarrhoea. There is impairment of function of the kidneys and other calcified soft tissues.

Vitamin D increases the absorption of calcium and secondarily of phosphorus in the small intestine. In vitamin D deficiency, large amounts of unabsorbed dietary calcium are detected in the faeces. In the absence of dietary calcium, vitamin D causes the mobilization of bone calcium and phosphorus into blood serum. Vitamin D improves the renal absorption of inorganic phosphate and calcium. In the absence of vitamin D or the absence of the parathyroid hormone, 99% of renal filtered calcium is reabsorbed, while the remaining 1% is reabsorbed if either of these two compounds is present.

7*

Vitamin D alters the permeability of the intestine to calcium and increases the rate of passage of calcium from the lumen. There is also evidence that vitamin D alters the permeability of subcellular membranes to calcium. Permeability is believed to take place by active transport, probably with a specific calcium-binding protein. Vitamin D has a marked protective effect on the structural integrity of mitochondria. Calcium is actively taken up by mitochondria and vitamin D has a marked stimulatory effect on the release of this calcium from mitochondria.

Evidence is now accumulating that vitamin D induces protein and enzyme synthesis in target organ cells in a manner similar to that of the hormonal steroids. The mode of action of vitamin D on calcium transport and bone mineral mobilization probably involves DNA transcription into mRNA and translation into functional proteins.

It is suggested that vitamin D is first taken up by the liver where it is transferred to a specific carrier protein which migrates with the α-globulin fraction and is picked up by many tissues, the highest concentrations appearing in bone cells and intestinal epithelium. Within 1-4 h most of this target organ vitamin is converted to 25-hydroxycholecaliciferol which is the biologically active form and it is this that induces transcription of a specific DNA into mRNA. This mRNA codes for a component(s) of the calcium transport system of the intestine and the mineral mobilization system of bone. The transport system then transports calcium and phosphorus from the lumen of the intestine and from bone mineral into blood, raising the serum product $(Ca^{2+}) (HPO_4^{2-})$ to levels supersaturating with regard to bone mineral.

C. PARATHYROID GLANDS

Parathyroid hormone is of basic importance to the fine control of serum calcium concentration and there are usually four parathyroid glands. The superior pair are situated on the medial part of the dorsal surface of each lobe of the thyroid gland and are often embedded in the thyroid, although separated by a connective tissue capsule. The inferior pair are found on the dorsal surface of the lateral lobes of the thyroid. As many as ten parathyroid glands have been found in man. The glands are brownish-yellow, oval (about 1.5 by 3.5 by 6.5 mm) and have a total weight of about 120 mg for four glands. Interspersed in the connective tissue are two main types of parenchymal cells which may be differentiated by staining reactions.

The primary function of the parathyroid glands is to participate in the mechanisms that maintain the constancy of calcium ion in the extracellular fluid. The most important effect is to promote the mobilization of calcium from bone. The level of ionized calcium in blood is the primary factor that regulates the secretory activity of the parathyroid glands. There appears to be no direct relation between extracellular phosphate levels and the secretion of the glands except that as plasma calcium concentration falls, plasma phosphate level rises. The parathyroid glands secrete "parathyroid hormone" (PTH) or "parahormone". This is a polypeptide of molecular weight about 9000. Bovine PTH contains 76-83 amino acid residues with no cystine. It has both bone-calcium mobilizing activity and phosphaturic activity. It increases the active absorption of calcium from the small intestine, for which action it requires the presence of vitamin D. The effect is not so marked as that produced by vitamin D alone and is probably less important than the effect of PTH on other target organs, e.g. bone and kidney.

The uptake of phosphorus by the intestine and its rate of flow from mucosa to serosa is also increased by parathyroid hormone. The primary effect on bone is to increase the rate of reabsorption of calcium and phosphate for which vitamin D is required. In the kidney, PTH increases the renal tubular reabsorption of calcium and increases the excretion of phosphorus. Both effects tend to raise extracellular calcium concentration. In the absence of vitamin D, parathyroid hormone still acts on phosphorus metabolism, but *not* on calcium metabolism.

D. THYROCALCITONIN

The thyroid gland secretes (thyro-) calcitonin, a hormone discovered in 1962. It is a polypeptide of molecular weight about 8700 that is very potent and rapidly lowers plasma levels of calcium and phosphorus. This effect seems to be due to a direct action on bone, producing deposition of calcium and phosphate. There is some evidence that steroid hormones can directly affect the rate of secretion of calcitonin. Estrogens appear to potentiate the action of calcitonin on bone.

8

CLINICAL ASPECTS OF THE PITUITARY-ADRENAL AXIS

I. ACTH IN BLOOD AND URINE

The first International Standard for ACTH was established in 1950 and the current (1962) standard contains 5 I.U./ampoule. Bioassays use hypophysectomized rats or mice and the most important and widely used assay uses the adrenal ascorbic acid-depletion (AAAD) caused by administered ACTH. Available radioimmune assays in plasma extracts are still relatively insensitive.

ACTH has a very short plasma half-life, about 1 min in the rat, and 5-15 min in man after intravenous injection. The fate of ACTH in man is unknown. There is no significant quantity of biologically active ACTH excreted in the urine. Biological assays use plasma from which the hormone has to be first extracted. It is resistant to low pH and high temperature and can be absorbed onto acidic resins in the presence of weak acid and eluted with strong acid. Normal average plasma ACTH values in man are about 0.25 mI.U./100 ml plasma at 6 a.m. and 0.11 mI.U./100 ml at 6 p.m. Routine clinical methods of estimation are not at present available.

II. URINARY CORTICOSTEROIDS

A. METHODS

(a) Definitions

Early methods of estimation of the urinary corticosteroids were colourimetric and utilized the properties of their 17-hydroxyl group. When this group remains unchanged in the estimation, the steroids are collectively known as 17-hydroxy-corticosteroids. In other estimations the 17-hydroxyl group is converted to a ketone and total 17-ketosteroids are determined before and after conversion. The difference between the two values is known as the 17-oxogenic-steroids and represents mainly corticosteroid metabolites. Later gas chromatography and radioactivity analysis enabled individual steroid metabolites to be determined.

(b) Porter-Silber reaction for 17-hydroxycorticosteroids

All corticosteroids possessing the side-chain:

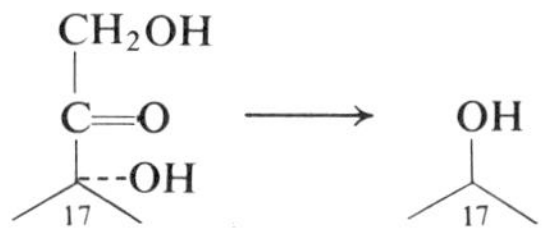

$$\underset{17}{\text{CH}_2\text{OH} \atop \text{C}=\text{O} \atop \text{---OH}} \longrightarrow \underset{17}{\text{OH}}$$

may be assayed by this method. Unfortunately any compound derived from dihydroxyacetone (HO . CH$_2$. CO . CH$_2$. OH) reacts similarly and may give falsely high values. To remove interfering substances a series of preliminary extractions are usually conducted according to the following scheme.

Neutralized urine is treated with the enzyme β-glucuronidase, which hydrolyses steroid conjugates and releases free steroids. These are then extracted from the urine by chloroform. The extract is washed with alkali and then with acid to remove strongly acidic and strongly basic steroids, dried, and then chromatographed on columns of magnesium trisilicate (florisil). The final extract is then treated with phenylhydrazine in concentrated sulphuric acid. Corticosteroids with a dihydroxyacetone side chain yield phenylhydrazones that may be determined quantitatively by colourimetry or spectrophotometry. The compounds determined by this method include: cortisol, cortisone, 11-deoxycortisol and the corresponding tetrahydroderivatives. This method is commonly used in the USA and results should be expressed as "Porter-Silber Chromogens" and not as "17-hydroxycorticosteroids".

(c) Norymberski method for 17-oxogenic-steroids

Sodium bismuthate (or preferably sodium periodate) will oxidize a number of 17-hydroxycorticosteroids to 17-oxosteroids (formerly called 17-ketosteroids). Consequently, if 17-oxosteroids are determined on a sample before and after bismuthate oxidation, the increase represents the amounts of 17-hydroxycorticosteroids originally present. The final estimation utilizes the Zimmerman reaction. The following side chains are all reduced to 17-oxosteroids by bismuthate:

$$
\begin{array}{cccc}
CH_2OH & CH_2OH & CH_3 & \\
| & | & | & O \\
C=O & CH.OH & CH.OH & \parallel \\
\text{—OH} & \text{—OH} & \text{—OH} & \longrightarrow \quad {}_{17} \\
{}_{17} & & &
\end{array}
$$

This method is not recommended as its error is large, depending on a difference value, and it gives misleading results in the presence of dehydroepiandrosterone. It also fails to estimate 21-deoxy-17,20-ketols which normally represent only a very small fraction of the 17-hydroxycorticosteroids.

(d) Appleby method

More accurate is to use a prior treatment with potassium borohydride which reduces 17-hydroxyprogesterone derivatives to the corresponding 17,20-glycols. If this reaction is conducted on urine, the 17-oxosteroids originally present are converted to 17-hydroxy compounds. The latter are not reduced by bismuthate, so that again by a difference method it is possible to obtain a value for 17,20-glycols (or 21-deoxyketols). A method using firstly reduction with potassium borohydride and secondly oxidation with sodium bismuthate determines the "total 17-oxogenic-steroids", i.e. 17,20,21-triols (e.g. cortols and cortolones); 17,21-diol-20-ones (e.g. cortisol and cortisone and their ring A dihydro- and tetrahydro-derivatives); 17,20-diols and 17-hydroxy-20-ketones (e.g. pregnanetriol and 17-hydroxypregnanolone). After extraction the steroids are estimated colourimetrically by the Zimmerman reaction. A formate is formed.

(e) Gas chromatography

Following hydrolysis of conjugates by β-glucuronidase and sulphatase the various corticosteroids may be extracted by suitable solvents. This mixture of steroids may be determined by gas chromatography and several alternate methods are at present being developed. Some methods require the preliminary separation of the ingredients by paper or thin-layer chromatography. Most authors also prepare derivatives of the steroids, such as acetates or halosilyl esters, to give better separations and more sensitive detection. At the present time gas-chromatographic assay of steroids in urine is conducted at only a few specialized research laboratories.

B. AMOUNTS PRESENT

Figure 8.1 shows the excretion values for the 17-oxogenic-steroids for normal adult males and females. In both there is a sharp rise at puberty and a maximum between 20 and 30 years. In women aged 20-40, excretion is 4-15 mg/24 h and in men 5-21 mg/24 h. Children excrete 2-4 mg/24 h. In pregnancy excretion may

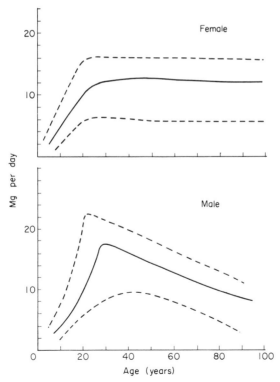

Fig. 8.1. Urinary 17-oxogenic-steroids.

Table 8.1. *Urinary excretion of fractionated corticosteroids (mg/24 h)*

Tetrahydrocortisol	1.0
Allotetrahydrocortisol	0.4
Tetrahydrocortisone	2.7
Cortisone	0.09
Cortisol	0.07
Tetrahydro-11-deoxycortisol	0.06
Tetrahydrocorticosterone	0.20
Allotetrahydrocorticosterone	0.20
Tetrahydro-11-dehydrocorticosterone	0.16
11-Dehydrocorticosterone	0.01
Corticosterone	0.02

rise to 100 mg/24 h. Table 8.1 shows the amounts of the individual steroids excreted per 24 h as determined by sophisticated fractionations. Urinary 17-hydroxycorticosteroids (Porter-Silber chromogens) are about 4-7.5 mg/24 h.

C. METABOLITES OF INDIVIDUAL CORTICOSTEROIDS

More than 90% of the radioactivity of injected cortisol, corticosterone and aldosterone appears in the urine within 24 h. With cortisol there is little or no radioactivity in the bile but with corticosterone a significant proportion of metabolites are secreted in the bile. Table 8.2 shows the urinary metabolites of cortisol and Table 8.3 the metabolites of corticosterone.

Table 8.2. *Urinary metabolites of cortisol*

(i) Unconjugated steroids:	
Cortisol, cortisone, Reichstein E and U, $11\beta,17\alpha,21$-trihydroxypregn-4-en-3-one	1%
(ii) Conjugated steroids:	99%
Tetrahydro metabolites:	
Tetrahydrocortisone, tetrahydrocortisol, allotetrahydrocortisol	50%
Hexahydro metabolites:	
β-Cortolone (30%), α-cortolone, β-cortol, α-cortol	30%
17-Ketosteroids:	
$3\alpha,11\beta$-dihydroxy-5β-androstane-17-one	
$3\alpha,11\beta$-dihydroxy-5α-androstane-17-one	
3α-hydroxy-5β-androstane-11, 17-dione	7%
3α-hydroxy-5β-androstane-11, 17-dione	
(iii) Unaccounted for:	12%

Table 8.3. *Metabolites of corticosterone*

(i) In urine:	
Unconjugated:	
Corticosterone	$< 1\%$
Conjugated:	
Tetrahydrocorticosterone, allotetrahydrocorticosterone, 11-deoxycorticosterone	} 50%
(ii) In bile:	
3α,20α-Dihydroxy-5β-pregnan-20-one	25%
(iii) Unaccounted for:	25%

About 55% of injected aldosterone activity is excreted as urinary glucuronosides, 5-10% being the 18-glucuronide of unchanged aldosterone, and about 0.1% is excreted as free unchanged aldosterone. About fifteen metabolites of aldosterone have now been isolated and the principal ones, with their percentage of radioactivity, are shown in Fig. 8.2.

III. BLOOD CORTICOSTEROIDS

A. PROTEIN BINDING

Corticosteroids occur in blood as "free" and "conjugated" forms, both of which are bound to plasma proteins in the albumin and globulin fractions. Bound and unbound forms are in dynamic equilibrium and only the non-protein-bound form can transfer across the cell semipermeable membranes of the target organ. It has been shown that 94% of unconjugated 17-hydroxycorticosteroids and 65% of 17-hydroxycorticosteroids glucuronosides are bound to plasma proteins; 72% of total plasma cortisol, 75% of plasma cortisone and 85% of plasma corticosterone and deoxycorticosterone are protein bound. Loose binding to albumin accounts for 11-20% of protein-bound cortisol and the rest is bound by a specific binding protein in the globulin fraction "transcortin". The normal plasma binding capacity is about 20-70 μg/100 ml. As total plasma cortisol rises, transcortin binding sites become saturated and more is bound to albumin and remains non-protein bound (Fig. 8.3).

In pregnancy there is a steady rise in plasma "transcortin", so that by the eighth and ninth months, the extra plasma cortisol associated with pregnancy is 95% protein bound instead of the normal 75%. In this way, the plasma unbound cortisol, which is probably the active form is little raised. Changes in protein binding capacity also occur in estrogen therapy and in some rare forms of Cushing's syndrome. In most clinical studies only total corticosteroids are estimated and protein-bound forms are usually ignored. The protein binding is broken by suitable extraction methods.

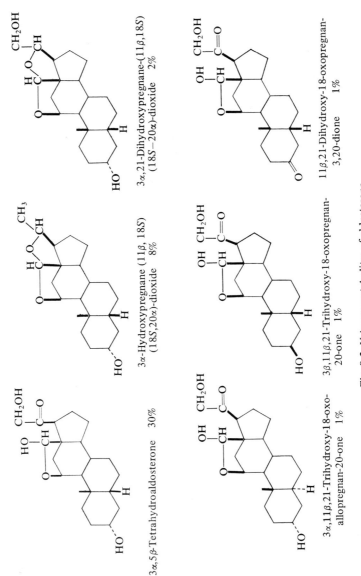

Fig. 8.2. Urinary metabolites of aldosterone.

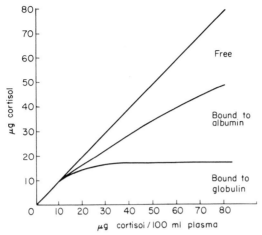

Fig. 8.3. Relationship between free plasma cortisol and protein-bound forms (from Cope, 1964).

B. METHODS

(a) Mattingly method (acid fluorescence)

Plasma is extracted with methylene chloride, and the extract shaken with a sulphuric acid-ethanol reagent. Both cortisol and corticosterone (i.e. 11-hydroxycorticosteroids) give a strong fluorescence that can be measured by fluorimeter. The fluorescence given by corticosterone is about four times as strong as that from cortisol. However, in human plasma the concentration of corticosterone is very much less than that of cortisol and the results are often (erroneously) expressed as "cortisol".

(b) Nelson and Samuels method

This is an adaptation of the Porter-Silber reaction for dihydroxyacetone side chains. The blood is first extracted by a chloroform-ether mixture, and the extracted substances are then partitioned between ethanol and hexane. The ethanol-soluble fraction is chromatographed on magnesium trisilicate (florisil) and the final extract treated with phenylhydrazine in sulphuric acid. A variety of modifications are in use in different laboratories.

(c) Norymberski method

This is an adaptation of the previously described method for 17-oxogenic-steroids of urine. Plasma is deproteinized by ethanol and then extracted by benzene. The extract is dissolved in aqueous ethanol and treated with potassium borohydride. The techniques described for urine are then applied.

C. LEVELS

Cortisol and corticosterone are the two major steroids found in human plasma and estimations of their concentration vary considerably with the method of determination used (Table 8.4).

Table 8.4. *Plasma corticosteroids, µg/100 ml*

Method	
Fluorescence	10.2 ± 3.6 cortisol, 1.3 ± 2.5 corticosterone
Isotope dilution	9.2 ± 1.5 cortisol, 1.2 corticosterone
Polarography	6.5-10.5 cortisol, 4.5-10.5 corticosterone
Porter-Silber chromogens	10.6-13.3 total
Tetrazolium salt chromogens	21.6 unconjugated, 75.0 conjugated

There is a definite diurnal (circadian, nyctohemeral) variation in plasma unconjugated corticosteroids, mainly accounted for by cortisol, with a peak of about 16 µg/100 ml occurring between 6 and 9 a.m. falling to about 5 µg/100 ml at midnight (Fig. 8.4). In depressive illness the diurnal variation is very abnormal. The diurnal variations of plasma ACTH and corticosteroids occur simultaneously. Diurnal variation does not become established in children until 2-10 years of age.

Corticosterone concentrations bear a constant relationship to those of cortisol throughout the 24 h with a maximum level of about 1.5 µg/100 ml. Conjugated corticosteroids vary similarly to the unconjugated steroids but lag by 2-4 h. This lag is also shown in urinary corticosteroids. Plasma disappearance rates are constant throughout the 24 h. During pregnancy there is a progressive rise in plasma corticosteroids to about three times normal in the last trimester. There is also a significant rise in stress conditions of all kinds.

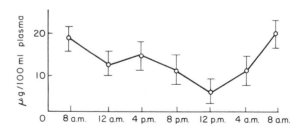

Fig. 8.4. Diurnal variation of 11-hydroxycorticosteroids in plasma (fluorimetric method).

IV. CORTICOSTEROID SECRETION RATES

The concentration of steroid in plasma depends upon its rate of secretion, its rate of removal and its distribution throughout the body. For short periods of time it is usual to assume that distribution volumes and rate coefficients for transfer between compartments remain constant. It is also assumed there is a steady state with constant pool sizes and constant rates of secretion and removal. Secretion rates are usually measured by determining the rate of disappearance (turnover time) of a labelled steroid from the plasma compartment. The metabolic clearance rate (MCR) is defined as that volume of plasma from which steroid is completely and irreversibly removed in unit time.

The simplest model has one compartment and if the MCR is constant the disappearance rate from the compartment will be proportional to the concentration in it. Thus a steroid load will decline exponentially. Analysis of serial data by first-order kinetics enables a clearance (or turnover) rate to be calculated. Extrapolation to zero time gives a theoretical concentration at the moment of injection of the steroid and a pool size can be calculated. Experimentally it has been discovered that, after injection of steroid into the plasma, there is a rapid decline in concentration for the first 20-30 min. This is followed by a slower decline which appears to obey the exponential law. Analysis of this latter part of the disappearance gives

$$\text{Turnover constant } K = \frac{1n_e 2}{\text{plasma half life } T\tfrac{1}{2}}$$

A single compartment, first-order kinetic model will not account for the observed disappearance of a cortisol load, but when a second compartment is introduced, the theoretical disappearance pattern follows closely that observed in practice after the first few minutes of immediate mixing. The first rapid decline is accounted for by equilibrium between the two compartments and the second slower decline after 30 min by the rate limiting exit from the

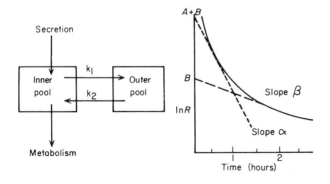

compartment. Solution of the appropriate differential equations shows that the concentration in the inner compartment (of radioactivity in the steady state or of non-isotopic steroid after the introduction of load) is given by

$$C = Ae^{-\alpha t} + Be^{-\beta t}$$

where A, B, α and β are obtained from the radioisotope data and the concentration in the inner compartment is known; the two pool sizes and the rates of entry and exit can then be calculated.

Steady states of entry and exit can only be assumed over short periods of time due to diurnal variation in secretion rates and kinetic results from plasma concentrations cannot be extrapolated. Satisfactory results can be obtained using 24-h urine specimens and estimating a "unique metabolite" (Table 8.5) of the steroid injected. Then

$$S = \frac{R}{SA}$$

where S is the secretion rate, A is the specific activity of the metabolite and R is the injected radioactivity. The collection of about 90% of the radioactive metabolite is usually considered sufficient. For corticosteroids this is achieved in 48 h.

Table 8.5. *"Unique" metabolites of steroid hormones*

Hormone	Metabolite(s)
Cortisol	Tetrahydrocortisol, tetrahydrocortisone
Corticosterone	Tetrahydrocorticosterone
Aldosterone	3-Oxoaldosterone
Testosterone	Testosterone
Dehydroepiandrosterone	Dehydroepiandrosterone
17α-Hydroxyprogesterone	Pregnanetriol

4-C^{14}-Cortisol (specific activity 20-30 mCi/mM) in alcohol is diluted with water or saline for oral or intravenous administration, respectively. The dose is in the 0.5-1.25 μCi range (3-4 x 10^6 cpm). Urine is collected for 24 h before the test and in two lots of 24 h after. Recovery of C^{14} in the first 24 h after the dose should be at least 65% for a valid estimation. Urine conjugates are hydrolysed with β-glucuronidase for 24 h at 37°C and free steroids extracted with methylene chloride. The extract is washed with alkali and water and concentrated under reduced pressure. Paper chromatography of a portion of the steroid extract separates tetrahydrocortisone (THE) and tetrahydrocortisol (THF) whose positions are identified on control strips by a blue-tetrazolium alkali reagent. The metabolites are eluted from the paper and portions used for the determination of the amount of steroid with the tetrazolium reagent and the amount of radioactivity present. The specific activity of the metabolite is then the mg/cpm for the total volume of eluate from the paper chromatogram and the cortisol secretion rate (mg/24 h) is the administered cpm/specific activity of the metabolite. It is not unusual to find discrepancies between the cortisol secretion rates determined separately for the two metabolites. In many laboratories only THE is isolated and estimated.

The cortisol secretion rate of normal women has been estimated as 6.3-28.6 mg/24 h with a mean of 16.2 mg, while normal men have a mean of 20.4 mg/24 h.

Aldosterone secretion rate is usually measured during bed rest on a normal diet of known salt content (120 meq.Na^+/day) and then with restricted salt. About 3 μCi of 1,2-H^3-aldosterone is injected intravenously and a portion of the subsequent 24 h urine extracted with chloroform at pH 1. The extract is washed with alkali and water, and evaporated under reduced pressure. It contains only the free aldosterone excreted which is only about 10% of the aldosterone secreted. This aldosterone is purified by paper chromatography, converted to the γ-lactone by periodic acid oxidation, further purified and its amount determined by gas chromatography.

Aldosterone secretion rate varies from 77-240 μg/24 h, and 90% of the activity of injected aldosterone appears in the urine in 48 h. It increases in pregnancy to about 1600 μg/24 h and decreases on a high salt diet (260 meq. Na^+/day). In a normal individual, salt restriction leads to an increase in aldosterone excretion by a factor of 2-5. The aldosterone secretion rate for normal women is about 140 μg/day in the follicular phase and about 233 μg/day in the luteal phase of the menstrual cycle. The rise in the second half of the cycle is abolished by the suppression of ovulation with oral contraceptives. About 16% of aldosterone is normally bound by plasma proteins, mainly albumin. Plasma renin is also elevated in the luteal phase of the menstrual cycle. These elevations of aldosterone and renin do not lead to retention of sodium and water (as measured by the urine concentrations).

V. CLINICAL TESTS FOR ADRENAL-PITUITARY-HYPOTHALAMIC FUNCTION

A. INTRODUCTION

The supposed sites of action of the various tests is shown in Fig. 8.5.

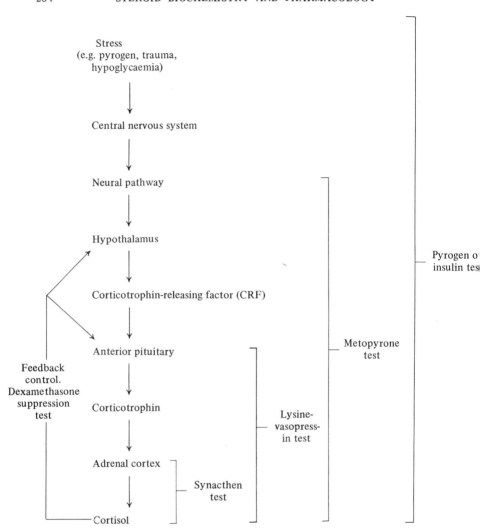

Fig. 8.5. Clinical tests for adrenal-pituitary-hypothalamic function.

B. STIMULATION BY ACTH (SYNACTHEN TEST)

For a hospitalized patient, 24-h urine samples are collected daily for about three days. These are analysed for 17-hydroxycorticosteroids or for 17-oxo-genic-steroids. The next day ACTH is given as an intravenous infusion over 4 h, the usual dose being 40 units. Blood samples are taken hourly during the infusion and plasma 17-hydroxycorticosteroids are measured. Intramuscular injections, each of 40 units of ACTH, are then given at 12-h intervals for a further 56 h. Synacthen (Ciba) is a synthetic corticotrophin supplied in ampoules of 0.25 mg. It contains the first twenty-four of the thirty-nine amino acids of natural ACTH as a zinc phosphate complex. It has high and consistent potency with freedom from protein reactions. In subjects with normal adrenal cortex function, plasma levels of 17-hydroxycorticosteroids (Porter-Silber reaction) increase from the normal range of 6-28 μg/100 ml to 35-55 μg/100 ml during the ACTH infusion. The urinary 17-hydroxycorticosteroids increase from 4-7.5 mg per day to 15-40 mg per day, while 17-ketogenic steroids rise from 4.6-19.0 mg per day to 30-65 mg daily. Where the response to ACTH is less than stated above, adrenocorticoid insufficiency may be assumed. Results may be unreliable if the patient is taking oral contraceptives, estrogens or Aldactone.

C. LYSINE-VASOPRESSIN TEST

Vasopressin probably acts as a corticotrophin-releasing factor, and causes the release of ACTH and hence a rise in plasma cortisol. The test is conducted by giving 10 units of lysine-8-vasopressin, either as a single intramuscular injection, or as an infusion over 2 h. The test is not popular because of the pain produced in smooth muscle. The response of plasma corticosteroids in a normal subject is similar to that following ACTH infusion. The response is almost abolished if 1.5 mg dexamethasone is given orally 2 h previously.

D. DEXAMETHASONE SUPPRESSION TEST

Suppression of plasma corticosteroid levels by short-term administration of potent synthetic steroids, which do not contribute significantly to plasma estimations, is used to investigate the feedback regulation of pituitary ACTH secretion. Dexamethasone is usually used and may be given intravenously or orally (2 mg). The suppressive effect of dexamethasone on plasma 17-hydroxysteroids varies according to the time of administration and it has been established that ACTH release is a cyclic phenomenon being initiated in the early morning. At this time a higher level of plasma steroid is needed for feedback inhibition. When given at midnight, 0.5 mg dexamethasone causes complete suppression of plasma 17-hydroxycorticoids throughout the following day (less than 12 μg/100 ml) and reduces the cortisol secretion rate to less than 2 mg/24 h.

E. METYRAPONE ("METOPIRONE") TEST

Metyrapone (Ciba) (Fig. 8.8) was discovered during a search for non-toxic analogues of D.D.T., following the discovery that these insecticides interfere with steroid hormone synthesis. Metyrapone specifically blocks 11β-hydroxylation and interferes with 19-hydroxylation. Consequently, the compound impairs the biosynthesis of both adrenal cortical hormones and estrogens. The blockage of 11β-hydroxylation leads to decreased circulating cortisol, which in normal individuals stimulates a release of ACTH. The latter triggers adrenal steroid biosynthesis and increased release of 11-deoxysteroids. In clinical practice the test is conducted by giving oral metyrapone, 750 mg every 4 h, or 250 mg every 2 h for 3-5 days. 17-Hydroxycorticosteroids or 17-ketogenic steroids are determined on 24-h urine samples collected for at least 2 days prior to the test, and then daily during the test. In normal subjects urinary 17-hydroxycorticosteroids increase to 15-35 mg per day. The maximum stimulation often occurs on the third day of metyrapone administration. Because of the effect on estrogen production, the test cannot be conducted during pregnancy. Meprobamate, chlorpromazine and some other drugs interfere with the test. Poor response to metyrapone occurs in patients with pituitary or hypothalamic tumours and in diabetic neuropathy, while in primary hypothyroidism, hypopituitarism, or in patients on long-term corticoid therapy, response may be delayed until the fifth day of the trial. This test has now been almost superseded by the Synacthen test which is biochemically more direct and less unpleasant to the patient.

F. PYROGEN TEST

Pyrogenic extracts of bacteria when injected into the body induce a stress condition to which the hypothalamus and pituitary should respond by releasing ACTH. The usual technique is to give 5 ng of pyrogen per kilogramme of body weight as a single intravenous injection. Plasma 17-hydroxycorticosteroids are measured before the injection, and then on blood samples taken hourly for 4 h. In a normal subject, plasma 17-hydroxycorticosteroids increase from the normal basal values to 40-50 μg/100 ml in the first 4 h of the test.

G. INSULIN STRESS TEST

Insulin (0.10 unit/kg body weight) is given intravenously and blood glucose estimated before and 30, 60 and 90 min after administration. A hypoglycaemia of about 40 mg glucose/100 ml blood should be obtained within 60 min. Some patients may require larger doses of insulin, depending upon body weight, etc. Plasma 17-hydroxycorticosteroids should rise by at least 7.5 μg/100 ml if the blood glucose falls to 40 mg/100 ml.

VI. SOME ABNORMALITIES

A. CUSHING'S SYNDROME

The primary disease usually lies in the hypothalamus or in the hypophysis and there is usually a basophil or a chromophobe tumour of the anterior lobe of the pituitary. The adrenals are stimulated to excessive cortisol production and are grossly enlarged. Autonomous biosynthetic activity is also usually associated with tumours of the adrenal cortex. Adrenal causes may account for 15% of the cases. Adrenal tumours may secrete large amounts of other adrenal steroids. Adrenocortical hyperplasia is associated with a variety of "non-endrocrine" tumours, e.g. bronchial carcinoma, which elaborate a substance with ACTH-like activity. Cushing's syndrome is most common in women of childbearing age. They exhibit a moon-face, obesity, acne, amenorrhea or menstrual irregularity, hirsuitism and male distribution of pubic hair. Urinary creatinine is decreased, 11-oxysteroids are very much increased while 17-ketosteroids are moderately increased (Table 8.6). There is a raised cortisol secretion rate and an exaggerated

Table 8.6. *Excretion of corticoids in Cushing's syndrome*

	mg/24 h		
	Normal	Cushings	Increase
Tetrahydrocortisol	1.0	8.7	x 9
Allotetrahydrocortisol	0.4	0.4	—
Tetrahydrocorticosterone	2.7	9.6	x 3
Cortisone	0.09	0.29	x 3
Cortisol	0.07	0.34	x 5
Tetrahydro-11-deoxycortisol	0.06	0.37	x 6
Tetrahydrocorticosterone	0.20	0.41	x 2
Allotetrahydrocorticosterone	0.20	0.17	—
Tetrahydro-11-dehydrocorticosterone	0.16	0.18	—
11-Dehydrocorticosterone	0.01	0.03	x 3
Corticosterone	0.02	0.08	x 4
Aldosterone (μg/24 h)	5	4	—

response of plasma corticosteroids to ACTH stimulation. Suppression of plasma cortisol with dexamethasone cannot be achieved. Location of the tumour and its removal or destruction are the necessary treatments and bilateral adrenalectomy is usually necessary.

B. ADDISON'S DISEASE (PRIMARY ADRENAL INSUFFICIENCY)

This condition, which is usually due to autoimmunity or tuberculosis, is characterized by anaemia, arterial hypotension, decreased metabolic rate, hypoglycaemia and decreased serum Na^+ and Cl^-. Pigmentary changes of external genitalia and mucous membranes frequently parallel the degree of hormone deficiency. More severe symptoms may not develop until 90% of the gland is non-functional. Stress, trauma or surgery may precipitate the condition. Urinary (Table 8.7) and blood corticosteroids are low and cortisol production rate varies from 0.6 to 19 mg/day. A value greater than 2.5 mg/day indicates some

Table 8.7. *Urinary corticoid excretion in Addison's disease*

Cortisol metabolite	mg/24 h	
	Normal	Addisons
Tetrahydrocortisol	1.0	0.15
Tetrahydrocorticosterone	2.7	0.5
Cortisone	0.09	0.02
Cortisol	0.07	0.01
Tetrahydro-11-deoxycortisol	0.06	0.08
Tetrahydrocorticosterone	0.20	0.02
Allotetrahydrocorticosterone	0.20	0.01
Tetrahydro-11-dehydrocorticosterone	0.16	0.02
11-Dehydrocorticosterone	0.01	0.0
Corticosterone	0.02	0.0
Aldosterone (μg/24 h)	4.0	0.0

remaining adrenal function. Diagnosis usually depends upon a poor or absent response to ACTH stimulation. Plasma ACTH is very high (> 400 pg/ml) but retains its diurnal variation. Acute adrenal insufficiency (Addisonian crisis) presents as nausea, vomiting, dehydration, prostration, with mental disturbances progressing to delirium, or to coma and shock.

C. SECONDARY ADRENAL INSUFFICIENCY (PITUITARY INSUFFICIENCY)

Secondary adrenal insufficiency results from failure of the pituitary. It may result from steroid therapy for other diseases, e.g. rheumatoid arthritis. The response to ACTH is often diminished or delayed and this distinguishes it from Addison's disease. There is no response to pyrogen or insulin stress. The response to vasopressin may differentiate pituitary from hypothalamic failure. Plasma ACTH is usually not detectable (< 10 pg/ml). Aldosterone production is normal.

D. CONN'S SYNDROME (PRIMARY ALDOSTERONISM)

Usually an adenoma of the adrenal cortex is present. Urinary aldosterone levels are abnormally high due to mineralocorticoids produced by the hyperplasia, or tumour, of the adrenal cortex. There is a disturbed electrolytic balance, impaired renal function and moderate to severe non-malignant hypertension. There is also severe vascular weakness, excessive thirst, headache, polyuria and nocturia. Removal of the tumour or hyperplastic gland effects an immediate and dramatic cure. Secondary aldosteronism results from cardiac, renal or hepatic insufficiency.

E. ADRENOGENITAL SYNDROME (CONGENITAL ADRENAL HYPERPLASIA)

Rarer diseases involving corticoids are congenital syndromes in which there is a block or partial absence of enzymes concerned with cortisol biosynthesis. So far four such enzyme deficiences have been discovered. The syndrome consists of varying degrees of masculinization in a genetic female or of precocious pseudopuberty in a genetic male. In each case the condition is produced by an excessive production of androgens by the adrenal cortex. If it begins in utero, congenital anomalies of the genito-urinary tract are present at birth, or may be accompanied by adrenal insufficiency of both glucocorticoids and mineralocorticoids. The output of cortisol is low, despite the enlarged adrenals.

1. 21-Hydroxylase deficiency

The enzyme lacking is the 21-hydroxylase necessary for the synthesis of both cortisol and aldosterone. In the presence of low levels of cortisol the pituitary responds by secreting high levels of ACTH. The endocrinological situation may be represented as in Fig. 8.6. The incidence is about 1:40,000.The blockage of normal pathways of corticoid production leads to high levels of metabolites available for pathways of synthesis to androgens and progestogens (mainly pregnanetriol). The excess production of androgens induces virilization in either sex. Steroid excretion measurements show high levels of 17-oxosteroids and of pregnanetriol which is produced from the accumulated 17α-hydroxy-progesterone, progesterone, 17α-hydroxypregnenolone and pregnenolone. As the amount of aldosterone produced by the normal adrenal is so low, the partial blockage of 21-hydroxylase has much less effect on aldosterone formation than on cortisol. Less than half the cases have the salt-losing form of the disease.

2. 11β-Hydroxylase deficiency

Another rare congenital syndrome appears to affect the two hormones to a much more severe degree. This is congenital lack of the 11β-hydroxylase enzyme. The endocrinological situation is shown in Fig. 8.7. In these patients the urine contains high levels of 17-oxosteroids and of the tetrahydrometabolite of the accumulated 17,21-dihydroxyprogesterone (11-deoxycortisol or Compound S). The latter gives a positive test in the Porter-Silber reaction. The urine also contains high levels of tetrahydro-21-hydroxyprogesterone (tetrahydro-deoxycorticosterone). Patients often have hypertension due to the action of accumulated 11-hydroxycorticosterone.

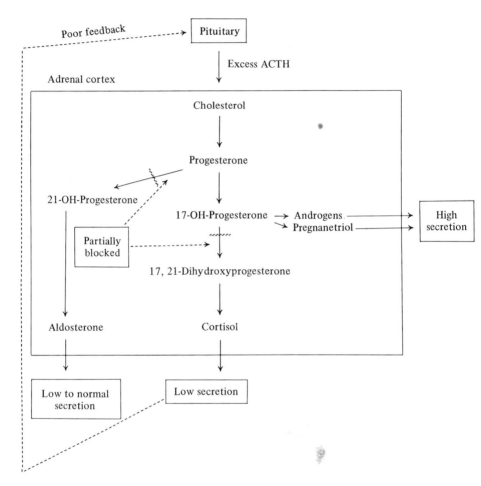

Fig. 8.6. Congenital 21-steroid-hydroxylase deficiency.

In both these conditions treatment with cortisone acetate is successful. The exogenous steroid not only supplies the lack of endogenous cortisol, but also suppresses the excess production of ACTH. Clinically, the dose of cortisone acetate required varies from 10-50 mg daily and is best regulated by following changes in 17-oxosteroid excretion. The maintenance dose is that which normalizes the androgen excretion.

3. 3β-Hydroxydehydrogenase deficiency

Even rarer is a deficiency of 3β-hydroxydehydrogenase activity much earlier in the biochemical adrenal pathway. The accumulated products are pregnenolone, 17α-hydroxypregnenolone and dehydroepiandrosterone and the urine contains metabolites derived from these. This is a salt-losing form of the disease.

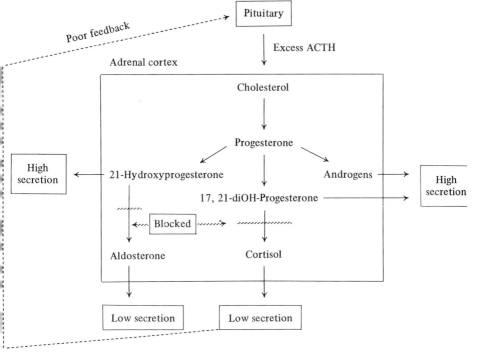

Fig. 8.7. Congenital 11β-steroid-hydroxylase deficiency.

4. 17α-Hydroxylase deficiency

So far only two cases have been described of a deficiency of 17α-hydroxylase in both the adrenal and the ovary. There was no auxiliary or pubic hair, high plasma ACTH, very high FSH and plasma corticosterone.

VII. CORTICOSTEROID THERAPY

A. REPLACEMENT THERAPY

The treatment for chronic adrenal insufficiency (in Addison's disease or in Cushing's syndrome after adrenalectomy) is 5-12.5 mg cortisone acetate (or

5-10 mg hydrocortisone) every 8 h, plus 0.05-0.15 mg fludrocortisone once a day. A normal diet is allowed and additional salt is added during excessive heat or humidity. If a maintenance dose of glucocorticoid is sufficient, it should result in a return of normal appetite, weight gain with subsequent weight stability, and elimination of asthenia, muscle weakness and gastro-intestinal symptoms. Pigmentation of the skin often lightens or disappears. Absorption of cortisone and hydrocortisone from the gastro-intestinal tract is rapid and the serum concentration reaches a peak promptly. It then declines with a half life of about 2 h. Thus the drug should be given every 6-8 h. Mineralocorticoid activity is provided by fludrocortisone. In secondary adrenal insufficiency, aldosterone production is usually normal and glucocorticoids only are required.

The usual treatment during Addisonian crisis is to give 134 mg intravenous hydrocortisone hemisuccinate (= 100 mg hydrocortisone), followed by one litre 5% dextrose in saline containing another 134 mg hydrocortisone hemisuccinate. If severe hyponatraemia is present, 3% saline is used initially. A switch is then made to 50 mg oral cortisone acetate every 6 h, giving 300-400 mg total steroid in the first 24 h and a total fluid of 2.5-3.5 litres 5% dextrose in saline. Doses of steroid are gradually reduced to maintenance level and fludrocortisone added to the regimen.

Adrenogenital syndromes are treated with oral cortisone acetate which supplies the missing glucocorticoids and suppresses ACTH secretion. Satisfactory suppression of androgen output usually begins 4-14 days after the initiation of treatment. The average patient requires a total daily dose equivalent to the usual physiologic output of the adrenal cortex (i.e. 20-40 mg cortisone, 15-35 mg hydrocortisone, 5-10 mg prednisone, etc.).

B. SUPPRESSION OF PATHOLOGICAL STATES

(a) General

Table 8.8 shows the relative doses of prednisone found valuable in the treatment of a variety of inflammatory, immune, allergic and possibly auto-immune diseases. Mechanisms of actions of anti-inflammatory steroids have been discussed previously. Steroids have proved of particular value in the treatment of rheumatoid arthritis and of some collagen diseases.

(b) Rheumatoid arthritis

Cortisone and related adrenal steroids have established a place in the treatment of some patients with rheumatoid arthritis because of the suppressive and anti-inflammatory effects on the measurable signs and symptoms of the disease. Initial dramatic improvement occurs in 62-95% of cases, but treatment has to be discontinued in 13-40% of cases because of undesirable side effects,

Table 8.8. *Uses of anti-inflammatory steroids*

Disease	Daily prednisone dose
A. Systemic administration	
Acute encephalomyelitis	60-80 mg
Acute lymphoblastic leukaemia	40-60 mg
Acute myeloid and monocytic leukaemia	40 mg
Acute polyneuritis	60-80 mg
Asthma	x 30 mg
Cholestatic hepatitis	40 mg
Chronic lymphatic leukaemia	40-80 mg
Cranial arteritis	30-40 mg
Haemolytic anaemia	200 mg
Herpes zoster	30 mg
Infantile haemolytic-uraemic syndrome	30-45 mg
Malignant exophthalmos	60-80 mg
Malignant lymphomas	40-80 mg
Nephrotic syndrome	40 mg
Periarteritis nodosa	30-40 mg
Pericarditis	40-60 mg
Polymyalgia rheumatica	30-40 mg
Polymyositis and dermatomyositis	60 mg
Refactory anaemia	60 mg
Regional ileitis	5-10 mg
Rheumatic fever	40-60 mg
Rheumatoid arthritis	5-10 mg
Sarcoidosis	20-40 mg
Scleroderma	40 mg
Severe ulcerative colitis	60 mg
Steatorrhoea	50-60 mg
Still's disease (Juvenile rheumatoid arthritis)	30 mg
Subacute hepatitis	40 mg
Systemic lupus erythematosus (SLE)	60-80 mg
Thrombocytopoenia	60 mg
Thyrotoxicosis	100-160 mg
B. Topical administration	
Allergic dermatitis	Neurodermatitis
Occupational dermatitis	Erythroderma
Acute and chronic eczema	Burns
Varicose eczema	Sunburn
Seborrhoeic eczema	Psoriasis
Infantile eczema	Pruritus vulvae et ani
Lichen ruber planus et verrucosus	

e.g. Cushingoid symptoms, lessened resistance to infection, osteoporosis, etc. Intra-articular injections of hydrocortisone acetate, prednisolone acetate or prednisolone *t*-butylacetate suppress the synovitis of the injected joint for 10-14 days or longer. The dose is usually 10-50 mg depending on the size of the joint. Doses of oral glucocorticoids for long-term treatment should be as small as possible, e.g. for men 50 mg cortisone, 7.5 mg prednisone or 1.25 mg dexamethasone; for post-menopausal women 30 mg cortisone, 4.5 mg prednisone or 0.75 mg dexamethasone (all per day). Doses should be divided and given every 8 h. Glucocorticoids are also recommended, together with penicillin, in cases of acute rheumatic fever.

(c) Collagen, or connective tissue diseases

The connective tissue, or collagen, diseases are a group of disorders that are loosely linked by the hypothesis that each is caused by a basic defect in some element of connective tissue. Usually included in the group are systemic lupus erythematosus (SLE), scleroderma, polymyositis (including dermatomyositis) and polyarteritis nodosa. Corticosteroids are powerless in scleroderma and of erratic effect in polyarteritis nodosa, but SLE and polymyositis are often improved.

Three types of lupus erythematosus are recognized: chronic discoid LE where the lesions are limited to the skin; intermediate or subacute LE where systemic systems also occur; and SLE where visceral lesions dominate the clinical picture and cutaneous lesions may be absent. Lupus erythematosus is the result of an abnormally reactive immunologic system. Numerous abnormal serum γ-globulins, that behave in many respects like auto-antibodies characteristic of LE cells, are found in the serum of patients with SLE, and sometimes in patients with dermatomyositis. In SLE, dermatomyositis and scleroderma, the fundamental pathologic lesion is the precipitation of fibrinoid material in the ground substance of connective tissue. In SLE there is associated mild inflammation and widespread lesions. In dermatomyositis there is pronounced degeneration and reactive inflammation within the striated muscles. Steroid therapy of SLE rapidly reduces a number of symptoms, e.g. fever joint pain, general malaise and serositis, but these return after 12-48 h. The renal lesion is notably resistant to steroid therapy. Cases that require steroid therapy are characterized by severe "toxicity", such as high fever and rapid progression of the disease with visceral lesions, when 60-80 mg prednisone should be given in four equal daily doses.

VIII. DRUGS AFFECTING ADRENAL STEROIDOGENESIS

A. 11β-HYDROXYLASE INHIBITORS

Metyrapone is one of a number of drugs which have been found to inhibit adrenal steroid biogenesis. Although now known through clinical use as an

11β-hydroxylase inhibitor, it acts perhaps even more sensitively on 18- and 19-hydroxylation systems. Another powerful 11β-hydroxylase inhibitor is 2-(*p*-aminophenyl)-2-phenylethylamine (Fig. 8.8).

B. *o,p'*-DDD

This was discovered to be the most active compound in the insecticide DDD causing cytotoxic adrenal atrophy in dogs. Mainly the inner layers of the adrenal cortex are affected, not the glomerulosa, and the secretion of all major corticoids is inhibited to some degree. It has been used in the treatment of adrenocortical carcinoma.

C. AMINOGLUTETHIMIDE

This has been used for several years as an anti-convulsant and has now been found to inhibit the synthesis of corticoids at some step(s) between the conversion of cholesterol to pregnenolone. Cholesterol accumulates in the adrenals of treated animals and there is compensatory hypersecretion of ACTH leading to adrenal hypertrophy. Large doses in animals have been shown to also inhibit gonadal steroidogenesis.

D. 17α-HYDROXYLASE INHIBITORS

Several active compounds are known, e.g. Su-8000, Su-9055. The secretion of cortisol is inhibited and there is compensatory hypersecretion of corticosterone and deoxycorticosterone.

E. MONOAMINE OXIDASE (MAO) INHIBITORS

Some of this class of drugs, commonly used in the treatment of depression to elevate mood, e.g. nialamide, Monase, Parnate, have some adrenal-inhibiting effects.

F. HEPARINOIDS

Heparin and related compounds are reducers of aldosterone secretion and appear to block some step between the conversion of corticosterone to 18-hydroxycorticosterone.

G. ORAL CONTRACEPTIVES

The effects of estrogens, progestogens (and androgens) on corticosteroid production, metabolism and function are complex. Progesterone is an inhibitor

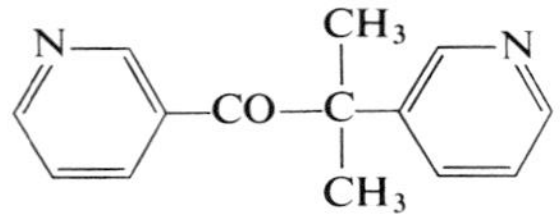

"Metyrapone" (CIBA)
Metopirone
2-Methyl-1,2-*bis*-(3-pyridyl)-1-propanone

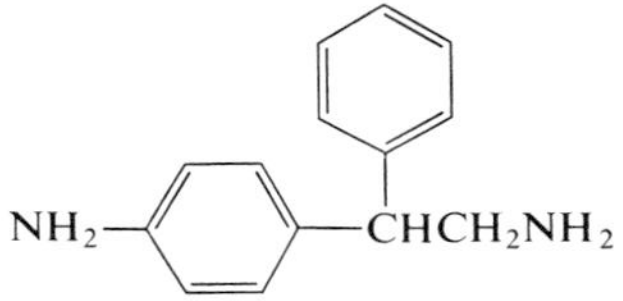

2-(*p*-Aminophenyl)-2-phenylethylamine

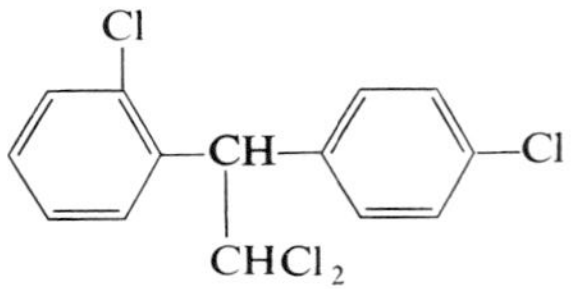

o, p′-DDD
1,1-Dichloro-2-(*o*-chlorophenyl)-2-(*p*-chlorophenyl)-ethane

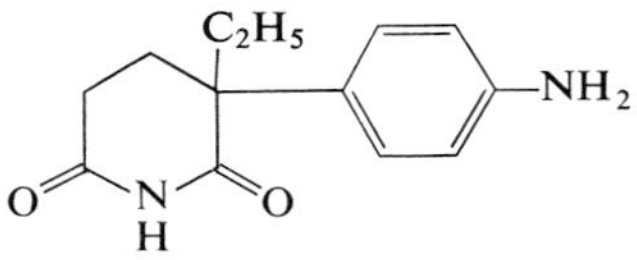

Aminoglutethimide
"Elipten" (CIBA)
α-Ethyl-α-*p*-aminophenylglutarimide

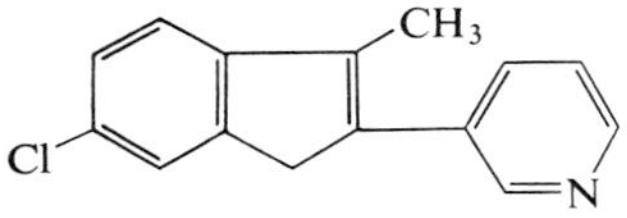

Su-8000

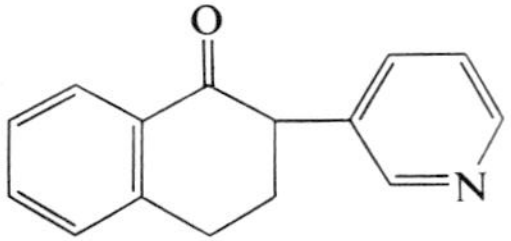

Su-9055

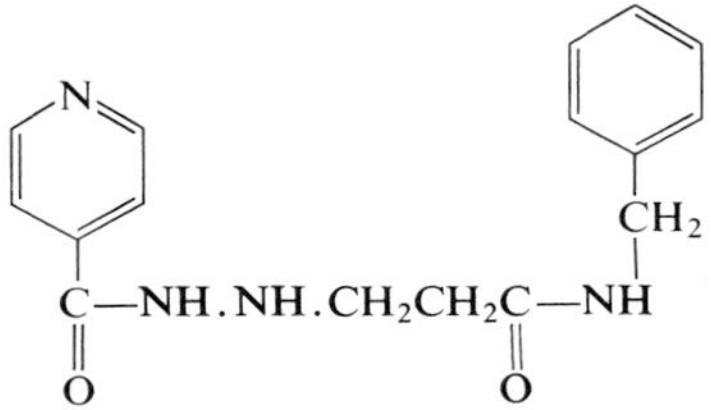

Nialamide
"Niamid"

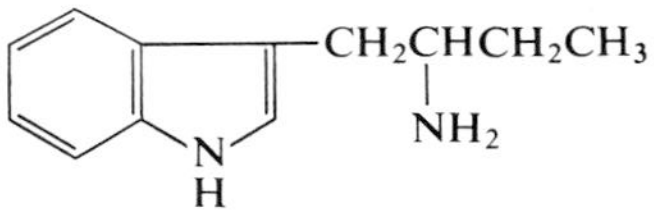

"Monase"
Etryptamine
α-Ethyltryptamine

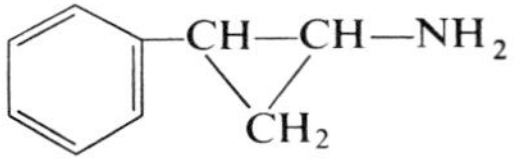

"Parnate"
Tranylcypromine

Fig. 8.8. Some inhibitors of adrenal steroidogenesis.

of the sodium-retaining effects of mineralocorticoids but the effects of synthetic progestogens vary unpredictably, some inducing adrenal atrophy and others adrenal hypertrophy with or without an alteration in corticosteroidogenic response to ACTH. In man, estrogens cause increased adrenal responsiveness to ACTH, decreased hepatic inactivation of corticosteroids and increased plasma protein binding of corticoids. Combined-type oral contraceptives have been found to cause an increase in plasma cortisol. There is some evidence that androgens depress plasma glucorticoid levels and inhibit ACTH secretion.

9

CLINICAL ASPECTS OF THE PITUITARY-GONAD AXIS

I. GONADOTROPHINS

A. UNITS

Human pituitary gonadotrophin (HPG) is a term used in a general sense to denote the gonadotrophic activity present in human body fluids. It has both follicle stimulating (FSH) and luteinizing (LH or ICSH) activity. When obtained from menopausal and post-menopausal women it is known as human menopausal gonadotrophin (HMG). The human chorionic gonadotrophin (HCG) of pregnancy is mainly luteinizing in action. All these substances can normally be assayed by biological methods, although immunological methods are under development. At present, immunological methods are used mainly for research purposes.

Arbitrary animal units for the measurement of gonadotrophins have now been superseded by the use of standard reference preparations, the first of which (HMG-20A) was unofficially available in 1956 and was prepared from the urine of menopausal and post-menopausal women. One unit was made equivalent to 1 mg of the standard preparation. The first official international standard preparation was introduced in 1960 (a variety of these are now available from the National Institute of Health, Bethesda, Maryland). The most recent are ovine preparations which separate the FSH and LH activities of the urinary gonadotrophins so that these can be estimated separately. All assays should now be expressed in terms of international units.

B. BIOLOGICAL ASSAY IN URINE

1. FSH: Augmentation tests

These methods depend on the ability of HCG to augment the action of normal FSH on the rat or mouse ovary, thus increasing the weight of the ovary. Mice are preferred for clinical estimations. Urine preparations are injected five times over 3 days giving a total dose of 40 I.U. The ovaries are weighed 72 h after the first injection.

2. LH: Ovarian ascorbic acid depletion (OAAD) test

This method is very sensitive and accurate but requires complicated purification of the urinary gonadotrophins before injection into female rats. The test depends on the ability of LH to deplete the ascorbic acid content of the ovaries of immature rats (21 days old) pretreated with pregnant mare's serum gonadotrophin (PMSG) and HCG. The rats are pretreated with a single injection of 50 I.U. PMSG, followed 56-65 h later by a single injection of 25 I.U. HCG. As a result of the pretreatment the animals show heavily luteinized ovaries each weighing about 100 mg. The bioassay is carried out 5-9 days after the HCG injection. Ovarian ascorbic acid is estimated 3 h after LH injection.

3. LG: Enlargement of the prostate in hypophysectomized, immature male rats

This method is applicable to cruder urinary extracts. Five days after hypophysectomy, the animals are injected with LH once or twice a day for 4 days and then the prostate is removed and weighed.

4. HCG: Prostate weight

Intact immature rats are injected subcutaneously once per day on three consecutive days, when the prostates are fixed for 24 h. On the fifth day the organs are freed from fat, dried and weighed.

C. IMMUNOLOGICAL AND RADIO-IMMUNOLOGICAL ASSAYS

The hormonal protein to be assayed is the antigen. Those whose antigenic activity is low can be enhanced by the addition of an adjuvent. Two types of adjuvent have been used, namely, absorption of the antigen to a particulate carrier (e.g. polystyrene particles) and the preparation of water-in-oil emulsions of the antigen with and without added mycobacteria (Freund's adjuvant).

Antibodies are produced by injecting the standard antigen into a suitable laboratory animal and the antiserum is isolated from the animal. The end-point of an immunological assay is the agglutination or precipitation caused by the mixing of the prepared antibody with different amounts of unknown antigen. The method is made much more sensitive if the antigen is radioactively labelled, e.g. with ^{131}I or ^{3}H, and becomes an exercise in saturation analysis or competitive protein binding. Labelled standard antigen is added to the antigen being measured and there is a redistribution of label. The higher the concentration of unlabelled antigen, the less activity will be bound to antibody. The antibody-bound and unbound hormones are then separated and estimated separately. The ratio of free : bound radioactivity is a measure of the original amount of hormone present.

A number of sensitive radio-immunoassays of gonadotrophic hormones have been described. There is a considerable degree of immunological cross-reactivity between HCG, LH and HMG and there is a reasonable supply of antigenic material available for the production of antibodies for the assay of LH and HCG. Difficulties in preparing FSH have limited the development of a specific radio-immunoassay.

D. NORMAL VALUES

Non-specific biological assays show that most normally menstruating women show a peak of HPG excretion in the urine at ovulation (Table 9.1). Specific biological assays show a sharp peak of LH excretion at ovulation. Normal males excrete 5-23 HMG units/24 h. The proportion of FSH and LH activities seems to be the same as that of post-menopausal urine. In menopausal women, the excretion of HPG is greatly elevated. A similar effect occurs after castration in both men and women and is believed to represent an attempt by the pituitary to stimulate unresponsive gonads. HPG in menopausal urine is about 35-158 HMG units/24 h.

Table 9.1. *HPG excretion in normal women (HMG units/24 h)*

	Non-parous	Parous
Menstruation	7.9	12.4
Follicular phase	7.9	12.7
Ovulatory phase	10.5	20.4
Luteal phase	7.7	9.8

HPG activity in blood of normal women is about 11-19 HMG units/100 ml plasma and in post-menopausal women above 100 HMG units/100 ml. Immunological assays have shown 0.8-3.2 mg LH/ml plasma in menstruating women not in the ovulatory phase and 4.6-12.2 mg/ml plasma in menopausal women. FSH activity has been quoted as 3.5-8.6 mI.U./ml in menstruating and 5.3-245.0 mI.U./ml in menopausal women.

Normal male serum contains 6-10 mI.U. of both FSH and LH/ml that is not subject to diurnal variation. Treatment with ethinyl estradiol causes a fall in both values and a rise in clominphene citrate. Testosterone propionate causes a fall in LH values.

There is a sharp mid-cycle peak in plasma LH during the normal ovulatory menstrual cycle which occurs either on the same day as the mid-cycle urinary estrogen peak or 1-2 days later. The initial increase in urinary estrogens precedes that of plasma LH. Plasma LH can rise to 40-160 mI.U./ml at mid-cycle from resting values of 1-20 mI.U./ml (Fig. 9.1). There is also a mid-cycle peak of FSH which probably very slightly precedes the mid-cycle peak of LH. There is another smaller peak of FSH during menstruation.

E. PREGNANCY TESTS

Human chorionic gonadotrophin occurs in urine as early as the twenty-third or twenty-fourth day of pregnancy, dated from the start of the last menstrual period, i.e. about 10 days after ovulation. There is a rapid increase in urinary HCG after about the fortieth day, a peak at the sixtieth day, and an abrupt fall to the eightieth day, when the level is maintained through the rest of the pregnancy. Peak values are 20,000 to 100,000 I.U./24 h and values for the second and third trimester of pregnancy are 4000 to 11,000 I.U./24 h.

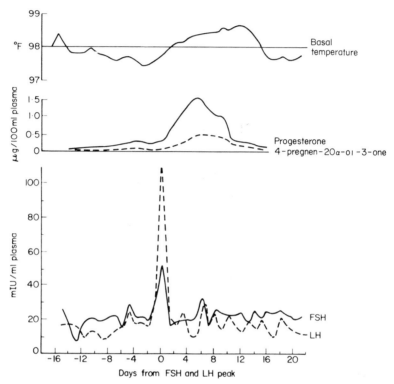

Fig. 9.1. Variation in plasma FSH and LH during the menstrual cycle (from Saxena *et al.*, 1968).

Pregnancy tests depend on the early detection of HCG in the urine. Early tests were all biological but have now been almost completely superseded by immunological tests. Tests have gradually become quicker and easier to perform.

1. Aschheim-Zondek (AZ) test

This involves the production of corpora hemorrhagia (fresh blood specks) or corpora lutea in the ovaries of infantile mice or rats 96 h after the first of a series of injections of urine or serum. The test is reliable but lengthy.

2. Friedman test

Here the corpora hemorrhagia are produced on the ovaries of young rabbits 48 h after intravenous injection of urine or serum.

3. Hogben test

This test depends on the extrusion of eggs from the female South African clawed toad, *Xenopus laevis*, within 12 h of the injection of urine into the dorsal lymph sac. The method is relatively insensitive and rather erratic. A variation uses the male North American frog, *Rana pipiens*, and stimulates release of spermatozoa.

4. Kupperman test

There is a hyperaemia (reddening) of the ovaries of infantile rats within 2 h after the intraperitoneal injection of serum or urine. The test tends to be erratic.

5. Gravindex test (Ortho Pharmaceuticals)

A drop of the urine specimen is placed on a glass slide against a black background and mixed with a drop of an antiserum containing antibodies to HCG. The urine of a pregnant female contains HCG and neutralizes the antibodies. Two drops of antigen are then added, consisting of latex particles coated with HCG. In pregnancy there is no agglutination, but in its absence the un-neutralized antibody agglutinates with the antigen. The concentration of HCG in urine needed to produce a positive reaction is about 5000 I.U./litre. The test is very sensitive and rapid (2 min). Positive results can be obtained by day 26 of the menstrual cycle, although negative results obtained prior to day 41 should be retested later. It is not possible to perform the test on serum, or on urine containing blood or large quantities of protein.

False positives are obtained where there is a cause other than pregnancy for large amounts of gonadotrophin in urine, e.g. menopausal women, young women with primary ovarian deficiency, chorionic tumours (hydatidiform mole, chorion-epithelioma), and in basophilic or eosinophilic tumours of the pituitary. There are also false positive reactions if placental tissue is retained after delivery or abortion. False negatives can be obtained in cases of intrauterine foetal death, threatened abortion, detached chorionic villi and in about 25% of ectopic pregnancies.

Other similar rapid slide tests are "Pregslide" (Denver Laboratories), the "Prepuerin" test (Burroughs-Wellcome), and the "Pregnosticon" test (Organon). The latter two can be adapted to the semi-quantitative estimation of urinary HCG by serial dilution of antisera and urine, when the tests take 24 h.

6. Direct agglutination test (DAP)

This test produces agglutination in the presence of HCG, *not* its absence as in the Gravindex test. It can be used for serum and for urine contaminated with blood. One drop of test reagent is added to a standard volume of urine and any agglutination observed after 2 min. Positive results can be obtained by day 32 of the menstrual cycle.

F. OVULATION INDUCTION

As early as 1931, only 4 years after the discovery of HCG by Aschheim and Zondek, preparations of HCG were used to induce ovulation in patients with anovulatory dysfunctional uterine bleeding. The ability of HCG to induce ovulation in the human in the presence of adequate FSH stimulation has been repeatedly demonstrated. HMG (Pergonal) has also been used. Later workers used pregnant mares serum (PMG), followed by HCG, but this causes anti-hormone formation and cannot be repeated indefinitely. Superovulation was reported in 1962. Human pituitary extracts, containing both FSH and LH activities, followed by HCG treatment, were found not to produce anti-hormones and ovulation could be induced repeatedly. FSH and LH are excreted in 24-48 h while HCG circulates for 5 days or longer. The exact dosage of FSH and LH necessary for the induction of ovulation depends on trials with individual patients and cases of superovulation have occurred.

The latest drug used for the induction of ovulation is clomiphene citrate which is an anti-estrogen with no estrogenic, androgenic, progestational or anti-androgenic activities. It apparently produces its major clinical effect by abolishing the inhibitory action of estrogen on the production of hypothalamic releasing factors, and hence on release of gonadotrophins. There is a marked increase in estrogen excretion shortly after treatment. The ideal patient for treatment has anovulation resulting from a hypothalamic defect, with a characteristic history of irregular menses from the outset. There is a high risk of multiple cysts and multiple pregnancies.

II. ESTROGENS

A. IN URINE

1. Metabolites present

The amount of estrogen measured in urine as estrone, estradiol, and estriol after the injection of estradiol or estrone represents only approximately 25% of the administrated material, the remaining 75% being eliminated from the body in other forms in urine, or by other routes of excretion (Table 9.2).

2. Methods of estimation

(a) General

Estrogens are present in human urine as water-soluble conjugates, e.g. estriol occurs mainly as the glucuronide with a little of the sulphate. Estrone is excreted mainly as the sulphate although some glucuronide is found in pregnancy urine. Prior to estimation these conjugates must be hydrolysed either by boiling the urine with acid, or by incubating it with enzyme mixtures of β-glucuronidase and sulphatases. Free estrogens are then extracted with ether or benzene. Washing of the extract with sodium bicarbonate removes the acid fraction leaving the total phenolic fraction.

(b) Brown method

A wide range of assay methods based on the Kober and allied reactions have been published. This method is one of the most widely used. The urine sample is

Table 9.2. *Estrogen metabolites*

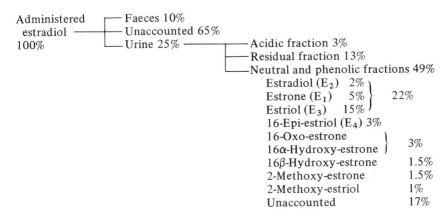

Administered estradiol 100%
— Faeces 10%
— Unaccounted 65%
— Urine 25% —
— Acidic fraction 3%
— Residual fraction 13%
— Neutral and phenolic fractions 49%

Estradiol (E_2) 2%	
Estrone (E_1) 5%	22%
Estriol (E_3) 15%	
16-Epi-estriol (E_4) 3%	
16-Oxo-estrone	
16α-Hydroxy-estrone	3%
16β-Hydroxy-estrone	1.5%
2-Methoxy-estrone	1.5%
2-Methoxy-estriol	1%
Unaccounted	17%

hydrolysed by acid, then extracted by ether. After washing with carbonate, the extract is partitioned between benzene-petroleum ether and water and alkali. The phenolic fraction is purified by a phase change depending on methylation. The estrogen methyl esters are then separated by chromatography on alumina columns and the fractions assayed separately by the Kober reaction. This consists of heating the estrogens with a mixture of phenol and sulphuric acid, diluting with water and reheating. The pink colour produced is measured at 520 mμ. A correction for interfering substances has been described. The method is sensitive (less than 5 μg/24 h), reproducible and recoveries are about 80%. Several drugs interfere with the assay, notably, cortisone, meprobamate, various aperients and most synthetic estrogens. Modifications of the method have been described to allow the specific assay of estriol, estrone and estradiol separately, after separation on an alumina column.

(c) Preedy-Aitken method (fluorimetric)

Acid-hydrolysed urine is extracted by ether, which is then extracted by saturated sodium bicarbonate solution. The residue is partitioned between toluene and N sodium hydroxide solution. The latter is neutralized and extracted by ether, the resulting extract chromatographed on celite columns and a fluorimetric assay conducted on each fraction using sulphuric acid. The method is accurate but tedious. Sensitivity is about 1 μg in a 24 h urine sample with recovery about 80%. A similar method employed by others uses paper chromatography in place of celite columns and phosphoric instead of sulphuric acid.

(d) Gas chromatography

Estrogens may be assayed by gas chromatography, but the success of the method depends on the previous extraction and purifications of the estrogens from the urine sample. Most published methods involve either acid or enzymic hydrolysis, followed by careful solvent extraction and partition. This extract is then further purified by paper or thin-layer chromatography. Most methods give recoveries of about 75%, with sensitivities down to 0.1 μg. All the major estrogen metabolites can be determined by these methods.

(e) Breuer method

This method was developed for the assay of the less abundant urinary estrogens and, in fact, is capable of determining about fifteen different metabolites. The sample is gel-filtered on Sephadex resins then hydrolysed by β-glucuronidase. By the use of the Girard reaction a ketonic and a non-ketonic fraction are obtained. Polar and non-polar fractions are separated by partition between water and benzene. The resulting extracts are then separated by paper chromatography and each metabolite separately estimated by a micro-Kober reaction. The method is reproducible and precise, but sensitivity is only 100-200 μg of each metabolite/litre of urine.

3. Amounts

(a) Children

Between the ages of 3 and 7 small quantities of estrogens are excreted by both boys and girls in approximately equal amounts, about 1 μg/24 h. In girls only, estrogen output rises sharply between the ages of 8 and 11 and after 11 a cyclic pattern emerges and precedes the menarche by as much as 1 or 2 years. The establishment of the cyclic pattern coincides with the first visible signs of secondary sexual development.

(b) Normally menstruating women

There are two peaks of excretion, one at or about the time of ovulation and the other during the luteal phase (Table 9.3). The amounts of estradiol, estriol and estrone rise and fall together. During the first 7-10 days of the cycle, about

5 μg of each compound is excreted per 24 h. Levels start to rise on or about the seventh day and reach a well-defined maximum at or about the thirteenth day, which is believed to coincide with the rupture of the follicle. There is then a rapid fall in the excretion of all three estrogens. The second rise starts on or about the twenty-first day and lasts until shortly before the start of menstruation. The pattern and amounts of estrogens are relatively constant for any individual, but there are large differences between individuals. Serial determinations are necessary to obtain a reliable estimate of ovarian function.

Table 9.3. *Estrogens in female urine, μg/24 h*

	Onset of menstruation	Ovulation peak	Luteal maximum
Estriol (E_3)	6 (0-15)	27 (13-54)	22 (8-72)
Estrone (E_1)	5 (4-7)	20 (11-31)	14 (10-23)
Estradiol (E_2)	2 (0-3)	9 (4-14)	7 (4-10)
Total	13	56	43

(c) Normal men

Small amounts of estrogens (5-20 μg), produced by the adrenal cortex and the testes, are excreted every 24 h. This is made up of about 55% estrone, 35% estriol and 10% estradiol.

(d) Menopausal and post-menopausal women

Compared with normally menstruating women only small amounts of estrogens are found and these are believed to be produced by the adrenal cortex. Total output is 5-15 μg/24 h, being mainly estriol and estrone in approximately equal amounts, with a small amount of estradiol.

(e) Normal pregnancy, labour, puerperium and lactation

Excretion of estrogens rises during pregnancy and reaches very high levels towards the end of gestation. There are wide fluctuations in individuals from day to day, and considerable variation in excretion between subjects at comparable stages in pregnancy. The amount of estrogens excreted acts as a measure of placental function, although it is necessary to perform serial estimations. Estrogens are necessary for the mother to maintain pregnancy, but the foetus lives in an environment virtually free from active estrogens as it metabolizes those of the mother's estrogens that reach it to sulphates and glucuronates which are excreted in the mother's urine.

There is a rise in estriol, estradiol and estrone excretion throughout pregnancy, the rate of increase being most marked between the sixth and twentieth weeks (Fig. 9.3). The increase in estrone and estradiol from the luteal maximum of the last menstrual cycle to the end of gestation is about 100-fold and the increase in estriol about 1000-fold. Usually only the excretion of the three "classical" estrogens, estradiol, estrone and estriol, have been studied, but at least eighteen estrogens have been isolated from human pregnancy urine (Table 9.4). A large fraction of the metabolites may be 2-hydroxy-estrone, which is

Table 9.4. *Urinary estrogens in late pregnancy, μg/24 h*

A. Non-ketonic fraction	
Non-polar fraction	
Estradiol	420
2-Methoxy-estradiol	200
Δ^{16}-Estratrienol	160
Total	780
Polar fraction	
Estriol	22,000 (range 12,000-40,000)
16-Epi-estriol	830
17-Epi-estriol	120
16,17-Epi-estriol	150
6-Hydroxy-estriol	1,000
2-Methoxy-estriol	300
6α-Hydroxy-estradiol	800
Total	25,200
B. Ketonic fraction	
Estrone	1,200
16α-Hydroxy-estrone	1,600
16β-Hydroxy-estrone	720
6α- and 6β-Hydroxy-estrone	750
2-Methoxy-estrone	600
16-Oxo-estradiol	1,100
Total	5,970

usually lost during the usual methods of estrogen estimation. After delivery there is a rapid fall in estrogen excretion; normal levels being reached in about 5 days. During lactation estrogen excretion is very low, for estrogens strongly inhibit prolactin secretion. In the placenta, estrone and estradiol form a much larger fraction of the total estrogens than they do in the body fluids and most is unconjugated. Any conjugated estrogen present is usually estriol.

B. IN BLOOD

1. Amounts

Estrogens are bound very tightly by plasma protein and about 95% of the circulating estrogens are bound. They are also conjugated, mainly as the glucuronosides and sulphates which are believed to render them inactive and more water-soluble. Table 9.5 shows some quoted mean values for estrogens in blood. The amounts are so small that they are at the limits of all methods of estimation. An ovulation peak has been detected in the blood estrogens of

Table 9.5. *Mean plasma estrogens (μg/100 ml)*

Normal women, menstrual cycle	Estrone	Estradiol	Estriol
Proliferative phase	0.023	0.01	
Ovulation peak	0.058	0.026	
Secretory phase	< 0.06	< 0.07	< 0.15
Normal males	< 0.06	< 0.07	< 0.15

normal menstruating women. In pregnancy there is a considerable rise in the concentrations of estrone, estradiol and estriol in blood, to a total of about 17 μg estrogens/100 ml plasma (Table 9.6 and Fig. 9.2).

Table 9.6. *Estrogens in pregnancy blood, μg/100 ml plasma*

	Estrone	Estradiol	Estriol
Free	1.42	0.80	0.36
Glucuronoside	0.44	0.69	2.88
Sulphate	4.10	1.57	4.40
Total	5.96	3.06	7.64

2. Methods of estimation

(a) Kober reaction

A variety of methods using the Kober reaction have been applied to blood. In one method the blood sample is extracted with a large volume of ethanol, the solvent evaporated and the residue dissolved in water and extracted with ether-toluene. This removes unconjugated estrogens. The aqueous phase is then hydrolysed by acid to release estrogens from their conjugates. Both fractions are then treated separately. After methylation, the mixture of estrogens is fractionated on alumina columns and each fraction assayed by a micro-scale Kober reaction.

(b) Fluorescence methods

Estrogens heated with strong sulphuric or phosphoric acids give an intense yellow-green fluorescence. This reaction is far less specific than the Kober reaction and many substances interfere. It is consequently important to ensure the removal of such substances before assay. Of the many variations of this

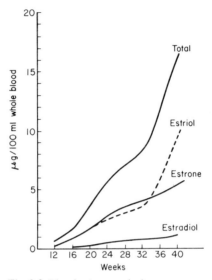

Fig. 9.2. Blood estrogens during pregnancy.

method that have been described, all involve solvent extraction of the acid-hydrolysed sample. The extract is then partitioned with an alkali (NaOH or NaHCO$_3$) then re-extracted with an organic solvent. The residue is partitioned on celite columns or by paper chromatography and the eluted estrogens assayed by the fluorescence reaction.

(c) Isotope methods

Plasma is extracted by chloroform, then partitioned between organic solvents. The estrogen fraction is then treated with ^{35}S-labelled pipsyl chloride (*p*-iodo-benzene sulphonyl chloride). This yields pipsyl esters of the estrogens (estrone and estradiol). Pipsyl esters of these two estrogens are prepared from laboratory samples using ^{131}I-labelled pipsyl chloride. These ^{131}I-esters are then added to the ^{35}S-esters and the mixture chromatographed on paper. The spots corresponding to the two esters are then separately counted for ^{131}I and ^{35}S. This allows a correction for losses and an estimate of estrogens in the original sample; recovery is about 65%. The method is specific and reproducible and exceedingly sensitive (limit about 5 ng/100 ml plasma).

III. PROGESTOGENS

A. PROGESTERONE METABOLITES

1. **Non-pregnant**

(a) In urine

Progesterone metabolites are excreted via the urine, bile and faeces, and are present in expired air and on the surface of the skin. Administration of radioactive progesterone has shown that 6-27% is excreted in the urine as pregnanediol, 1.5-5% as pregnanolone and 0.5-2% as pregnanediones; about 0.01% is excreted unchanged. Pregnanediol is present conjugated with glucuronic acid at C-3 forming sodium pregnanediol glucuronoside. Pregnancy urine also contains small amounts of allo-pregnanediol and 5α-pregnane-3β,20α-diol. The formation of C-6 and C-16 oxygenated derivatives are important pathways in the metabolism of progesterone. The compounds formed are mainly the 5α-pregnanes with 6α-hydroxyl groups, e.g. 5α-pregnane-3α,6α-diol-20-one, and 5α-pregnanes with 16α-hydroxyl groups, e.g. 5α-pregnane-3α,16α,20α-triol. After the administration of ^{14}C-progesterone, urinary metabolites are as shown in Table 9.7. Urinary pregnanediol estimations are undertaken to obtain

Table 9.7. *Urinary metabolites of progesterone*

	Total %	% Of each fraction containing 3,6,20-oxygenated pregnanes
Pregnanediol	28.5	8.7
Less polar than pregnanediol, e.g. pregnenolones, pregnanediones	23.1	19.2
More polar than pregnanediol, ketonic	22.5	54.9
More polar than pregnanediol, non-ketonic	9.0	47.6

information regarding the production of progesterone by the ovary or placenta, but results should be used with caution due to the small and variable proportion of progesterone metabolites appearing in the urine.

Children, regardless of sex, aged between 3-15 and post-menopausal women excrete about 750 μg pregnanediol/24 h. In normally menstruating women, the excretion per 24 h is at, or below, 1000 μg and probably arises mainly from the adrenal cortex. Following ovulation a rise occurs and during the luteal phase excretion is 2000-5000 μg/24 h and is mainly derived from the progesterone secreted by the corpus luteum. Pregnanediol output begins to fall several days before the onset of menstruation and continues to decline for the first two or three days of bleeding. The output in the luteal phase varies greatly between individuals. In anovulatory cycles, the cyclical pattern of pregnanediol excretion does not occur and values remain constant throughout the cycle. Normal men excrete about 900 μg pregnanediol/24 h, arising from the adrenal cortex.

Pregnanetriol is also frequently estimated in urine. This compound is secreted mainly by the adrenal cortex but is probably also synthesized by the ovaries. Radioactivity studies have shown that 30% of 17α-hydroxyprogesterone appears in the urine as pregnanetriol glucosiduronide. Normal women excrete about 1 mg/24 h in the follicular phase, rising to about 1.8 mg at ovulation and falling in the luteal phase. In pregnancy, values can rise to 7 mg/24 h. Children excrete about 0.3 mg/24 h and normal men 1-2 mg.

(b) In plasma

Plasma progesterone in normally menstruating women is low during menstruation and the follicular phase (0.1 to 0.5 μg/100 ml), but rises markedly at mid-cycle in association with the rise in the luteal phase.

Plasma 17-hydroxyprogesterone can be used as a measure of corpus luteum function both in a normal cycle and in pregnancy, as in pregnancy the placenta produces only progesterone. In the normal cycle, there is a plasma peak of both 17-hydroxyprogesterone and progesterone beginning at mid-cycle, indicative of ovulation, reaching a maximum in the middle of the luteal phase and falling prior to menstruation. In pregnancy plasma 17-hydroxyprogesterone rises to a peak of about 2 μg/100 ml at about 4 weeks and then falls, while plasma progesterone has a similar peak, of about 10 μg/100 ml, falls slightly and then rises greatly to term. These results indicate that the life of a functional corpus luteum in pregnancy is relatively short.

Normal males show a plasma progesterone of about 0.045 μg/100 ml.

2. In pregnancy

In pregnancy there is a steady rise in urinary pregnanediol from the progesterone produced by the placenta. At the twelfth week it is about 5-15 mg/24 h and by the thirty-sixth week about 45 mg, when it then remains constant until delivery, when there is a rapid fall. The excretion of pregnanediol mirrors the increase in mass of the placenta. About 15% of the progesterone produced daily (about 300 mg, of which 20-25 mg comes from the ovaries) is excreted in the urine. Blood progesterone shows a gradual rise throughout pregnancy (from about 3μg/100 ml) to about 15 μg/100 ml at term. The measurement of urinary pregnanediol has for long been used as a measure of placental function, but it has been suggested that urinary estriol is more useful as it also gives evidence of a satisfactory foetal circulation (Fig. 9.3).

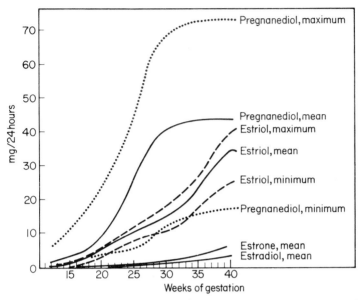

Fig. 9.3. Urinary pregnanediol and estriol during pregnancy.

B. METHODS OF ESTIMATION

1. Progestogens in urine (pregnanediol)

(a) Klopper-Strong-Cook method

The urine is hydrolysed by acid, then extracted with toluene. The extract is treated with permanganate to destroy an interfering metabolite, and purified by chromatography on alumina columns. The product is then acetylated and further purified by chromatography. The final product is determined by colorimetry with a sulphuric acid reagent. Recovery with this method is better than 90%.

(b) Goldzieher-Nakamura method

The urine is treated with β-glucuronidase, then extracted with chloroform. The extract is purified by chromatography on silica gel, then acetylated. The acetylated products are further purified by chromatography then determined colorimetrically by a sulphuric acid reagent. This method, which measures pregnanetriol plus pregnanediol, gives recoveries of almost 100%.

(c) Gas chromatography

After acid hydrolysis of the urine, a toluene extract is prepared and pregnanediol is obtained by thin-layer chromatography on silica gel. The spot is eluted with ethanol and injected into a gas-liquid chromatograph. Recovery with this method is about 80-90%, but its sensitivity is much greater than any other method. In some published methods, the pregnanediol is acetylated prior to gas chromatography.

2. Progestogens in blood

(a) Zander and Simmer method

Progestogens (mainly progesterone) are extracted from blood by an ethanol-water mixture. This extract is concentrated, then partitioned with ethyl acetate and water. The organic phase is separated and a dry residue obtained. This is dissolved in methanol, cooled to $-15°C$ and solid impurities removed. The methanol extract is diluted with water and the mixture extracted by petroleum ether. The final extract is separated by paper chromatography and the progesterone spot eluted and determined by UV spectrophotometry. Sensitivity of the method is about 0.05 μg and recovery about 80%. A variety of modifications to the original technique have been published.

(b) Heap method

Progesterone is extracted from alkali-treated plasma by ether. The extract is separated by paper chromatography and the progesterone spot eluted. This material is then used as a substrate for a 20β-dehydrogenase, which yields 20β-hydroxypregn-4-en-3-one. This product is purified by paper chromatography, then assayed by fluorimetry.

(c) Gas chromatography

Progesterone may be determined by extracting alkali-treated plasma with ether, purifying the extract by paper or thin-layer chromatography, then using gas-liquid chromatography. The sensitivity of the method is about 0.01 μg of progesterone and recoveries are about 80%.

(d) Isotope dilution

Several methods have been described. In one, ^{14}C-progesterone is added to plasma, progesterone is then extracted from the plasma, purified by paper or thin-layer chromatography, then reduced by ^{3}H-borohydride. The resulting products are purified by chromatography and counted separately for ^{14}C and [3]H. The ^{3}H count gives an estimate of the progesterone content that can be corrected by the recovery of [14]C.

C. METABOLISM OF ORAL CONTRACEPTIVES

After injection of ^{14}C-labelled norethisterone or norgestrel into rabbits, 45% and 57.4% of the radioactivity appears in the urine, mostly within 2 days. Small amounts of the activity from norgestrel are excreted in the expired air. Less than 0.5% of the dose remains in the plasma 24 h after injection. Up to 5 h after injection, large amounts of the activity are found in liver, kidney, intestine and bile, while a large proportion of the dose appears to undergo an entero-hepatic circulation. The uterus takes up a high concentration of the activity. At 24 h the amount of radioactivity in the tissues has decreased markedly. Metabolites of norethisterone are mainly polar compounds (indicating hydroxylation) while metabolites of norgestrel show partial or complete reduction of the α, β-unsaturated ketone group in ring A. There is little or no metabolism of the ethinyl group. About 10% of the dose is excreted in the faeces.

In man, 30-60% of oral or intravenous 4-^{14}C-lynestrenol is excreted in the urine within 5 days with 50-60% as conjugated metabolites. Metabolites in the unconjugated fraction are almost entirely polar compounds and hydroxylation occurs at two points in the molecule. Again there is little or no metabolism of the ethinyl group. It has been suggested that a minor metabolite of these synthetic progestogens is ethinyl estradiol and that this partially accounts for the oral contraceptive activity of such progestogens when administered alone.

IV. THE MENSTRUAL CYCLE

Simultaneous assays of LH, FSH, estriol, estrone, estradiol, pregnanediol and pregnanetriol on 24-h urine samples are frequently performed throughout the menstrual cycle in fertility studies. In addition, estimations of total 17-hydroxy-corticoids, 17-oxosteroids and dehydroepiandrosterone are sometimes performed. Typical results are shown in Table 9.8 and Fig. 9.4. The ovulatory phase

Table 9.8. *Typical urine hormone concentrations per 24 h throughout the menstrual cycle*

	Menstruation	Follicular phase	Ovulatory phase	Luteal phase
Gonadotrophins (HMG units)	3.0	2.8	2.8	2.9
Pregnanediol, mg	0.3	0.5	0.4	0.7
Pregnanetriol, mg	0.4	0.36	0.45	0.57
Estriol, μg	2.1	1.5	2.7	4.0
Estrone, μg	1.2	1.4	2.5	2.2
Estradiol, μg	0	0	1.0	0

is considered to extend over 6 days. A normal menstrual cycle is judged by the presence of ovulatory peaks of the various hormones.

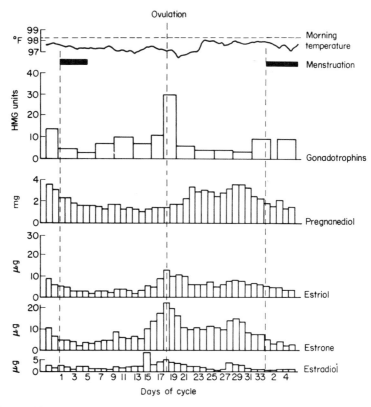

Fig. 9.4. Hormone assays during the menstrual cycle in 24-h urine samples (from Brown, J. B., Klopper, A. and Loraine, J. A. (1958). *J. Endocr.* **17**, 401).

V. ENDROCRINE RELATIONS BETWEEN MOTHER, FOETUS AND PLACENTA

A. GONADOTROPHINS

In addition to chorionic gonadotrophin, the placenta synthesizes and excretes another protein hormone of molecular weight 20,000-30,000. This was first identified in 1962 and named "human placental lactogen (HPL)". It appears to be very similar in composition to human growth hormone. HPL can be detected in maternal plasma as early as the sixth week of pregnancy and reaches 3-5 μg/ml at term. It has a half-life of 15-30 min. This means that the placenta secretes 300-1000 mg/day at term (Fig. 9.5).

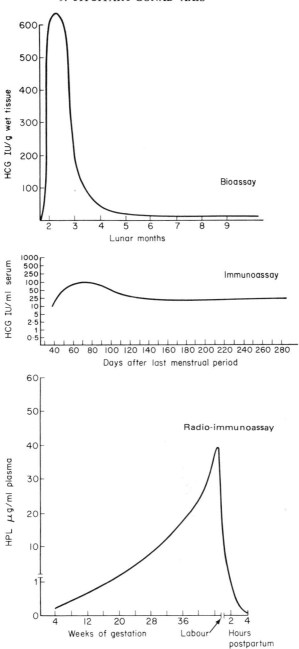

Fig. 9.5. Protein hormone secretion by the placenta.

During pregnancy, a large number of metabolic adjustments occur which favour anabolic processes and it is possible that HPL brings about some of these. It may also play a part in regulating foetal growth.

HPL has a profound effect on the mammary gland, inducing growth and lactation. It also has luteotrophic, erythropoietic and aldosterone-stimulating actions. The concentration of HPL in blood begins to rise rapidly only after the corpus luteum is no longer necessary for maintenance of the pregnancy.

B. PROGESTERONE

The placenta elaborates large amounts of pregnenolone and progesterone, but mostly not directly from acetate. Maternal cholesterol is probably the major precursor. Neutral steroids formed in the foetus are the metabolic products of progesterone and pregnenolone reaching it from the placenta.

The concentration of progesterone in the blood of the umbilical cord vein at term has been estimated as 72 μg/100 ml plasma and 44 μg/100 ml plasma in the umbilical arteries. Maternal blood progesterone rises to a very high level (25 μg/100 ml plasma) with progressing gestation, but falls immediately after delivery.

The foetal liver is the most active site for the metabolism of progesterone reaching the foetus from the placenta. A large number of metabolites have been isolated, e.g. pregnanolone, pregnanediol, pregnanediol sulphate and glucuronate.

The mid-term foetus does not appear to be able to utilize pregnenolone. Foetal adrenals can produce hydrocortisone and its sulphate, deoxycorticosterone sulphate, corticosterone sulphate and 11-dehydrocorticosterone sulphate.

C. ANDROGENS

Dehydroepiandrosterone sulphate is formed in the foetus (indicated by differences in the concentrations in cord arteries and veins). In addition 16α-hydroxy-dehydroepiandrosterone has been found in venous cord blood which represents an extensive 16α-hydroxylation mainly in the foetal liver. Because of the large amount of sulphatase and 3β-steroid-dehydrogenase present in placental tissue, dehydroepiandrosterone can be readily converted to androstenedione and testosterone and hence to estrone and estradiol. These products then return to the foetus.

Recently it has been shown that the concentration of urinary testosterone sulphate is increased in women carrying a male foetus only, indicating the activity of the male foetal testes. There were no differences in the mother's peripheral plasma testosterone for male and female foetuses, both values being higher than in the non-pregnant state.

D. ESTROGENS

It has been well established that the greatly increased amounts of estrogens elaborated during pregnancy are formed in the placenta and are transported mainly to the maternal circulation and then excreted in the urine. It is believed that products secreted by the maternal adrenals, e.g. dehydroepiandrosterone

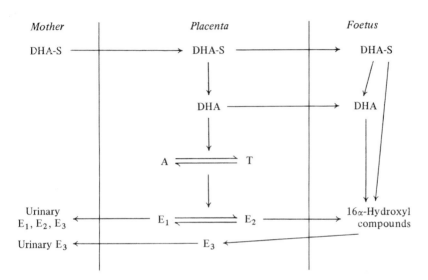

DHA-S	Dehydroepiandrosterone sulphate	
DHA	Dehydroepiandrosterone	
A	Androstenedione	
T	Testosterone	
E_1	Estrone	
E_2	Estradiol	
E_3	Estriol	

Fig. 9.6. Conversion of dehydroepiandrosterone sulphate to estrogens in the foetal placental unit (from Wang and Bulbrook, 1968).

and its sulphate, serve as precursors for the estrogens formed by the placenta (Fi. 9.6). As the pregnancy progresses, the dehydroepiandrosterone formed by the foetus becomes a more important precursor of placental estrogens. Estriol seems to be synthesized from 16α-hydroxylated precursors made by the foetus and not from estrone and estradiol. The 16α-hydroxylation of dehydroepiandrosterone takes place in the foetal liver where small amounts of estrogens can also be produced from testosterone and androstenedione. Estrogens originating from the placenta or formed in the foetus are extensively conjugated by various foetal tissues which may be a detoxification mechanism. Double sulphate-glucosiduronate conjugates are known.

E. MINERALOCORTICOIDS

The secretion of aldosterone is elevated in pregnancy and there is a progressive rise in the rate of secretion as the pregnancy progresses. This comes from the maternal adrenals, but appears to be stimulated by the foetus. Progesterone has a natriuretic action, possibly by inhibiting the action of aldosterone at the renal tubular level. The foetus synthesizes 15α-hydroxy-progesterone and this may stimulate maternal adrenal aldosterone production. Maternal plasma renin is also elevated in pregnancy.

F. IMMUNOLOGY

Early in the development of the mammalian foetus, the trophoblast becomes intimately associated with the uterine epithelium but is not rejected, although it is virtually a homograft. It has been suggested that local production of immunosuppressive steroids by the placenta and their release in high concentrations may interfere with local immunological reactions but the latest view is that there is some form of barrier separating the foetal antigens from the maternal competent circulating lymphocytes which have been induced by them. It has been suggested that this barrier is an early deposit of sialomucin on the outer surface of the trophoblast which may prevent activated maternal lymphocytes gaining attachment to it and hence penetrating into the trophoblast to destroy their "target cells".

VI. ANDROGENS

A. IN URINE

1. Amounts

17-Oxosteroids (or 17-ketosteroids) is a term often used in clinical studies to indicate urinary androgens, as most androgenic steroids in urine are 17-oxosteroids. But there are some androgens which are not 17-oxosteroids and some 17-oxosteroids that are not androgenic. Estrone, for example, is a 17-oxosteroid, but it can be separated from the others because of its phenolic properties, leaving the neutral fraction which is more nearly representative of the urinary androgens.

The 17-oxosteroids are excreted in urine in the conjugated form, mainly as glucuronosides and sulphates, and it is necessary for most assays to carry out an initial hydrolysis. In normal males about two-thirds of the total 17-oxosteroids arise from the adrenals and only a third from the testis. In women these compounds arise almost entirely from the adrenals. Individual 17-oxosteroids can be estimated by fractionation. Originally this was done with digitonin, but is done now, almost exclusively, by chromatography, either on paper or on alumina columns.

In normal men, aged 20 to 40, total urinary 17-oxosteroids/24 h is 12-17 mg. with a maximum at 25 years. There is a steady rise at puberty and a decline in middle and old age to about 5 mg/24 h (Fig. 9.7). Females show slightly lower values, being 7-12 mg/24 h at ages 20-40. A considerable overlap with normal male values occurs. There is no fluctuation with the phases of the menstrual cycle, but there is a diurnal variation, values being lower during the night.

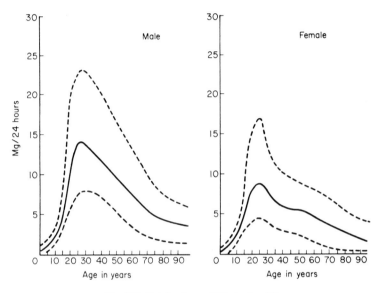

Fig. 9.7. Total urinary 17-ketosteroids.

In young children below the ages of 6, excretion is very low, about 1 mg/24 h. From this age until puberty there is a gradual rise in both sexes. The average value at puberty in either sex is about 9 mg/24 h. Table 9.9 shows some values for the individual 17-ketosteroids in adults. The urine of males contains 5-200 µg testosterone/24 h.

2. Methods of estimation

(a) Zimmermann method

Urine is treated with acid to hydrolyse 17-oxosteroid conjugates. The free compounds are then extracted by chloroform, carbon tetrachloride or benzene. The extracts are washed with alkali, then the residues treated with m-dinitrobenzene in alkali. The colour is then estimated by colorimeter. The method is reliable and has a high percentage recovery and reproducibility. Its lack of specificity can be a danger when applied to urines containing novel metabolites.

(b) Polarographic method

A variety of workers have applied polarography to the determination of 17-oxosteroids in urine. The method, which is reliable and has high reproducibility, correlates well with results from the Zimmermann method, but has been little used in clinical laboratories.

Table 9.9. *Individual urinary 17-ketosteroids (mg/24 h)*

| | Adults | |
	Female	Male
Androsterone[a]	1.6	2.1
Etiocholanolone[a]	1.9	2.1
Dehydroepiandrosterone[a]	0.4	0.6
11-Oxo-androsterone[b]	0.5	0.7
11-Oxo-etiocholanolone[b]	0.5	0.6
11-Hydroxy-etiocholanolone[b]	0.9	0.7
Epiandrosterone[a]	–	–
11-Hydroxy-androsterone[b]	–	–
Total 17-ketosteroids	7.7	10.7

[a] 11-deoxy-steroids
[b] 11-oxy-steroids

(c) Vestergaard method

This is probably one of the best methods for determining separately in urine the amounts of the major androgen metabolites: dehydroepiandrosterone, androsterone, etiocholanolone, 11-oxoetiocholanolone and 11β-hydroxyandrosterone. The urine is first hydrolysed by β-glucuronidase, then the free steroids extracted with ether and benzene. The extract is evaporated and the residue fractionated on alumina columns by gradient elution chromatography with ethanol and benzene. The resulting fractions are then separately estimated by a modified Zimmermann reaction. A variety of modifications to the method have been developed in a number of laboratories. Some workers separate the metabolites by thin-layer chromatography, while others determine the final amounts by gas chromatography of trimethylsilyl ethers of the various compounds.

(d) Ismail-Harkness method

This method is particularly good as it separates testosterone and epitestosterone in urine. The method uses an ether extract of an acid-hydrolysed urine.

Ketonic and non-ketonic fractions are separated by the Girard-T reagent using Amberlite IRC-50 resin as a catalyst. The resulting material is then separated by chromatography on alumina, then on paper. The testosterone eluted from the chromatograms is then determined by gas chromatography.

B. IN BLOOD

1. Amounts

Both androstenedione and testosterone exist in plasma in a directly extractable form and these are estimated by most of the published methods. Unconjugated testosterone is transported strongly, but non-specifically, bound to serum albumin and weakly but specifically bound to a β-globulin. Additional testosterone is liberated by hydrolysis with β-glucuronidase. Adult males have 0.2-1.7 μg testosterone/100 ml plasma and adult females 0.05-0.10 μg/100 ml. Androstenedione levels for adult males are 0.06-0.10 μg/100 ml (representing a plasma androstenedione to testosterone ratio of 1:13), while adult females have 0.1-0.3 μg/100 ml (representing an androstenedione to testosterone ratio of 3:1). Prepubertal males have about 0.042 μg testosterone/100 ml and prepubertal females about 0.019 μg/100 ml and a similar difference in androstenedione levels occurs. The ratios of androstenedione to testosterone are very similar in prepubertal males and females. At puberty, males show a 20-fold rise in plasma testosterone, but no change in androstenedione levels, whereas females show only a 2-fold rise in plasma testosterone with a 5-fold rise in androstenedione.

About 85% of the total plasma 17-oxosteroids exist in blood as sulphate esters, tightly bound to protein, mainly albumin. Dehydroepiandrosterone and then androsterone are the principal compounds (Table 9.10). There is a gradual decline with age. Recently a double isotope dilution derivative technique has been used to measure testosterone and a number of 17-oxosteroids in the plasma of both men and women (Table 9.11).

Table 9.10. *Plasma 17-oxosteroids in adults (μg/100 ml)*

	Male	Female
Total 17-oxosteroids	80-275	90-190
Dehydroepiandrosterone	70-230	40-140
Androsterone	10-60	20-50
Epiandrosterone	13	—
Androst-5-en-3β,17β-diol	27	—

Table 9.11. *Plasma androgens, µg/100 ml*

	Males	Females
Testosterone	0.67	0.035
Dehydroepiandrosterone	0.51	0.48
Δ^4-Androstenedione	0.13	0.13
Etiocholanolone	0.07	0.056
Androsterone	0.16	0.07
11-Hydroxy-Δ^4-androstenedione	0.20	0.18

2. Methods of assay

(a) Zimmermann reaction

Steroids containing the group $-\overset{\overset{\textstyle O}{\|}}{C}-CH_2-$ react with *m*-dinitrobenzene in the presence of alkali to give a purple colour. Under the conditions of assay normally employed, the reaction is given mainly by 17-oxosteroids, though 3-oxo and 20-oxo compounds also react and give low intensity colours. Due to the low concentration of testosterone in blood, this method has been applied mainly to the assay of dehydroepiandrosterone and androsterone. A plasma sample is extracted with ethanol then continuously extracted by ether. The extract is washed with alkali and chromatographed on florisil columns. Phenolic compounds (estrogens) are removed by washing with sodium hydroxide, then by water. The resulting extract is then separated by paper chromatography and the eluates containing dehydroepiandrosterone and androsterone separately estimated colorimetrically with the Zimmermann reaction applied on a micro-scale. Recoveries are 70-90%, but reproducibility is poor.

(b) Finkelstein-Forchielli-Dorfman method

Developed specifically for testosterone, this method relies on an enzymic conversion of testosterone to estrone plus estradiol. These compounds can then be assayed fluorimetrically as usual. The method is difficult to use and recoveries and reproducibility are only moderate.

(c) Isotope dilution

This method is similar in principle to that described for progesterone. ^{14}C-Testosterone is added to the plasma which is then acetylated by ^{3}H-acetic anhydride. The testosterone acetate so formed is separated from the plasma by paper or thin-layer chromatography and ^{3}H and ^{14}C are separately counted. The ^{3}H gives an estimate of the testosterone and the ^{14}C recovery provides a correction factor. Recovery is of the order of 85-95% and sensitivity is of the order of 0.05 μg/100 ml plasma. Alternatively, testosterone 2,4-diacetyl-thiosemicarbazone is formed with ^{35}S-thiosemicarbazide (method of Riondel).

(d) Gas chromatography

A variety of methods have been described and all rely on the initial separation of a plasma extract by thin-layer or paper chromatography. The resulting eluates are injected into the instrument. Recovery is 80-90% and sensitivity is good. Specificity has been questioned, as 17-epitestosterone may not be completely removed.

VII. SECRETION RATES OF ANDROGENS AND ESTROGENS

The secretion of estrogens and androgens is much more complicated than that of corticoids and it is not possible to use the same simple one- and two-compartment models. Only a small proportion of metabolites occur in the urine and methods using blood estimations after the injection of a radioactive steroid have to be used. The situation is further complicated by androgens and estrogens being secreted by more than one gland and by the secretion of prehormones.

A prehormone has been defined as a substance which exerts its biological effect by peripheral conversion to a more active compound and then contributes significantly to the overall biological effect. Peripheral conversion could be in any tissue, including those of the larger organs. In the human body a number of biologically inactive prehormones are secreted by the endocrine glands, the most important being dehydroepiandrosterone sulphate, pregnenolone and pregnenolone sulphate. The principal precursors of testosterone appear to be androstenedione and dehydroepiandrosterone with minor amounts coming from androstenediol and 17-hydroxyprogesterone. Metabolic clearance studies have shown that in the adult male androstenedione and dehydroepiandrosterone contribute only a negligible proportion to circulating testosterone, whereas in the adult female and the prepubertal male, about one-half of the circulating testosterone is formed from blood androstenedione and about 15% from blood dehydroepiandrosterone.

The total steroid entering the circulation from both secretion and conversion from precursors is the blood production rate and this can be estimated from the metabolic clearance rate of injected radioactive steroid. The proportion of the blood production rate not formed from precursors is the secretion rate. In the adult male the blood production rate of androstenedione is about 2.8 mg/24 h and of testosterone about 7.2 mg/24 h, of which about 1 mg and 0.3 mg respectively comes from prehormones. In the adult female blood production of androstenedione is about 3 mg/24 h and of testosterone about 0.3 mg/24 h, of

9

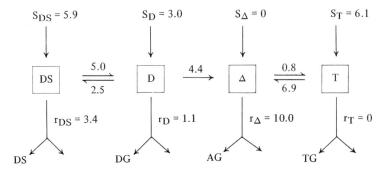

A. Normal Male

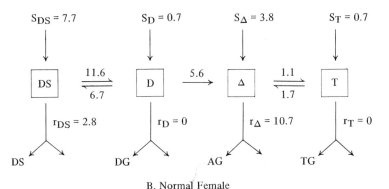

B. Normal Female

DS = Dehydroepiandrosterone sulphate
D = Dehydroepiandrosterone
Δ = Δ^4-Androstenedione
T = Testosterone
DG, AG, TG = Glucuronosides
A = Androsterone
S_{DS} = Secretion rate of dehydroepiandrosterone sulphate
All amounts in mg./24 hours

Fig. 9.8. Secretion and interconversion of the androgens.

which about 0.3 mg and about 0.25 mg respectively comes from precursors. In females, large amounts of androstenedione are secreted by the adrenals.

A four-component model which has been used in calculating androgen secretion rates is shown in Fig. 9.8. The adrenal secretion of dehydroepiandrosterone sulphate has been calculated as 5.9 and 7.7 mg/24 h in normal adult men and women respectively. The metabolic clearance rates of the sulphates in man are generally much lower than those of the corresponding free compounds (Table 9.12).

Table 9.12. *Metabolic clearance rates of androgens in man (litres whole blood/24 h)*

	Free	Sulphate
Dehydroepiandrosterone	1000	16-30
Testosterone	1000	20-35

A similar complicated system exists for the estrogens. In the luteal phase of the menstrual cycle, the blood production of estradiol and estrone is about 260 and 240 μg/day respectively, of which about 20 and 60 μg arise from prehormones. In males, the blood production rate of estrone is about 160 μg/day, of which about 40 μg comes from precursors, possibly dehydroepiandrosterone sulphate. All the blood estradiol (40 μg/day) of the male comes from prehormones. The adrenal is believed to secrete estrone sulphate and this is the source of blood estradiol in the male and in the follicular phase of the female.

VIII. ABNORMALITIES OF GONADAL AND PITUITARY FUNCTION

A. CHROMOSOME ABNORMALITIES

The determination of genetic sex is very important in the investigation of disorders of the gonad-pituitary axis. Several human "intersexes" are possible due to non-dysjunction of the chromosomes of either parent during meiosis in the gonads (Table 9.13).

Many persons with numerical alterations involving sex chromosomes have been found to be mosaics and for some conditions mosaicism is almost as common as the purely aneuploid condition. Many of these aberrations are believed to occur in the early postzygotic mitoses. Mosaicism may be manifest in

Table 9.13. *Human sex chromosome types*

XX	Normal female	XXXY ⎫	due to non-
XY	Normal male	XXO ⎬	dysjunction by both
XXX	Super female	XYO ⎭	parents, extremely rare.
XO	Turner's syndrome, gonadal dysgenesis		
			Mosaics, a variety of mixtures of
XXY	Klinefelter's syndrome		XX, XY, XYY, or XXX, are
YO,OO	Non-viable		known to occur.
XYY	"Aggressive male"		

all organs and tissues of the body, or there may be variations in cell percentages from organ to organ. Relative percentages tend to vary with age, one cell line being gradually eliminated. The large number and variety of sex chromosomal abnormalities that develop into adulthood, as opposed to autosomal abnormalities which are much more lethal, indicates the relative inertness of both the X and Y chromosomes. About seventy genes which show sex-linked inheritance have now been described, of which four variants occur with sufficient frequency to make them useful markers. There are now two clusters of genes, one of which shows linkage with the Xg blood group and the other with colour blindness. Another important sex-linked gene is that for the glucose-6-dehydrogenase type. The Y chromosome probably carries few genes, although it is strongly masculinizing. The manner in which the XX and XY chromosome constitutions bring about female and male phenotypes is unknown.

1. Super Female, Polysomy-X syndrome

The Super Female has a female phenotype, usually with normal external genitalia. Most subjects menstruate normally at first. Some have small breasts and infantile external genitalia with a small vagina. In some cases the menopause occurs very early and ovaries then have a post-menopausal appearance; some cases are fertile. When secondary amenorrhea has supervened, the urinary gonadotrophins occur in the menopausal range and estrogen supplementation is advised. The majority of cases are mentally retarded, especially the variants with four or even five X chromosomes.

2. Turner's syndrome (gonadal agenesis or dysgenesis)

Cases of Turner's syndrome also have a female phenotype, but the ovaries fail to develop and no ova are present. Usually ovarian remnants (streaks) are present containing only stroma. There is short stature, a small uterus, barrel chest, cubitus valgus, neck webbing and failure to menstruate. There is an absence of breast development, absent or scanty pubic hair and mental retardation. Some cases may have menstruated sometime and these usually have high urinary gonadotrophins, in the menopausal range. Other cases have never menstruated and have low urinary gonadotrophins indicating poor function of the hypophysis. Estrogen supplementation is usually advised.

In addition to the pure XO genotype, several other genetic variations exhibit the clinical picture of Turner's syndrome. These are mainly represented by structural alterations in one of a pair of X chromosomes and by mosaics. Structural alterations in one of the X chromosomes are not uncommon. One important aberration is partial deletion or loss of a portion of the X chromosome. Cases have been reported involving the long arm (designated "Xq-"), the short arm (designated "Xp-") or both arms. Rarely, an X chromosome may be in the form of a ring (designated "Xr") or the long arms may be abnormally long so that a large metacentric chromosome is produced (an isochromosome, designated "Xqi").

The Barr bodies in resting nuclei, the number of which indicate one less than the number of X chromosomes, are areas of heterochromatin representing those regions of chromosomes which remain in a tightly coiled physiochemical status throughout interphase. Only one of the two X chromosomes manifests heterochromatic behaviour, whereas the other X and the single X of the male are always euchromatic, i.e. they are uncoiled at interphase. It is believed that the heterochromatic X chromosome is genetically inactive, being rendered so soon after fertilization. In different cells from the same animal, the inactive X (of X's) can be either the maternal or paternal one. The heterochromatic X chromosome is pyknotic at mitotic prophase and replicates DNA late. When a structurally abnormal X chromosome is present, it always becomes heteropyknotic. The Barr body, or sex chromatin, probably consists almost entirely of all or most of the long arm of the X chromosome and may be small when shortening of this arm is present.

A number of mosaics also present the clinical picture of Turner's syndrome. The most common mosaic is XO/XX, while others are XO/XX/XXX, XO/XXX, XO/XY and XO/XYY. In addition an XO line may be associated with any of the structural abnormalities, the most common being XO/XXqi. Patients with pure genotype XXp- (i.e. a short arm deletion of one of the X chromosomes) are more severely affected than those with genotype XXq-. Patients with an XXqi genotype who are trisomic for the long arm and monosomic for the short arm are about as severely affected as patients with an XO genotype. The proportion of patients with mosaicism increases with increasing age of the patient material and is accompanied by progressively milder clinical manifestations. Occasionally, gonadal streaks retain a few follicles and menstruation occurs. It is believed that the incidence of XO conceptions is about 1:400 and live births about 1:5400. It is possible that pure XO is universally fatal and that all live births may be hidden XO/XX mosaics.

3. Male Turner's syndrome, Noonan's syndrome, "pure" gonadal dysgenesis

Much more rare are cases of male gonadal dysgenesis. Here the testes atrophy at the foetal stage and in the absence of male hormone the foetus, despite its XY chromosomes, develops female characteristics. It is known from animal experiments that androgens are required by the male foetus for the development of male characteristics. Cases are caused by a developmental abnormality rather than from abnormal chromosome complement. The presence or absence of active testes may be detected by measurements of circulating testosterone. In cases of gonadal dysgenesis very low levels are present, while in testicular feminization both testosterone and estrogens in plasma are in the normal ranges for male and female, respectively. As these patients are at high risk from malignancy, orchidectomy is usually conducted and the patients maintained on exogenous estrogens.

In 1963 Noonan recognized that this syndrome could occur in females as well as males. In general, severely affected patients present the clinical picture of Turner's syndrome, e.g. short stature, frequent congenital heart disease and a complex of anatomical abnormalities. Gonadal dysgenesis may vary from essentially normal gonadal size to complete testicular absence. There are usually well-developed secondary sexual characteristics in males. Webbing of the neck is sometimes present and mild to moderate mental retardation is frequently observed. It is believed that some females previously believed to have Turner's syndrome, but with sex positive chromatin or normal chromosome complement, actually have Noonan's syndrome. Cases of "pure" gonadal dysgenesis with XY chromosomes are usually designated as Swyer's syndrome. In this condition there are no other abnormalities although the dysgenesis has such an early prenatal onset and is so severe that the resulting individual's internal and external genitalia are completely feminized.

4. Testicular feminization

In cases of testicular feminization there is a female phenotype with well-developed breasts and female external genitalia, but little or no axillary or pubic hair. Chromosome studies show a normal male genotype and surgical examination shows poor development of the female organs and the presence of two, usually undescended, testes in the abdomen or elsewhere. There is usually no uterus, while vas deferens or epididymus are usually present bilaterally. Urinary gonadotrophins are usually normal or very slightly raised.

It has been postulated that there is a genetically produced failure of end-organ response to androgens, as the testes secrete both androgens and estrogens. This also applies to the hair follicles as cases are not hirsuit. Because of the increased risk (10% of cases) of gonadal cancer, the testes of such patients should be removed and estrogen replacement therapy started. The patients are a (sterile) female to all appearances. An artificial vagina can be constructed in those cases who wish to marry.

Incomplete testicular feminization also exists as a separate syndrome. The body build is slightly more masculine and there is a slightly enlarged phallus. Further degrees of masculinization appear to merge into Reiferstein's syndrome.

5. Aggressive male

The XYY syndrome, here called the "aggressive male", appears as a normal, very tall male with an aggressive personality, and probably a history of civil misdemeanours. Some are normally fertile, although chromosome abnormalities may occur in their children. In others, testicular atrophy occurs after puberty. Estrogen or anti-androgen treatment may be indicated.

6. Klinefelter's syndrome

Male hypogonadism is conveniently considered in two sections. Firstly, there are primary cases of testicular failure where, due to the failure of the normal feedback mechanism, there is excess production and excretion of gonadotrophins. There are also secondary cases of hypogonadism due to pituitary or hypothalamic insufficiency, and in such cases gonadotrophin excretion is low or absent.

The hypergonadotrophic syndromes are by far the commonest. They are characterized by varying degrees of seminiferous tubule failure and decreased Leydig cell function. The classical form is the Klinefelter's syndrome, which is now known to be associated with chromosome abnormalities of the cells of the testicular tissues, which possess abnormal numbers of the female X chromosome. In most cases, other tissues of the patient (i.e. skin, blood, etc.) also share the abnormality. The commonest type is XXY, but variants with XXYY, XXXYY, XXXY and XXXXY have been reported. Mosaics of XX/XXY and XY/XXY also occur. There is a male phenotype with small female breasts, no sperm and often some mental retardation. In these cases, as has been stated, urinary gonadotrophins are high, being mainly FSH activity not LH. Plasma and urine testosterone levels may be lower than the normal range, but are more frequently in the low normal. The patient with Klinefelter's syndrome is in a state of androgen insufficiency arising partly from low production, partly from tissue insensitivity, and partly from estrogen antagonism. Adequate sexual maturation can be achieved by androgen treatment, though the infertility is irreversible and the gynecomastia does not usually regress. The usual treatment is to give i.m. 200 mg of testosterone in the form of a long-acting ester (e.g. enanthate), initially weekly, then monthly as the treatment progresses. In the older patients failing testicular function leads to increased nitrogen and calcium loss. These can be at least partially restored by the use of a weak androgen with strong myotropic properties.

The hypogonadotrophic syndromes are all cases of testicular failure secondary to hypothalamic or pituitary failure, but such cases are rare.

7. Mongols (Down's syndrome)

Here there is an extra autosome and females menstruate but only rarely reproduce. It is possible that other abnormalities in non-sexual chromosomes may cause infertility.

8. Hermaphrodites

A number of patients with XO/XY mosaicism have been described. The most commonly reported clinical type has intersex genitalia with a more or less hypodysplastic testis on one side and a streak gonad on the other. Their internal genitalia usually consist of an infantile uterus with Wolffian duct derivatives on the testicular side and a fallopian tube on the gonadal streak side. Patients may be reared as females, in which case both gonadal rudiments are usually removed, or as males if it is possible to bring gonads down to the scrotum. Other clinical types may appear as a female with Turner's syndrome or as a hypogonadal male. These variations seem to depend on the relative amounts of the two cell lines.

Several reports have been published of phenotypic females with some evidence of masculinization, and of intersex individuals who seem to possess some Y chromosome material. They may represent Y chromosome deletions, either as pure Xy genotype or as mosaics, e.g. XO/Xy.

Mosaic hermaphroditism of XX/XY genotype has also been reported. This may be caused by the same process that produces chimerism in cattle twins or by diaspermy.

B. DISEASES OF THE PITUITARY GLAND OR HYPOTHALAMUS

This section does not include diseases where the secretion of these tissues is suppressed by diseases occurring elsewhere in the body. Once such a secondary cause has been removed, it is usual for the hypophysis and/or the hypothalamus to resume normal secretion.

1. Anorexia nervosa

The fact that amenorrhea may appear before the anorexia becomes marked, and always before emaciation is extreme, refutes the assumption that the amenorrhea is the result of wilful starvation and points to a psychogenic origin for both the hypothalamic-induced pituitary deficiency and the patients inability to eat. Treatment with gonadotrophins may be of value.

2. Frohlich's syndrome, adiposogenital dystrophy

There is pituitary hypofunction, with secondary hypogonadism and obesity of the typical mammary-mons-girdle type. The primary lesion may be in the hypothalamus as destruction of the pituitary usually leads to underweight. The uterus is small, the external os of the cervix is pinhole in size and the vagina is short and narrow. There is usually a delayed menarche and then secondary amenorrhea. Urinary gonadotrophins and 17-oxosteroids are very low. Replacement therapy with cyclic estrogen and progestogen is recommended, together with gonadotrophins or clomiphene. After surgical correction of the lesion (usually a cranio-pharyngioma), androgen therapy should start at puberty. This syndrome also occurs in males—the "Billy Bunter" or "Dicken's fat boy" syndrome. It has been suggested that the Emperor Napoleon I acquired symptoms of this syndrome about the age of 40.

3. Glinski's or Simmond's or Sheehan's disease; pituitary cachexia

In this condition there is pituitary insufficiency, due to ischemic neuroses of the gland, often occurring after parturition. The disease is characterized by amenorrhea, loss of axillary and pubic hair, signs of hypothyroidism and asthenia. When massive, the lesion causes a syndrome resembling Addison's disease. In its milder form, it mimics non-endocrine wasting diseases. Women are more susceptible than men. A variety of deficiency symptoms occur, due to dysfunction of all the endocrine glands under the control of the pituitary, e.g. genital atrophy, hypotension, hypothermia, hypoglycaemia, a very low basal metabolic rate, high blood cholesterol, low urinary 17-oxosteroids. The meto-pirone test may help to distinguish dysfunction of the hypothalamus, as in anorexia nervosa, and dysfunction of the pituitary gland. Ovulation and subsequent pregnancy have been successfully induced with gonadotrophin replacement therapy.

4. Pituitary adenoma

Adenomas may occur in the chromophobe (neutrophil), basophil or acidophil cells of the pituitary. Basophil adenomas produce the characteristic signs of Cushing's syndrome. Chromophobe adenomas are usually composed of non-secreting cells and mainly cause symptoms of pressure. Acidophil adenomas produce acromegaly.

Acromegaly is characterized by hypersecretion of somatotrophin which causes overgrowth of bone, connective tissue and viscera; there is also typical enlargement of hands, feet, face and head. It usually starts in the third or fourth decade and effects both sexes equally. An eosinophilic adenoma is found in 75% of cases, rarely eosinophilic hyperplasia, and malignancy almost never. The overgrowth of eosinophils may later obliterate other normal cells in the hypophysis and cause other symptoms of hypopituitarism. The gonads may be large but function subnormally. The adrenal cortex is hypertrophied but does not oversecrete. While high levels of urinary 17-oxosteroids have been occasionally reported in individual cases, the majority show normal or subnormal values. Hypercalciuria is common and diabetes occurs in about a sixth of the cases.

Giantism is a rare genetic variation of the normal and is produced by high secretion of somatotrophin in youth. There may be delayed puberty with consequent prolongation of the period of linear growth.

5. Chiari-Frommel syndrome

This is characterized by amenorrhea, prolonged galactorrhea and moderate obesity and is the result of a variably induced hypothalamic dysfunction that inhibits the release of gonadotrophins from, and permits excessive production of, lactogenic hormone by the anterior pituitary. The amenorrhea is associated with marked secondary atrophy of both the uterus and ovaries. There is an absence of urinary pregnanediol, low urinary FSH and high urinary lactogenic hormone.

Cyclic uterine bleeding is obtainable by cyclic administration of estrogen and progestogen, while clomiphene has restored ovulatory cycles and led to pregnancy. The syndrome usually appears in post-partum, poorly nourished young women. Even after breast feeding has been discontinued for several months, amenorrhea and lactation continue. It is suspected that there is an increase in secretion of prolactin by the pituitary, possibly associated with an adenoma of the pituitary eosinophils. Some cases also have acromegaly.

6. Hypopituitarism

The pituitary dwarf, or midget, has been discussed previously.

7. Fertile Eunuch syndrome

Spermatogenesis is normal but androgen secretion, and hence masculinization, is poor. The secretion of FSH appears to be normal but that of LH absent.

C. DISEASES OF THE GONADS

1. Reiferstein's syndrome

This is an hereditary testicular disorder somewhat resembling Klinefelter's syndrome and is known as Reiferstein's syndrome, only here there is no evidence of abnormal chromosomes and the basis of the condition is uncertain. In some adult males, no recognizable testicular tissue can be found and the condition has a variety of causes. In certain cases there may be a congenital absence of testicular tissue, while in others it may have been destroyed by a disturbance in embryological development, or by an infection. Traumas, including accidental surgical interference, may also contribute, though in most cases the etiology is obscure. This condition of anorchia (or functional prepubertal castrate syndrome, or testicular agenesis) produces patients with sexual infantilism in whom puberty cannot occur. Androgen replacement therapy can produce full sexual maturation, though the patient is naturally sterile.

2. Male climacteric

Unlike the female, there is no clear-cut climacteric in man. Nevertheless adult Leydig cell failure can occur in some individuals, and the presenting withdrawal symptoms are very analogous to those seen at the menopause in women (i.e. irritability, hot flushes, depression, etc.). The commonest cause is probably Klinefelter's syndrome and true idiopathic Leydic cell failure is probably rare. Another cause is infectious atrophy of the testes. Whatever the cause, androgen therapy is usually of value in restoring well-being, though it is without value in the equally common condition of psychogenic impotence, and a differentiation between the two can be made by comparing the effects on the patient of an androgen with those of a placebo, such as sesame oil.

3. Stein-Leventhal syndrome; bilateral polycystic ovaries

This is a clinically heterogeneous condition in which the cardinal symptoms are amenorrhea (which may be primary or secondary) or oligomenorrhea with sterility, hirsutism and moderate obesity. The ovaries are much enlarged and have a white shiny coat beneath which there are numerous large cysts. The secondary amenorrhea is gradual in onset. In about 20-30% of patients, the urinary excretion of 17-oxosteroids is raised but adrenal and ovarian suppression tests suggest that the excess androgen comes from the adrenals in some patients and from the ovaries in others. This divides the cases into the "ovarian type" and "adrenal type" whose responses vary to the different forms of treatment. It is believed that there is an altered biochemical pathway for estrogen synthesis that results in excessive secretion of androgens. High levels of androstenedione have been found in ovarian vein blood, usually with normal levels of estrogen. The androgen:estrogen ratio is several times normal. It is not known which androgen is responsible for the hirsutism and virilization occurring in the syndrome, but androstenedione or dehydroepiandrosterone from the ovaries or adrenals is more likely than testosterone. There is high blood testosterone in most cases, possibly by conversion from secreted dehydroepiandrosterone (sulphate). The fluid collected from the ovarian cysts contains very high levels of androstenedione with little or no estrogen or progesterone. This contrasts markedly with other types of ovarian cysts.

In vitro studies have found two types of enzyme deficiencies in the ovaries. In some cases a deficiency in 3β-hydroxysteroid dehydrogenase, e.g. the conversion of pregnenolone to progesterone, has been found. This would account for the high levels of urinary Δ^5-pregnanetriol found in some cases, as this is the theoretically accumulated product of such a blockage. In other cases a deficiency in the aromatization system, e.g. the conversion of androstenedione to estrone, has been found. Some cases have increased urinary 11-oxo-pregnanetriol which is thought to be an adrenal metabolite.

Plasma and urinary estrogens and progesterone are in the normal range for the follicular phase but all the signs of ovulation are absent. Urinary FSH and LH appear to be normal but without the mid-cycle peak. The universal treatment is bilateral wedge resection of the ovaries but only cases of the "ovarian type" show consistent and maintained improvement. It is believed that this treatment reduces the feedback on the hypothalamus and restores the cyclic secretion of gonadotrophins. Amenorrhea tends to recur after a few years. After wedge resection about 30-40% of cases, in whom menstruation is restored, become pregnant. Treatment with gonadotrophins and/or clomiphene can also be used to induce ovulation. The pregnancy rate with clomiphene is about the same as with wedge resection.

4. Primary ovarian failure

There is increased secretion of gonadotrophins, but the ovaries do not respond. Subjects have a soft skin, small larynx, high-pitched voice, underdeveloped breasts, hypoplastic generative organs, gastro-intestinal spasticity and bladder irritability. Estrogen treatment relieves the deficiency syndromes, as in the menopause, and cyclic menstruation can be established with estrogen and progestogen.

5. Ovarian tumours

Ovarian tumours, creating pelvic congestion, more often cause abnormal uterine bleeding, but rare cases are masculinizing and produce amenorrhea. There is regression of the female secondary sexual characteristics, hirsutism, partial alopecia, deepening of the voice and hypertrophy of the clitoris. Excretion of 17-oxosteroids may not be raised. Studies of individual urinary androgens usually show increased androsterone, with little change in etiocholanolone and dehydroepiandrosterone.

There are three main varieties of masculinizing tumours—arrhenoblastoma (the most common), adrenal rest tumour and hilus cell tumour. The ovarian hilus cells closely resemble the testicular Leydig cells. Tumours of the granulosa cells (thecal cell tumour) appear to secrete estrogens while the very rare luteomas secrete pregnanediol. There are several other extremely rare types of ovarian tumours.

6. Chorionepithelioma of the testis

High levels of urinary estrogens have been reported in this condition. High levels of HCG occur in blood and urine.

D. MENSTRUAL DISTURBANCES

1. No menstruation (amenorrhea)

Natural causes are youth, pregnancy, lactation and menopause. Primary amenorrhea is defined as present when menstruation has not occurred by 18 years of age. Among the possible causes are Turner's syndrome and testicular feminization. Secondary amenorrhea may be due to a variety of environmental and emotional causes, malnutrition and severe systemic disease. Among the endocrine causes are Stein-Leventhal syndrome and Sheehan's syndrome. Nearly half the women presenting with primary amenorrhea have either a genetic disorder or some type of hermaphoditism.

2. Too little menstruation

(a) Hypomenorrhea

This is scanty menstruation at normal cyclical intervals. It is seldom possible to find an endocrine cause and ovulation occurs. If currettage shows a poorly developed endometrium, cyclical therapy should be used.

(b) Oligomenorrhea

This is scanty menstruation at extended intervals. It is the follicular phase which is usually prolonged while the luteal phase is of normal length. In most cases there is no indication for therapy.

3. Too many menstruations

(a) Polymenorrhea

This is shortened regular intervals between menstruations. When this is due to a short follicular phase, there is no infertility and no treatment is usually required. When this is due to a short luteal phase (less than 14 days), showing lack of enough progesterone, infertility is nearly always present. The luteal phase can be prolonged by an injection of 250 mg 17α-hydroxyprogesterone caproate plus 10 mg estradiol benzoate on the fifth or sixth day after the first rise in basal body temperature. Normal menstruation can also be delayed in this way or by three tablets of 100 mg norethisterone daily from the twenty-first or twenty-sixth days of the cycle. In both cases there is a delay of about 5 days.

(b) Bleeding at ovulation

This probably represents a form of estrogen withdrawal bleeding due to transient reduction in the secretion of estrogens.

4. Too much or excessive menstruation

(a) Hypermenorrhea and menorrhagia

This is excessive blood loss at normal cyclical intervals. In the young, heavy bleeding (hypermenorrhea) is usually also prolonged (menorrhea) and is due to an incompletely developed cycle with deficient progesterone secretion; also the immature uterine muscle lacks contractability. In adults, increased bleeding is often due to fibroids, polyps, pelvic congestion with a retroverted uterus or atherosclerosis.

(b) Metrorrhagia (dysfunctional uterine bleeding)

This is irregular, prolonged bleeding with very variable intervals of freedom between them. In pubertal cases the condition has usually self-corrected by the age of 20 years. It is known as metropathia haemorrhagica at the menopause. There is a failure of ovulation and Graafian follicles do not rupture but go on producing ever larger amounts of estrogens, which cause cystic glandular hyperplasia of the endometrium. Eventually the follicle degenerates, the estrogen level falls and only the surface of the endometrium bleeds heavily, eventually leading to necrosis and complete shedding of the endometrium. These functional cases comprise about 60% of juvenile cases, 10% of sexual mature cases and 35% of premenopausal cases. Urinary estrogens are very high but fall when bleeding begins. Pregnanediol excretion is usually of the anovulatory type.

Threatened abortion is another important cause (20% of juveniles and 40% of mature cases). Carcinoma and fibroids account for about 30% of sexual mature cases and 45% of the premenopausal cases. Functional metrorrhagia can be very satisfactorily corrected by hormone treatment, although this is not recommended for the juveniles, e.g. 3 x 100 mg oral norethisterone for 10 days to produce withdrawal bleeding.

5. Painful menstruation (dysmenorrhea)

Secondary dysmenorrhea may be due to fibroids, endometriosis or cervical stenosis. Endometriosis is a local lesion involving numerous organs and arises from the development of ectopic endometrial tissues. These tissues frequently follow the normal cyclical pattern of the uterine epithelium and by virtue of repeated bleeding and incapsulation of the affected tissues, give rise to the formation of cysts which are often brown or purple in colour. Endometriosis occurs commonly in the myometrium where it may be called adenomyosis. Other common sites are the cervix, vagina and other pelvic organs. At a later stage endometrial tissue disappears completely and is replaced by fibrosis. Early treatment with oral norethisterone daily for at least 6 months causes lesions to rapidly disappear.

E. TESTS OF GONADAL FUNCTION

1. Testes

Measurements of 17-oxosteroid excretions are of no value, as about 70% of these compounds arise from the adrenal cortex. Surprisingly, estrogen excretion is a more reliable measure, as about 80% of the urinary estrogens of a normal man are formed by the Leydig cells. Another test of value, but difficult to perform, is basal plasma testosterone. It must be remembered that both testosterone and estrogens may be formed by adrenal carcinoma. Where hypoactivity of the testes is suspected, evaluation of pituitary gonadotrophins may be conducted best by radioimmune assay on urine and blood. Exogenous gonadotrophins stimulate androgen production in the normal male.

2. Ovaries

(a) Urinary hormones

In contrast to the male situation, measurements of urinary estrogens are of value in assessing ovarian function. In cases of ovarian dysgenesis, or of hypopituitarism, estrogen excretion is reduced well below the normal range. Adrenal estrogens account for only a small proportion of the estrogens of normal female urine. Urinary androgen levels may be high in secondary amenorrhea with hirsutism and may indicate an androgen secreting adrenal or ovarian tumour. Gonadotrophic activity is assessed as for the male. Exogenous gonadotrophins stimulate estrogen production and, indeed, may induce ovulation.

Urinary excretion of pregnanediol is frequently measured as a test of corpus luteum function in non-pregnant women, and of placental function during pregnancy. In amenorrheic women there is a low excretion with no definite cyclic pattern during the month. Most of the pregnanediol in these subjects arises from the adrenals. For menstruating women with anovular cycles, again the typical monthly variation in urinary pregnanediol is lacking; the luteal peak particularly is absent. No abnormalities in pregnanediol excretion occur in dysmenorrhea.

Abnormal pregnanediol excretion has been observed in a variety of pregnancy disorders. In pre-eclamptic toxaemia, urinary pregnanediol levels are usually lower than the normal range during the third trimester. In threatened or habitual abortion the position is less clear. While some subjects show low values of pregnanediol outside the normal range, others appear normal. Serial measurements are of value as a consistent decline is often associated with foetal death.

(b) Challenge tests

Ovarian function in (non-pregnant) amenorrhea can be assessed by progestogen-estrogen challenge tests. The progesterone test is carried out by the injection of 20 mg progesterone, or of 20 mg progesterone plus 2 mg estradiol benzoate, on two successive days. Alternatively, one tablet for 2 days of 10 mg norethisterone acetate plus 0.2 mg ethinyl estradiol may be given. If progestogen withdrawal bleeding occurs within 10 days, it can normally be assumed there is adequate estrogen secretion by the ovaries and that the endometrium is present and capable of functioning. This occurs in most cases of short duration secondary amenorrhea. An improvement in living conditions, treatment of systemic disease and emotional problems may bring about regular cycles. Cyclical progesterone treatment may help. It is unusual to obtain progestogen withdrawal bleeding in cases of long-standing secondary amenorrhea as the endometrium may have become markedly atrophic and incapable of responding to progesterone without preliminary estrogen treatment. It is rare to obtain progestogen withdrawal bleeding in primary amenorrhea.

The estrogen test is performed with an injection of 20 mg estradiol valerate. If estrogen withdrawal bleeding occurs within 4 weeks, it indicates that the endometrium has undergone proliferative changes, having been atrophic prior to the test. This type of bleeding is given in cases of primary amenorrhea if an endometrium is present. If no estrogen withdrawal bleeding takes place, it is probable that there is no functional endometrium.

F. HYPERSECRETION OF SEX HORMONES

The following human conditions are associated with excess production of one or more of the sex hormones.

1. Adrenal hyperplasia and tumours

In adrenal hyperplasia there is high urinary excretion of 17-oxosteroids and pregnanetriol. High levels of urinary pregnanediol have been reported in both hyperplasia and malignancy, but the assay methods used were relatively non-specific and the high levels of other urinary steroids probably interfered with the assay methods used. Very high levels of all three major urinary estrogens have been reported for some patients with either condition.

2. Adrenogenital syndrome

Large increases in blood and urine androgens occur in this syndrome. Some increase may also occur in excretion of corticosteroid metabolites, though normal blood cortisol is usually found.

3. Cushing's syndrome

This condition, which may be due to either an adrenocortical tumour or to hyperplasia, leads to the excessive production of corticoids. Blood cortisol is high, and the normal diurnal variation is absent. All urinary corticoid metabolites are increased, though those showing the most marked changes are cortisone, cortisol, corticosterone and their tetrahydro-metabolites. The excretion of 17-oxosteroids is also usually increased, especially when a maligant adrenal tumour is present.

4. Diabetic pregnancy

Abnormally high levels of HCG have been found in the blood and urine of about one-third of pregnant diabetics. Blood estrogens may be raised and the urinary output, particularly of ring D-ketolic estrogens, is also increased. In contrast, pregnanediol in urine is within the normal range.

5. Gynaecomastia

Estrogen excretion somewhat higher than the normal male level has been reported for some adult patients suffering from exfoliative dermatitis and gynaecomastia. However, no increased estrogens could be found in cases arising at puberty. Levels of urinary pregnanediol in these latter patients were also normal. Gynaecomastia is a common side-effect in male patients given long-term estrogen therapy (for prostatic carcinoma, etc.). It has also been reported occasionally as a side-effect in patients on steroids with no estrogenic properties.

6. Hirsutism

Most hirsute women excrete significantly higher levels of 17-oxosteroids than similar non-hirsute women of comparable age. The severity of the hirsutism is not correlated with the amount of 17-oxosteroids excreted. Of individual urinary androgens, increase in dehydroepiandrosterone, etiocholanolone and androsterone have been demonstrated. Pregnanetriol excretion in hirsute women with irregular menstrual cycles shows no significant difference from the normal.

7. Hydatiform mole

In this condition there is usually a very marked increase in urinary HCG; however, blood levels of progesterone are normal, while both urinary pregnanediol and estrogens are either normal or low.

8. Hyperemesis gravidarum

While urinary 17-oxosteroids are usually within the normal pregnancy range, the excretion of dehydroepiandrosterone is increased.

9. Hypertrophic pulmonary osteoarthropathy

Estrogen excretion in men with this disease is about double the normal. Some cases show gynaecomastia, but no demonstrable relationship exists between this symptom and the level of urinary estrogen.

10. Liver diseases

Increased levels of urinary estrogens have been reported in a variety of liver diseases. Estriol appears to be the metabolite most commonly increased. In contrast, the excretion of androgens is reduced.

11. Mammary carcinoma

While no significant changes in 17-oxosteroid or corticosteroid output have been found, it has been suggested that measurements of urinary etiocholanolone and 17-hydroxy-corticosteroids are significantly altered in some patients and that a knowledge of this change is of considerable value for predicting the future clinical course of the disease. Patients with recurrent or metastatic mammary carcinoma who fail to respond to adrenalectomy or hypophysectomy show higher pre-operative values of urinary etiocholanolone and lower 17-hydroxy-corticosteroids. It has been reported that urinary excretion of estriol by these patients is often somewhat higher than the normal.

12. Obesity

While urinary 17-oxosteroids are in the normal range for most obese subjects, it has been found that a sudden weight loss induced by starvation leads to a marked reduction in 17-oxosteroid output. A significant correlation has also been reported between urinary estriol and body weight.

13. Prostatic carcinoma

Excretion of 17-oxosteroids is not abnormal in these patients; however, excessive excretion of 11-oxo-etiocholanolone, but not of other metabolites, has been reported for some patients.

14. Steroid fever

Some patients with fevers of obscure etiology, usually in association with joint pains, have been reported to excrete high levels of etiocholanolone. It is known that when administered in a high dose, this compound will induce fever in the human, but the clinical reality of "steroid fever" still remains to be demonstrated.

15. Stress conditions

Many types of stress, including surgery, burns, infections, cold and low oxygen tension, are known to lead to an increase in blood cortisol and in the excretion of urinary corticoids. Increases in the output of 17-oxosteroids have also been noted.

IX. SEX HORMONE THERAPY

A. HORMONE-DEPENDENT CANCER

A variety of human tumours regress when exogenous steroid hormones are given. The classic examples of such tumours are disseminated cancer of the breast, cancer of the uterine endometrium and cancer of the prostate. The approach to the treatment and understanding of these diseases is fraught with difficulties and cannot be more than outlined here. Basically, it is believed that both breast and endometrial cancer tend to be stimulated by estrogens, whilst androgens stimulate prostate cancer. More accurately it should be said that sex hormones stimulate some cells in some tumours. Taking breast cancer as an example, it is found that less than 40% of patients show objective responses to any form of hormone manipulation. Those that do respond, do so for only a limited time and the disease always recurs. The remission time may be as long as 3 or 4 years, but usually it is only a matter of months. Despite these facts, hormone treatment of advanced breast cancer is the most successful treatment available.

General schemes for the treatment of breast cancer are shown below:

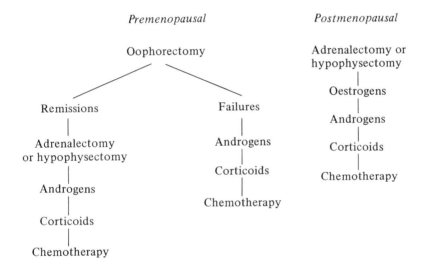

In this chart the sequence of treatments is shown. A patient is held on a particular treatment until evidence of disease progression becomes apparent. The treatment is then changed and again held until further progression occurs. Alternative approaches to hormone therapy include "medical hypophysectomy" by giving hormones that strongly suppress the pituitary secretion of gonadotrophins. The selection of androgen used has proved largely irrelevant. An extremely weak androgen like Δ^1-testololactone gives just as good responses as testosterone propionate. For endometrial cancer, potent progestogens produce temporary remissions in about 30% of cases. Estrogens, or non-estrogenic anti-androgens, produce temporary remissions in a high percentage of cases of prostatic cancer. The mechanism of action of steroids in the treatment of these cancers is not known. It is likely that the exogenous compounds have a cytotoxic effect on certain especially sensitive cells of the tumour. This produces a regression of the tumour mass. However, continued growth of the non-sensitive cells eventually leads to continued progression of the disease.

B. OTHER SEX HORMONE TREATMENTS

Sex hormones are routinely used for the suppression of various pathological conditions and the following is a selection of indications:

Estrogens	*Androgens*	*Progestogens*
Acne vulgaris	Uterine fibroids	Metrorrhagia
Senile vaginitis	Osteoporosis	Dysmenorrhea
Senile pruritus	Cachexia	Mastitis
	Prostate hypertrophy	Endometriosis
	Myomas	Prostate hypertrophy
	Nephrosis	Uterine hypoplasia
		Dysfunctional uterine bleeding
		Menorrhagia

Estrogens inhibit prolactin secretion and exogenous estrogens, such as stilbestrol, and are still the best suppressives of lacation. Recommended regimes give 3 x 15 mg on the first day postpartum, 3 x 10 mg on the second day, 3 x 5 mg on the third day, 2 x 5 mg on the fourth day and 5 mg on the fifth and subsequent days. Recently "Estrovis", a single tablet of 4 mg ethinyl estradiol cyclopentyl ether, has been found very effective in the suppression of lactation.

Estrogen replacement therapy is of benefit for the vasomotor syndrome of menopausal women, i.e. hot flushes, outbreaks of sweating, attacks of dizziness and secondary disturbances of sleep. Ethinylestradiol (0.01-0.02 mg/day), mestranol or quinestradol are now the preferred oral estrogens in interrupted doses. Many preparations also contain a mild sedative and/or a muscle relaxant. A number of mixtures of 0.004-0.02 mg ethinylestradiol and 2.5-5 mg methytestosterone are also available. The addition of androgen was developed to counteract the side effects produced by the too large doses of estrogens formerly used, i.e. withdrawal or breakthrough bleeding. Although androgens are very effective themselves in suppressing the vasomotor disturbance, their use is not recommended because of irreversible virilism produced by long-term use.

Threatened abortion due to hormonal deficiencies may be treated with weekly depot injections of 250 mg 17α-hydroxyprogesterone caproate.

10

PLANT STEROIDS

I. C-28 AND C-29 STEROLS

A. OCCURRENCE AND STRUCTURE

A variety of C-28 and C-29 sterols are present in nature (Table 10.1) and many have now been isolated from both plant and animal sources. The additional carbon atoms are in the side chain as either methyl or ethyl groups and there may also be an additional double bond, usually in the side chain. Nomenclature is based on cholestane, ergostane and stigmastane all of which are defined as having a 20R-configuration. Ergostane has a 24S-configuration and stigmastane a 24R-configuration (Fig. 10.1).

265

Most of the common sterols of the marine invertebrates contain 28 or 29 carbon atoms, the main exception being 24-dehydrocholesterol which comprises 34% of the sterols of the barnacle. In the sponges are found clionasterol and

Table 10.1 *Sterols of plants, fungi, algae and marine invertebrates*

Compound and source	Configuration and side chain substituents	Double bonds
Plants		
Brassicasterol	24*S*-methyl	5, 22
α-Spinasterol	24*R*-methyl	5, 22
β-Sitosterol (cinchol)	24*R*-ethyl	5
Stigmasterol	24*R*-ethyl	5, 22
Campesterol	24*R*-methyl	5
γ-Sitosterol (clionasterol)	24*S*-ethyl	5
Fungi		
Ergosterol	24*S*-methyl	5, 7, 22
Fungisterol	24*S*-methyl	6, 8, 22
Zymosterol	–	8, 24
Ascosterol	24-methyl	8, 23
Episterol	24-methylene	7
Fecosterol	24-methylene	8
Algae		
Fucosterol	24-ethylene	5
Sargasterol	21α-methyl, 24-ethylene	5
Marine invertebrates		
Chondrillasterol	24*S*-ethyl	7, 22
Poriferasterol	24*S*-ethyl	5, 22
Spongesterol	24*S*-ethyl	22
Clionasterol (γ-sitosterol)	24*S*-ethyl	5
Desmosterol (24-dehydrocholesterol)	–	5, 24
Chalinasterol (24 (28)-methylenecholesterol)	24-methylene	5
Stellasterol	21α-methyl, 24*R*-methyl	7, 22

poriferasterol (Fig. 10.1), while 24-methylenecholesterol has been found to comprise 36% and 53% of the sterols of oysters and clams respectively. Marine algae contain the two isomeric sterols fucosterol and sargasterol (Fig. 10.2).

The most abundant sterols of the higher plants (phytosterols) are β-sitosterol and stigmasterol. Major sources of β-sitosterol are cotton seed oil and sugar cane wax. The principal sterol of soya bean oil is γ-sitosterol (clionasterol). Four

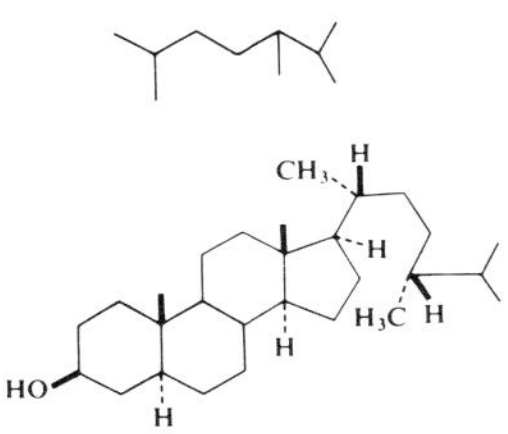

Fig. 10.1. Some naturally occurring derivatives of campestanol, stigmastanal and ergostanol.

Campestanol
(24S)-24-Methyl-5α-cholestan-3β-ol
24α-Methyl-5α-cholestan-3β-ol

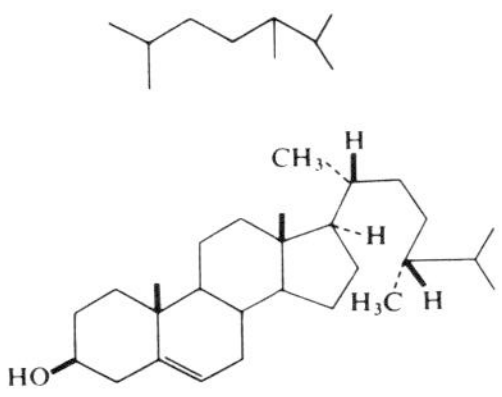

Campesterol
(24R)-24-Methyl-5-cholesten-3β-ol
24α-Methyl-5-cholesten-3β-ol

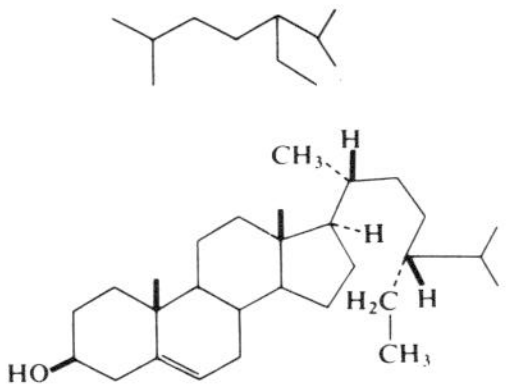

β-Sitosterol, Cinchol
(24R)-24-Ethyl-5-cholesten-3β-ol
5-Stigmasten-3β-ol
22,23-Dihydrostigmasterol

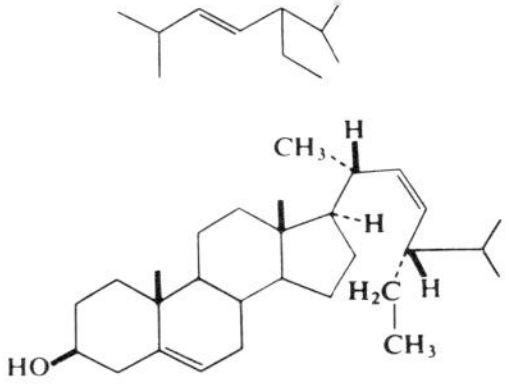

Stigmasterol
(24R)-24-Ethyl-5,22-cholestadien-3β-ol
5,22-Stigmastadien-3β-ol

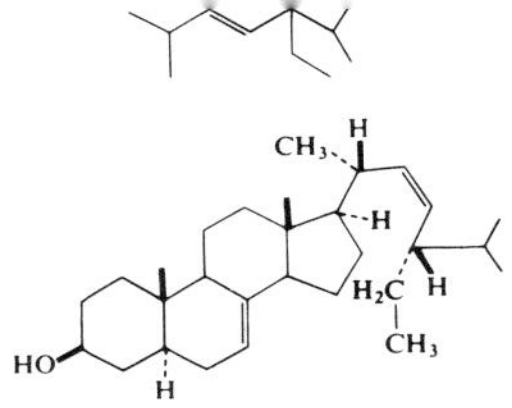

α-Spinasterol
(24R)-24-Ethyl-7,22,(5α)-cholestadien-3β-ol
7,22-Stigmastadien-3β-ol

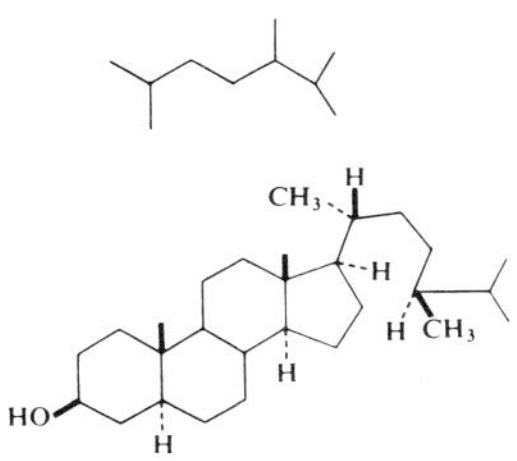

Ergostanol
(24S)-24-Methyl-5α-cholestan-3β-ol
24β-Methyl-5α-cholestan-3β-ol
5α-Ergostan-3β-ol

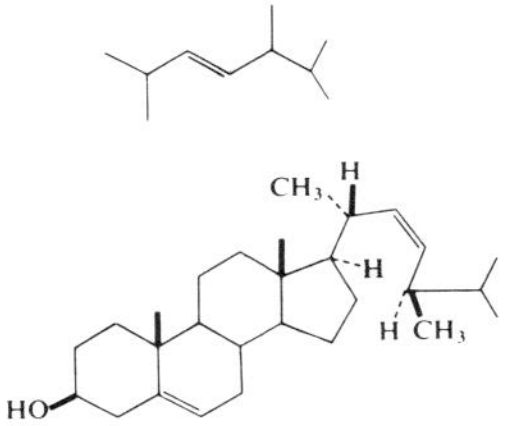

Brassicasterol
(24S)-24-Methyl-5,22-cholestadien-3β-ol
5,22-Ergostadien-3β-ol

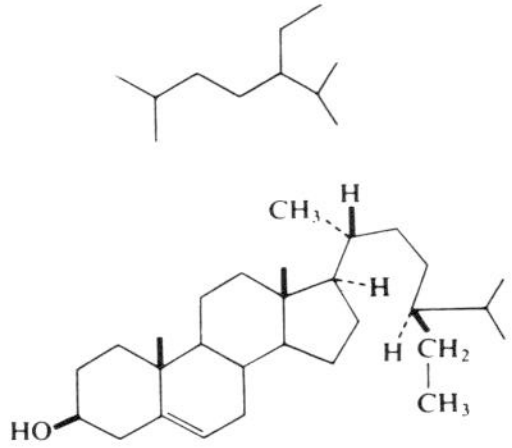

Clionasterol
γ-Sitosterol
(24S)-24-Ethyl-5-cholesten-3β-ol

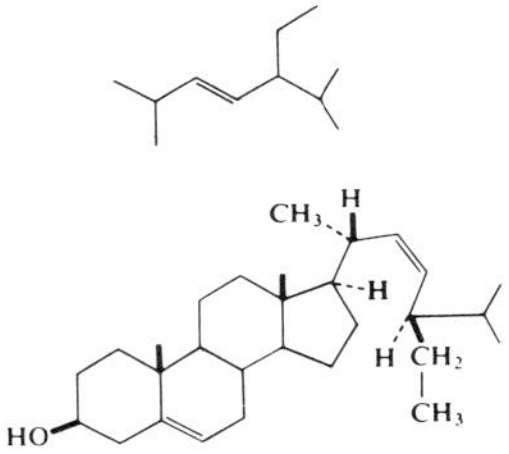

Poriferasterol
(24S)-24-Ethyl-5,22-cholestadien-3β-ol

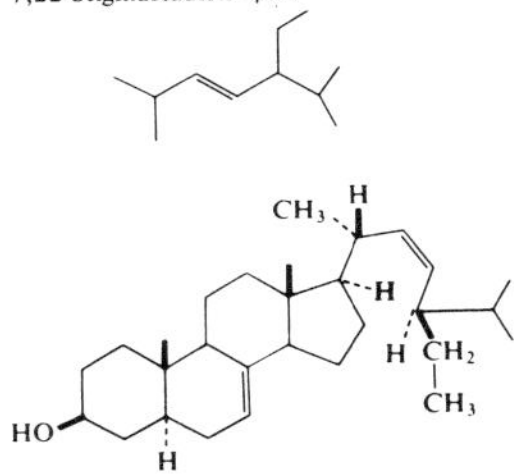

Chondrillasterol
(24S)-24-Ethyl-7,22,(5α)-cholestadien-3β-ol

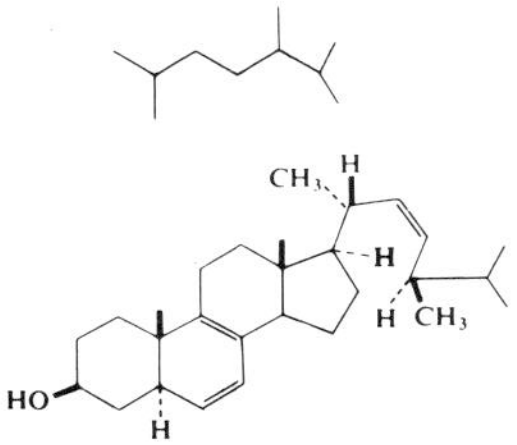

Fungisterol
(24S)-24-Methyl-6,8,22,(5α)-cholestatrien-3β-ol
6,8,22,(5α)-Ergostatrien-3β-ol

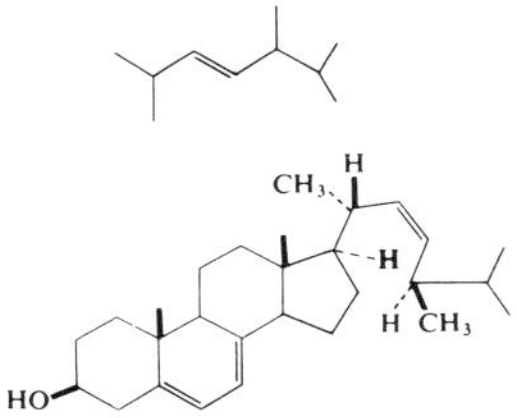

Ergosterol
(24S)-24-Methyl-5,7,22-cholestatrien-3β-ol
5,7,22-Ergostatrien-3β-ol

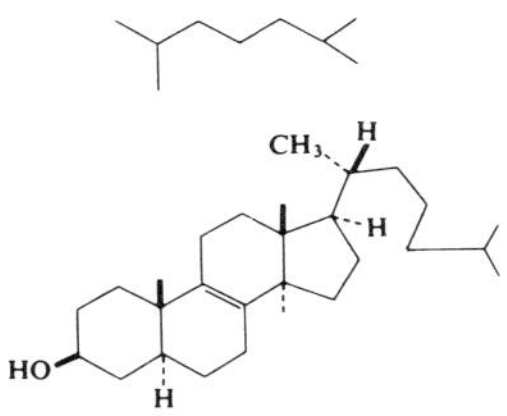

Macdougallin
14α-Methyl-8,(5α)-cholesten-3β-ol

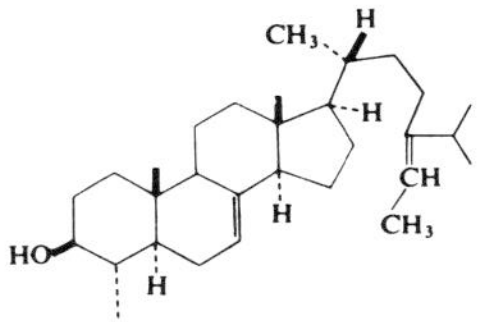

Citrostadienol
4α-Methyl-7-Z-24(28),(5α)-stigmastadien-3β-ol

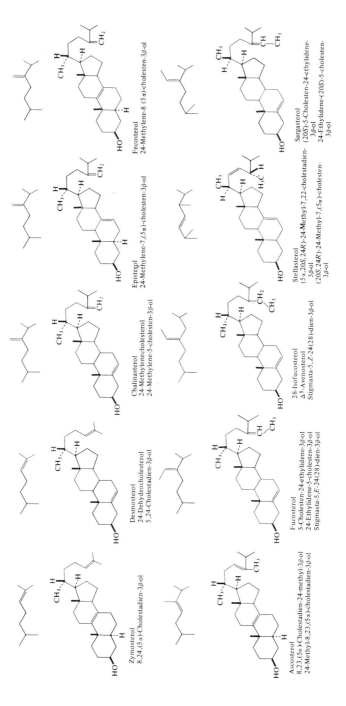

Fig. 10.2. Some naturally occurring derivatives of cholesterol and 20-epicholesterol.

isomeric spinasterols have been isolated from spinach or alfalfa, e.g. α-spina-sterol. The major sources of stigmasterol are the calabar bean and soya bean oil. Stigmasterol is important as a precursor for the synthesis of progesterone in commercial quantities. Two less common phytosterols which occur in rapeseed oil are brassicasterol and campesterol. Macdougallin is a 14α-methyl sterol isolated from the Mexican cactus, *Peniocereus macdougallii*.

Recently 28-isofucosterol (Fig. 10.2) has been isolated from higher plants, e.g. oat seeds. This compound is different from the fucosterol found in marine algae in the configuration of the ethylidene side chain. Full stereochemical description of fucosterol and 28-isofucosterol requires the introduction of another system of nomenclature which was introduced by the Chemical Abstracts Service in 1968. This applies to the completely general situation represented by a pair of doubly bound atoms A and B, and their nearest neighbours, 1, 2 and 3, 4 respectively. Since the molecular configuration of this system is such that all of the atoms lie in the same plane, P, the necessary and

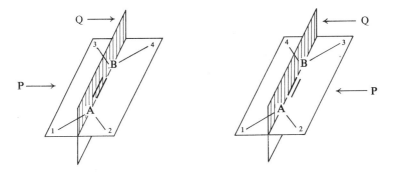

sufficient condition for stereoisomerism is that the atoms or groups attached to A (1 and 2) and B (3 and 4), respectively, be unequal. Thus the two possible configurations shown can be differentiated by indicating that groups 1 and 3 are on the same or the opposite side of the reference plane Q. The rules for specifying these configurational differences are that it is first necessary to determine which of the two groups attached to each of the doubly bound atoms has the higher priority according to the Sequence Rule system of nomenclature. Then that configuration in which the two groups of higher priority are on the *same* side of the reference plane is assigned the stereochemical descriptor Z (German: zusammen) while that configuration in which these groups are on *opposite* sides is assigned the descriptor E (German: entgegen). Other plant sterols, besides 28-isofucosterol, which have been identified as belonging to the Z series are Δ^7-avenosterol (stigmasta-7,Z-24(28)-dien-3β-ol) and citrostadienol (α-or α_1-sitosterol or 4α-methyl-5α-stigmasta-7, Z-24(28)-dien-3β-ol).

The most common yeast sterols are ergosterol and zymosterol. Minor sterols are ascosterol, fecosterol and fungisterol. Cholesterol, the characteristic mammalian sterol, is also present in small amounts in higher plants and is the major sterol in some red algae. The function of these C-28 and C-29 sterols appears to be the same as in animals, i.e. they form part of the structure of cell membranes. Sterols are also required for the sexual phase of some fungi and are required as growth factors for some micro-organisms.

B. BIOSYNTHESIS

There is no reason to suppose that the mechanisms of squalene biosynthesis in plants differ from those in animals, but later stages have been shown to be different. Mevalonic kinase, the first enzyme in the sequence from mevalonate to squalene has been demonstrated in a number of plants. Degradation of eburicoic acid and the biosynthesis of ergosterol from ^{14}C-acetate reveals that the labelling pattern of the side chain is the same as that of cholesterol, but that the extra methylene or methyl group does not arise from acetate. Incubation with ^{14}C-formate gives a label specifically at C-28 in both eburicoic acid and ergosterol. S-Adenosylmethionine is probably the intermediate methyl donor. It has been suggested that the alkylation mechanism is that a Δ^{24}-steroid intermediate is methylated to give a carbonium ion which may be stabilized by

the addition of a hydride ion to give a 24-methyl steroid, or by the loss of proton from the introduced methyl group, a 24-methylene steroid. In the latter case a second transmethylation will produce a further carbonium ion, which can then give either a 24-ethyl or a 24-ethylidene steroid.

It is believed that 24-ethyl steroids can also arise by the reduction of 24-ethylidene steroids, and 24-methyl steroids by the reduction of 24-methylene steroids. The 24-ethyl steroids of higher plants and marine invertebrates appear to arise from isomeric ethylidene steroids, e.g. fucosterol is a precursor of clionasterol while 28-isofucosterol is a precursor of β-sitosterol. Details of the introduction of the *trans* double bond at C-22 into sterols such as ergosterol and stigmasterol have not yet been elucidated.

There have been few reports of lanosterol in higher plants and evidence is now available which indicates that lanosterol may not play such an important role in sterol biosynthesis in plants. More frequently, cycloartenol has been

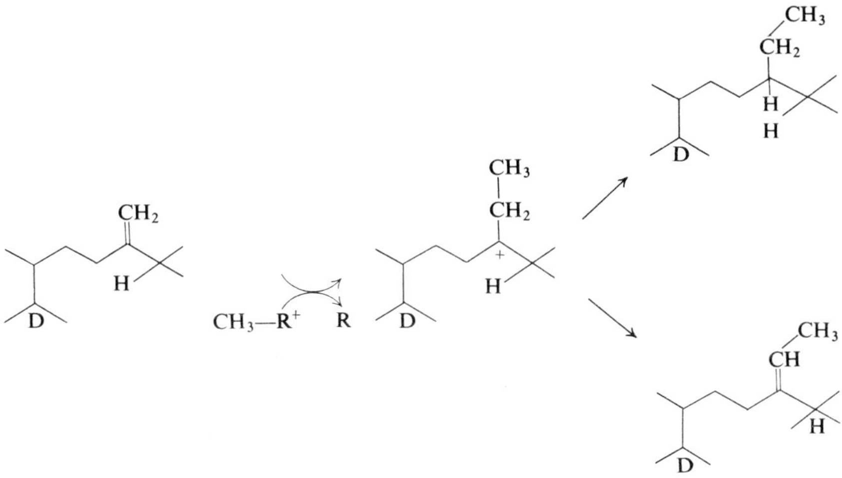

CH_3
CH_2
H
H
D

CH_3
CH_2

CH_2
H
H
D
CH_3—R^+ R   D
+
H

CH_3
CH
H
D

isolated and it is probable that this is the cyclization product of squalene epoxide in the higher plants. Lanosterol is produced by the cyclization of a chair-boat-chair-boat folded squalene chain followed by rearrangements. A series of hydrogen and methyl migrations with proton loss from C-9 gives lanosterol, but if the hydrogen from C-9, instead of being lost, migrates to C-8 and a 9β, 19-cyclopropane ring is formed with loss of a proton from C-19, cycloartenol is formed (Fig. 10.3). It would appear that there are two pathways of sterol biosynthesis in plants, one via lanosterol and the other via cycloartenol. The formation of cycloartenol apparently requires the involvement of some non-bridged intermediate, since the migrating C-10 methyl group is on the same side of the molecule (*cis*) as the migrating C-9 hydrogen.

Alkylation is believed to occur at a late stage, e.g. lanosterol → desmosterol → 24-methylenecholesterol → 28-isofucosterol → β-sitosterol.

II. C-30 STEROLS

A. PARENT HYDROCARBONS

The cyclic C-30 compounds containing 6-isoprene units may be divided into the pentacyclic triterpenes proper, e.g. α-amyrin, which occurs together with β-amyrin as the acetates in the latex of rubber trees, and the tetracyclic triterpenes (trimethyl-steroids) which are derivatives of 5α-cholestane. This latter group may be further divided according to the structure of the C/D ring fusion and of the conformation at C-17 and C-20. The three additional methyl groups in the trimethyl-steroids are numbered 30 (attached to C-4 with α-configuration), 31 (attached to C-4 with β-configuration) and 32 (attached to C-14).

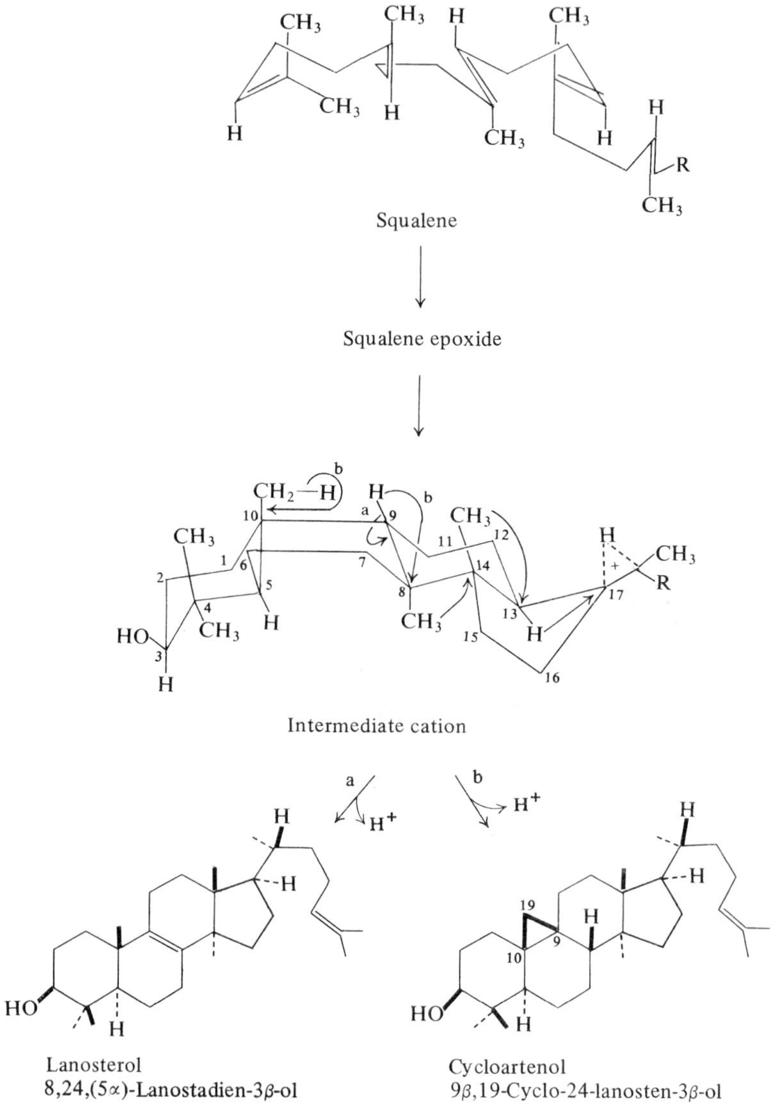

Fig. 10.3. Cyclization of squalene to lanosterol or cycloartenol.

Figure 10.4 shows the parent hydrocarbons of the naturally occurring C-30 trimethyl-steroids. The configurations in 5α-lanostane are the same as in

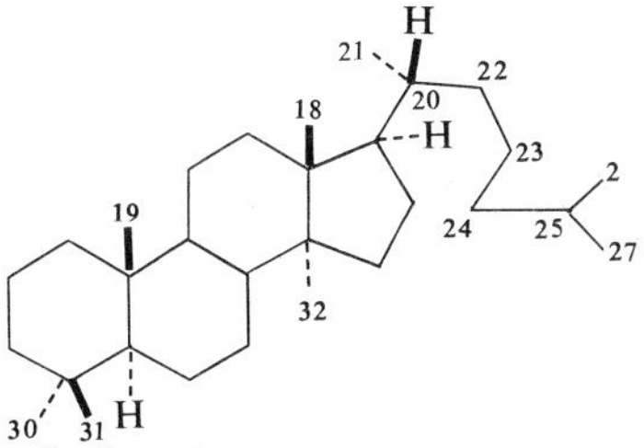

5α-Lanostane
4,4,14α-Trimethyl-5α-cholestane
(14α,20R implied in the name)

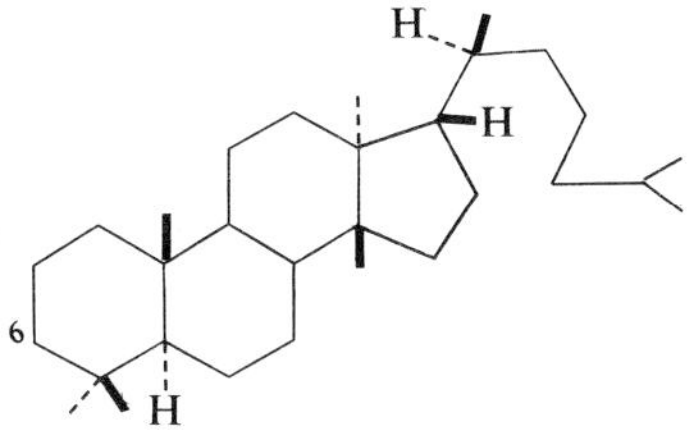

5α-Tirucallane
5α,13α,14β,17α,20S-Lanostane

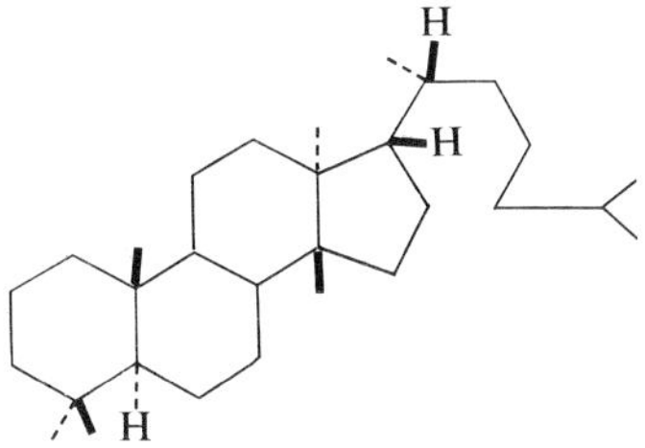

5α-Euphane
5α,13α14β,17α-Lanostane
(20R implied in the name)

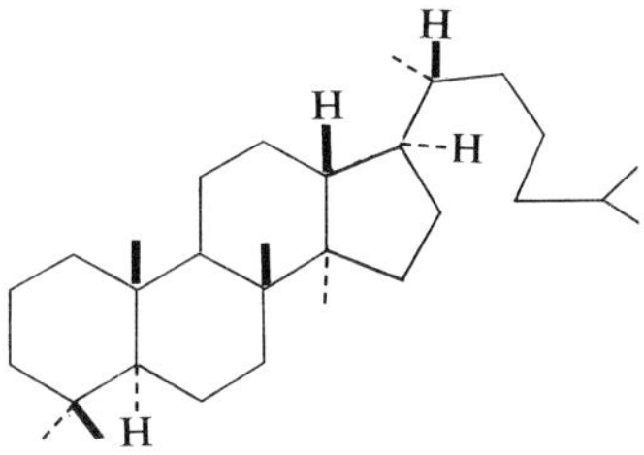

5α-Dammarane
8-Methyl-18-nor-5α-lanostane
(all configurations except 5α implied in the name)

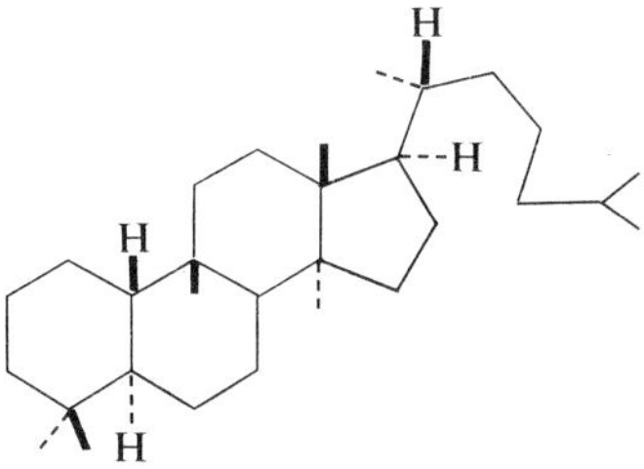

5α-Cucurbitane
19(10-9β)-abeo-5α-Lanostane

Fig. 10.4. Parent hydrocarbons of the trimethyl-steroids.

cholestane and 5α-lanostane is 4,4,14α-trimethyl-5α-cholestane. In 5α-tirucallane and 5α-euphane the C/D ring fusions are *cis* which reverses the configurations of the substituents at C-13 and C-14. In both cases the side chain at C-17 is inserted in the α-configuration but the configuration at C-20 differs. Two additional parent hydrocarbons are 5α-dammarane, which is 8-methyl-18-nor-5α-lanostane, and 5α-cucurbitane, which is 19(10-9β)-*abeo*-5α-lanostane, i.e. there is a β-hydrogen atom at C-10 and a β-methyl group at C-9. The *abeo* system of nomenclature is used for bond migrations. It has recently been discovered that ring A of the 4,4-dimethyl-3-oxo-Δ^5-steroids exists in a conformational equilibrium with a boat and chair ratio of about 4:1, while ring A in the 4,4-dimethyl-3-oxo-5α-steroids is a flattened chair. These conformational effects are due to non-bonded interactions between the axial β-methyl substituents at C-4 and C-10 in the chair conformation of ring A.

B. TRITERPENES

Acyclic squalene was originally isolated from the liver oil of sharks but was later found to occur in other fish oils and animal products, e.g. ovarian dermoid cysts, human ear wax and sebum; it has also been found in vegetable oils and fungi. A related triterpene is ambrein, which is found in ambergris and is used in the perfume industry. Onocerin is obtained from *Onosis spinosa* and is of interest as a product of incomplete cyclization of squalene. It is believed that variations in the cyclization of squalene account for the different types of steroid triterpenes of the lanostane, euphane, tirucallane, dammarane, etc. series.

The true triterpenes can be divided into the hydropicene type and the lupane type. The former are derived from a hydropicene substituted with eight methyl groups and the parent hydrocarbons are α- and β-amyrane. The latter are derived from a cyclopentenobenzophenanthrene ring system and lupane is a parent hydrocarbon.

Of the true triterpenes related to β-amyrin, 18β-glycyrrhetic acid (enoxolone) and its water soluble derivative, carbenoxolone, are important as anti-inflammatory compounds and have been employed in Addison's disease and rheumatoid arthritis because of their cortisone-like effects. Large doses are required and cortisone is more reliable. Glycyrrhetinic acid (Fig. 10.5) occurs conjugated with two molecules of glucuronic acid as glycyrrhizic acid, which constitutes some 6-14% of the dried rhizome and roots of the liquorice plant, *Glycyrrhiza glabra*. Liquorice is a demulcent and mild expectorant. Extracts are used in cough lozenges and pastilles and in cough syrups. It is also used as a flavouring agent to disguise the taste of bitter medicines. Unlike cortisone, glycyrrhetinic acid gives symptomatic relief of peptic ulcer pain and there have been numerous claims that it causes peptic ulcers to heal. Again large doses are needed, e.g. 20-25 g of liquorice extract a day for 6 weeks in conjunction with a salt-limited diet. In large doses it may cause salt and water retention leading to hypertension and severe electrolyte imbalance.

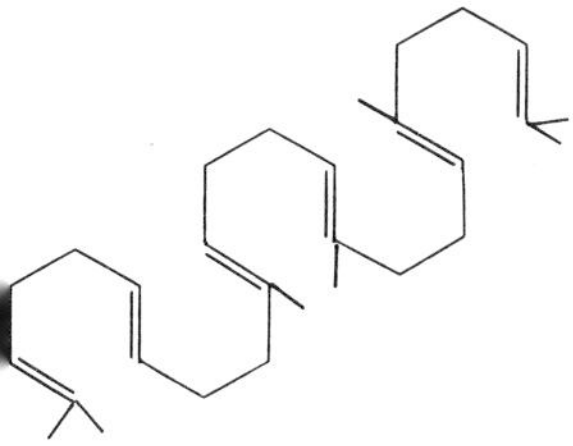

Squalene

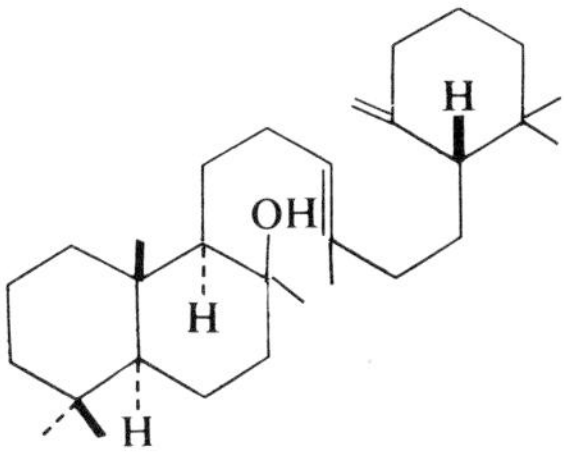

Ambrein

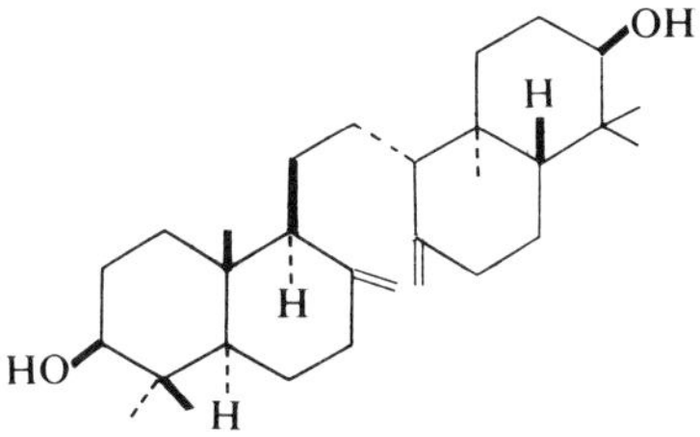

Onocerin

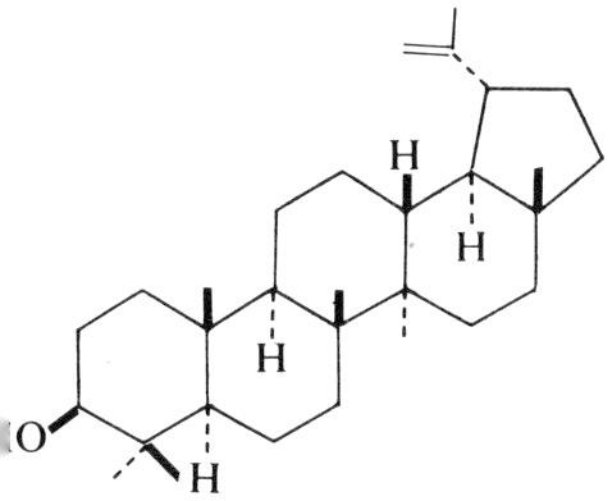

Lupeol

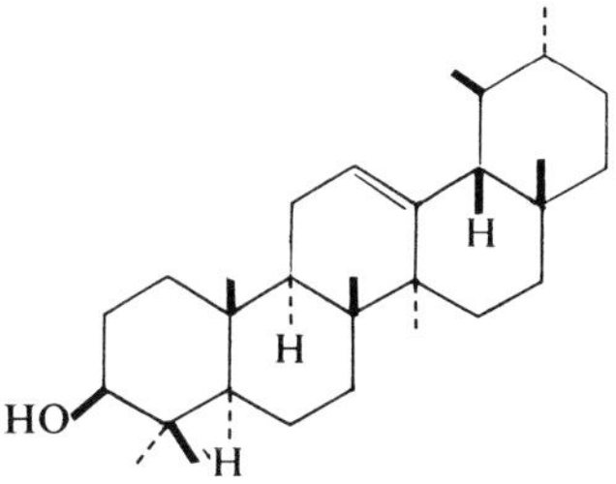

α-Amyrin

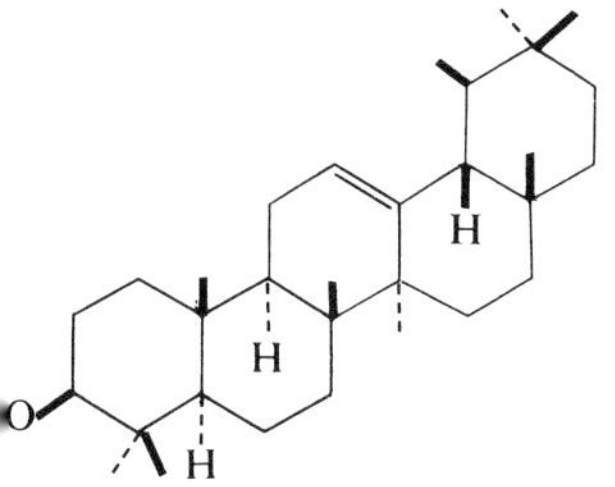

β-Amyrin
18β-Oleanane

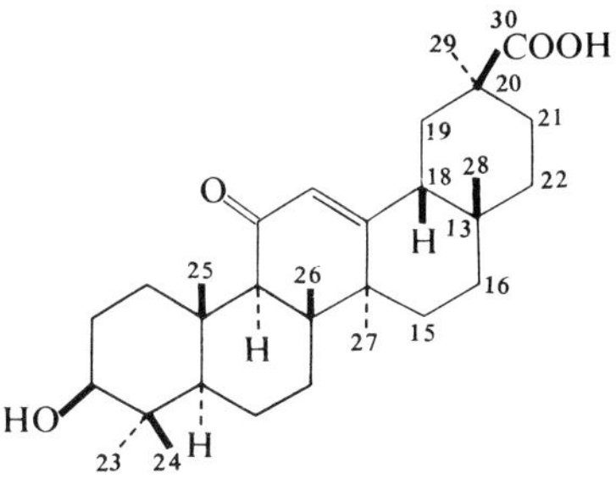

18β-Glycyrrhetic acid, Glycyrrhetinic acid
Enoxolone
3β-Hydroxy-11-oxo-18β-olean-12-en-30-
oic acid

Fig. 10.5. Some non-steroidal triterpenes.

C. LANOSTANES

Lanosterol is the principal constituent of the unsaponifiable fraction of wool fat, which also contains a number of other C-30 steroids. One of the most abundant is agnosterol (Fig. 10.6) and other important compounds are the 24,25 dihydro-derivatives of lanosterol and agnosterol. After saponification, some 53 lb of wool fat yields about 37 lb of fatty acids, 4 lb cholesterol, 14 lb oil and 9 lb of wax of which the major component is lanosterol. Other members of the lanostane series have been isolated from several species of wood rotting fungi, e.g. eburicoic acid and polyporenic acid A both of which are C-31 compounds.

In the sea cucumbers (family *Holothuriodeae*) (marine invertebrates) have been found a number of steroids with a lactone ring between C-18 and C-20 which have been designated as holothurinogenins. Recently these compounds have been found to have the same configuration as lanostane, with the exception that the configuration at C-20 remains unknown.

Griseogenin   Seychellogenin

D. EUPHANES AND TIRUCALLANES

Euphol and its 20α-methyl epimer, tirucallol, were isolated from a commercial resin (latex) from species of Euphorbia. Elemolic acid occurs in elemi resin from Manila. These resin compounds are very interesting stereochemically but nothing is known about their function (Fig. 10.7). Dammarane derivatives occur in dammar resin, also from species of Euphorbia.

III. CARDENOLIDES, CARDIAC GLYCOSIDES

A. OCCURRENCE AND STRUCTURE

A large number of plant extracts containing cardiac glycosides have been used by the natives in certain parts of the world as arrow poisons. The preparations most commonly used today are obtained from digitalis, strophanthus and squill (sea onion). Official digitalis is the dried leaf of the common purple foxglove, *Digitalis purpura*. The seeds and leaves of a white flowered variety, *Digitalis lanata*, are widely used in Europe and for commercial production of derivatives

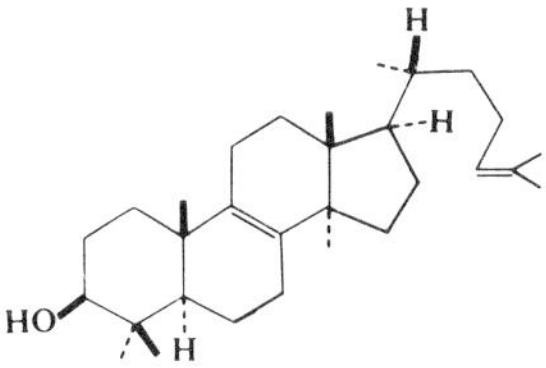

Lanosterol
8,24,(5α)-Lanostadien-3β-ol
4,4,14α-Trimethyl-8,24,(5α)-
cholestadien-3β-ol
(from wool fat)

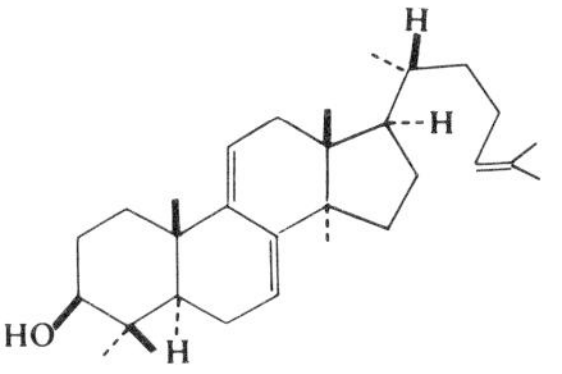

Agnosterol
7,9(11),24,(5α)-Lanostatrien-3β-ol
4,4,14α-Trimethyl-7,9(11),24,(5α)-
cholestatrien-3β-ol
(from wool fat)

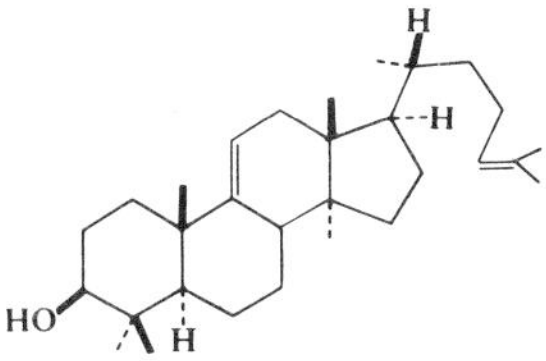

Parkeol
9(11),24,(5α)-Lanostadien-3β-ol
4,4,14α-Trimethyl-9(11),24,(5α)-
cholestadien-3β-ol
(from shea nut fat)

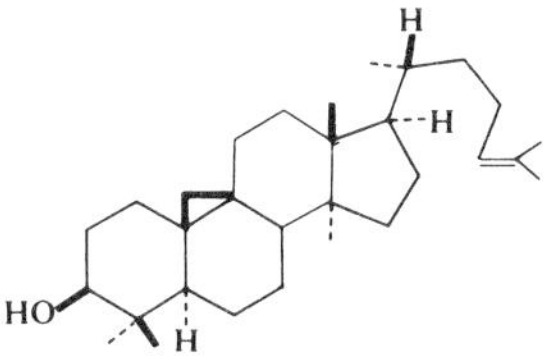

Cycloartenol
9β,19-Cyclo-24-lanosten-3β-ol
24-Cycloarten-3β-ol
(from *Artocarpus integrifolia*)

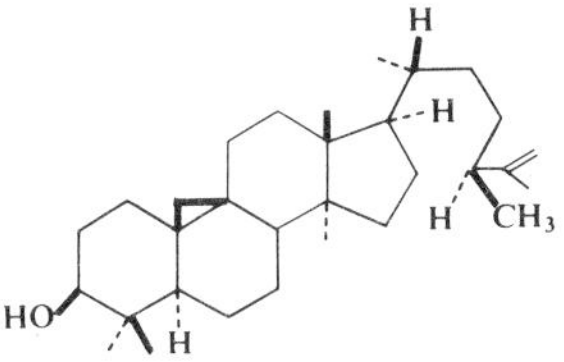

Cyclolaudenol
(24S)-24-Methyl-9β,19-cyclo-5α-lanost-
25(26)-en-3β-ol
4,4,14α-Trimethyl-9β,19-cyclo-25(26),
(5α)-ergosten-3β-ol
(24S)-24-Methyl-25,(5α)-cycloarten-3β-ol
(from opium)

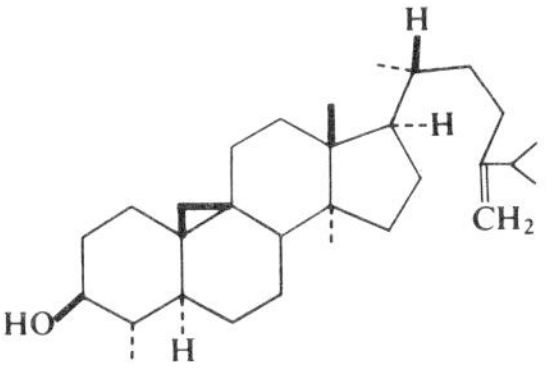

Cycloeucalenol
4α,14α-Dimethyl-24-methylene-9β,19-
cyclo-5α-cholestan-3β-ol
24-Methylene-31-nor-5α-cycloartan-3β-ol
(from Australian tallow wood)

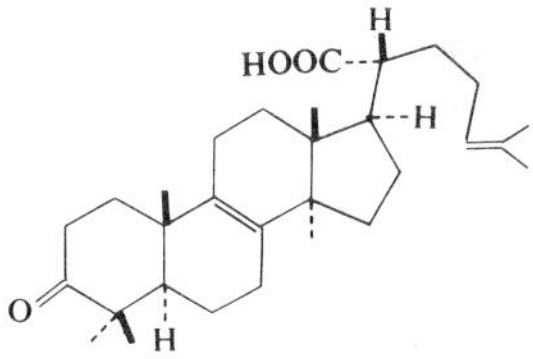

Pinicolic acid A
3-Oxo-4,14α-trimethyl-8,24,(5α)-
cholestadien-21-oic acid
8,24,(5α)-Lanostadien-3-one-21-oic acid
(from the fungus *Polyporus pinicola*)

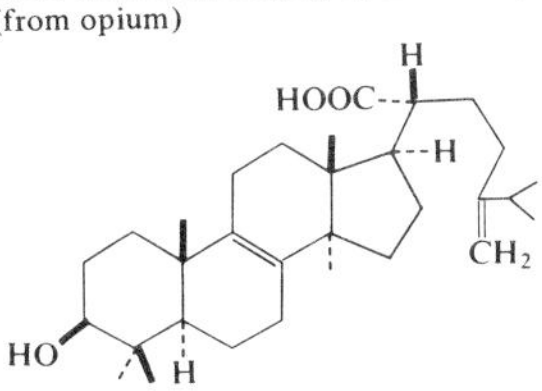

Eburicoic acid
3β-Hydroxy-4,4,14α-trimethyl-8,24(28),
(5α)-ergostadien-21-oic acid
24-Methylene-8,(5α)-lanosten-3β-ol-21-
oic acid
(from several species of fungi)

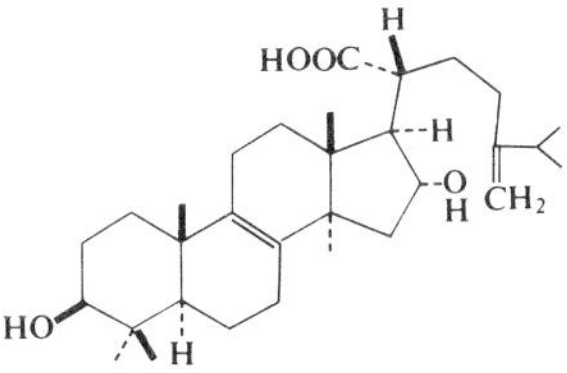

Tumulosic acid
16α-Hydroxyeburicoic acid
24-Methylene-8,(5α)-lanosten-3β,16α,diol-
21-oic acid
(from the fungus *Polyporus tumulosus*)

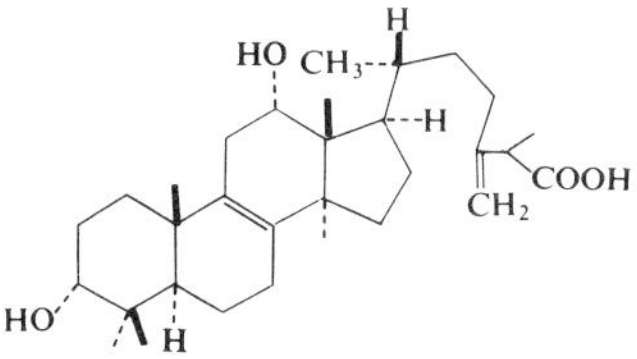

Polyporenic acid A
Ungulinic acid
3α,12α-Dihydroxy-8,24(28), (5α)-
ergostadien-27-oic acid
24-Methylene-8,(5α)-lanosten-3α
12α-diol-27-oic acid
(from the fungus *Polyporus betulinus*)

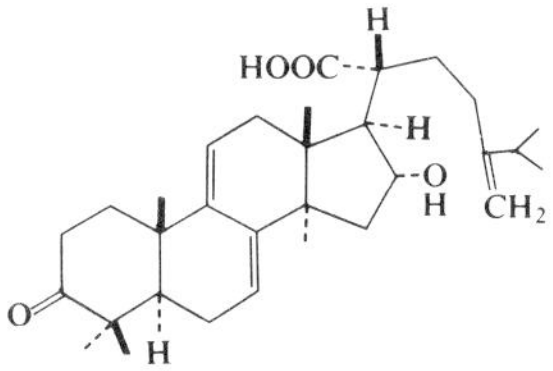

Polyporenic acid C
16α-Hydroxy-3-oxo-4,4,14α-trimethyl-
7,9(11),24(28),(5α)-ergostatrien-21-oic
acid
24-Methylene-7,9(11),(5α)-lanostadien-
16α-ol-3-one-21-oic acid
(from the fungus *Polyporus betulinus*)

Fig. 10.6. Some naturally occurring derivatives of lanostane.

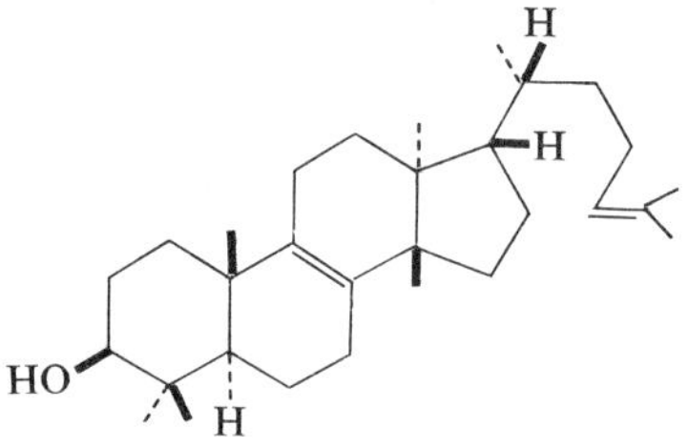

Euphol
8,24,(5α)-Euphadien-3β-ol
4,4,14β-Trimethyl-5α,13α,14β,17α-
cholesta-8,24-dien-3β-ol
(from dried *Euphorbia* latex)

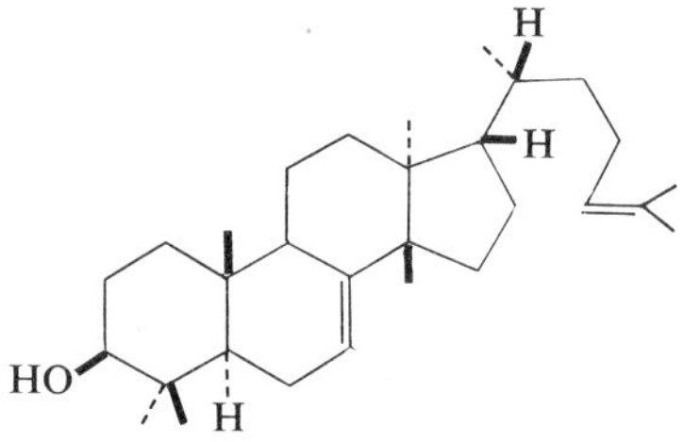

Butyrospermol
Basseol
7,24,(5α)-Euphadien-3β-ol
(from the nut fat of the shea tree,
Butyrospermum parkii)

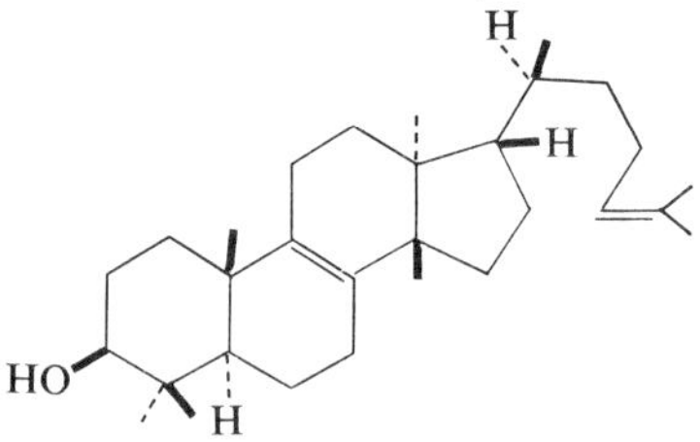

Tirucallol
8,24,(5α)-Tirulcalladien-3β-ol
(from the resins of *Euphorbia tirucalli*
and *E. triangularis*)

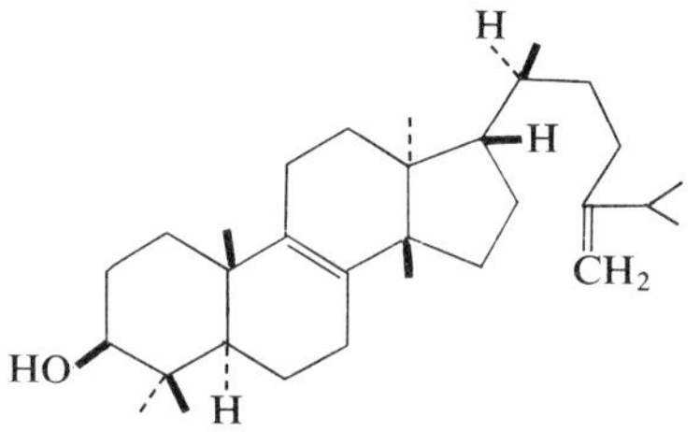

Euphorbol
4,4,14β-Trimethyl-5α,13α,14β,17α,20-*iso*-
ergosta-8,24(28)-dien-3β-ol
24-Methylene-8,(5α)-tirucallen-3β-ol
(from *Euphorbia* resins)

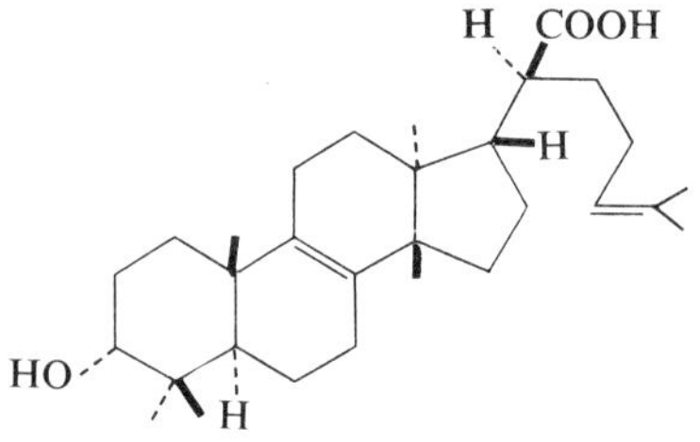

Elemolic acid
3α-Hydroxy-4,4,14β-trimethyl-5α,13α,14β,
17αcholesta-8,24-dien-21-oic acid
8,24,(5α)-Tirucalladien-3β-ol-21-oic acid
(from elemi resin, from Manila)

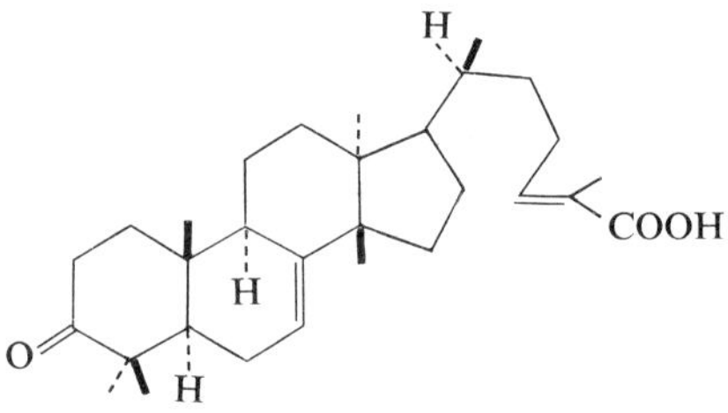

Masticadienoic acid
3-Oxo-4,4,14β-trimethyl-5α,13α,14β,17α,
cholesta-7,24-dien-26-oic acid
7,24,(5α)-Tirucalladien-3-one-26-oic acid
(from gum mastic)

Fig. 10.7. Some naturally occurring derivatives of euphane and tirucallane.

Plant source	Precursor glycoside in plant	Split off by enzymic or mild alkaline hydrolysis	Cardiac glycoside extracted	Split off by acid hydrolysis	Aglycone or genin
D. purpurea leaf	Purpurea glycoside A	Glucose	Digitoxin	3 mols. Digitoxose	Digitoxigenin
	Purpurea glycoside B	Glucose	Gitoxin	3 mols. Digitoxose	Gitoxigenin
Digitalis					
D. lanlata leaf	Lantoside A	Glucose and acetyl	Digitoxin	3 mols. Digitoxose	Digitoxigenin
	Lantoside B	Glucose and acetyl	Gitoxin	3 mols. Digitoxose	Gitoxigenin
	Lantoside C	Glucose and acetyl	Digoxin	3 mols. Digitoxose	Digoxigenin
S. Kombé seeds	K-strophanthoside	Glucose	Strophanthin	Glucose and cymarose	Strophanthidin
	K-strophanthoside	2 mols. Glucose	Cymarin	Cymarose	Strophanthidin
Strophanthus					
S. gratus seeds			Ouabain (G-strophanthin)	Rhamnose	Ouabagenin (G-strophanthidin)
Convellaria majalis Lily of the Valley, leaves and flowers			Convallotoxin	Rhamnose	Strophanthidin
Nerium oleander Oleander			Oleandrin	Oleandrose	Oleandrigenin
Uzara root			Uzarin	2 mols. Glucose	Urzarigenin
Strophanthus sarmentosus seeds			Sarmentocymarin	Sarmentose	Sarmentogenin

in the USA. It gives a higher yield of glycosides (about 0.2-0.3% of dry weight). The drug strophanthus is obtained from the seeds of *Strophanthus gratus* and was long used as an arrow poison. Squill is the dried fleshy pulp of the sea onion and comes from *Urginea (Scilla) maritima* which belongs to the lily family (Table 10.2). Many other cardenolides are known but have not found a medicinal use (Table 10.3).

Table 10.3. *Some naturally occurring cardenolide aglycones*

Derivatives of 3β,14-Dihydroxy-20(22),(5β,14β)-cardenolide

Digitoxigenin					
Acovenosigenin	1β-ol				
Gitoxigenin		16β-ol			
Gitaloxigenin		16β-formoxy			
Oleandrigenin		16β-acetoxy			
Cannogenin			19-one		
Sarmentogenin				11α-ol	
Sarmutogenin				11-one,12β-ol	
Caudogenin				11-one,12α-ol	
Sinogenin				11α-ol,12-one	
Decogenin				11-one,12-one	
Saverogenin				11α-ol,12-one,7α,15α-epoxide	
Leptogenin				11-one,12β-ol, 7α,15α-epoxide	
Inertogenin				11-one,12α-ol, 7α,15α-epoxide	
Chryseogenin				11-one,12-one,7α,15α-epoxide	
Tanghinigenin				7α,15α-epoxide	
Periplogenin		5β-ol			
Strophanthidin		5β-ol	19-one		
Bipindogenin		5β-ol		11α-ol	
Sarmentologenin		5β-ol	19-ol	11α-ol	
Ouabegenin	1β-ol	5β-ol	19-ol	11α-ol	
Antiarigenin		5β-ol	19-one		12β-ol
Adynerigenin		16β-ol	8(14)-ene		
Neriantogenin		16β-ol	14-ene		

Derivatives of 3β,14-Dihydroxy-20(22),(5α,14β)-cardenolide

Uzarigenin	
Corotoxigenin	19-one
Coroglaucigenin	19-ol

The active constituents of these drugs are glycosides but they are usually found in association with saponins of similar structure. Each glycoside is a combination of aglycone or genin together with one to four molecules of sugar.

The pharmacological activity lies in the aglycone. The sugars are thought to confer water solubility and cell permeability, and are important in determining the relative potency of the aglycone.

Some twenty sugars have been isolated as hydrolysis products of the plant heart poisons, but only D-glucose, L-rhamnose and D-fucose have been isolated from other plant sources. Eleven of the sugars are 3-methyl-ethers and eight are

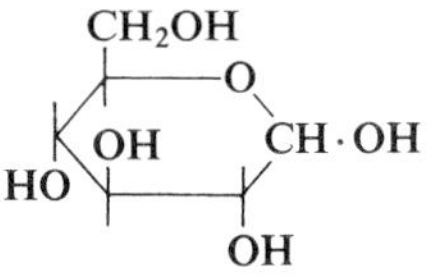

D-Glucose

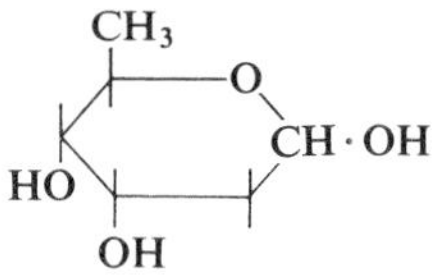

D-Digitoxose
2,6-Dideoxy-D-ribohexose

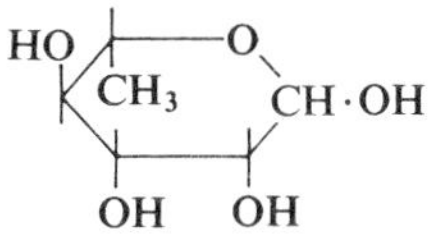

L-Rhamnose

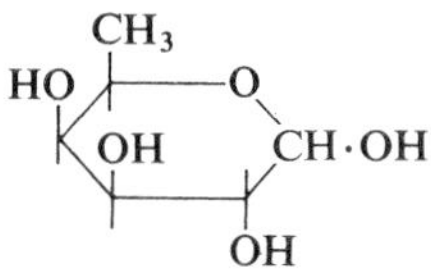

D-Fucose

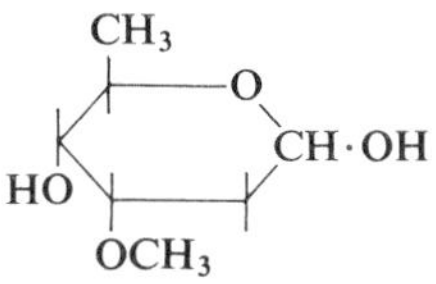

D-Cymarose
3-O-Methyl-D-digitoxose
2,6-Dideoxy-3-methoxyaldohexose

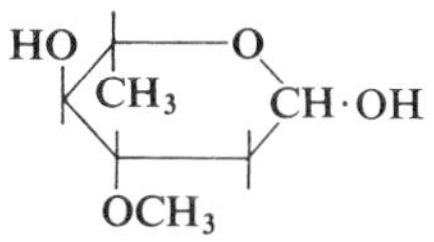

L-Oleandrose

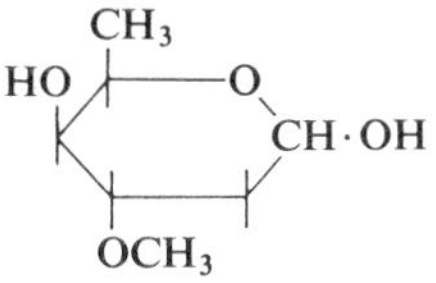

D-Sarmentose
2-Deoxy-hexomethylose

Digilanidobiose   = 4-O-β-D-Glucopyranosyl-D-digitoxose
Strophanthobiose = 4-O-β-D-Glucopyranosyl-D-cymarose
Scillabiose   = 4-O-β-D-Glucopyranosyl-L-rhamnose

Fig. 10.8. Some glycosides isolated from the cardiac glycosides.

2,6-dideoxy-compounds (Fig. 10.8). These sugars form di-, tri- and tetra-saccharides which are all conjugated onto the 3β-hydroxyl group of the aglycone. All the D-sugars are joined by a β-glycosidic linkage and all the L-sugars by an α-glycosidic linkage. The conformational formula shows that the sugars are linked to the aglycone in the same steric sense in each series and that in the β-D series, the 6-methyl group is "up" while in the α-L-series it is "down". The 2-deoxy sugars have characteristically high reactivity and glycosides in which a 2-deoxy sugar is attached directly to the aglycone undergo mild acid hydrolysis very easily. When a 2-hydroxy sugar, e.g. glucose, rhamnose, digitalose, is attached directly to aglycone, fission can only be achieved under conditions of hydrolysis so drastic that tertiary hydroxyl groups in the aglycone are also eliminated. In these cases alcoholysis often proceeds more rapidly and more smoothly than hydrolysis, e.g. by standing for several days at 35°C in 2%

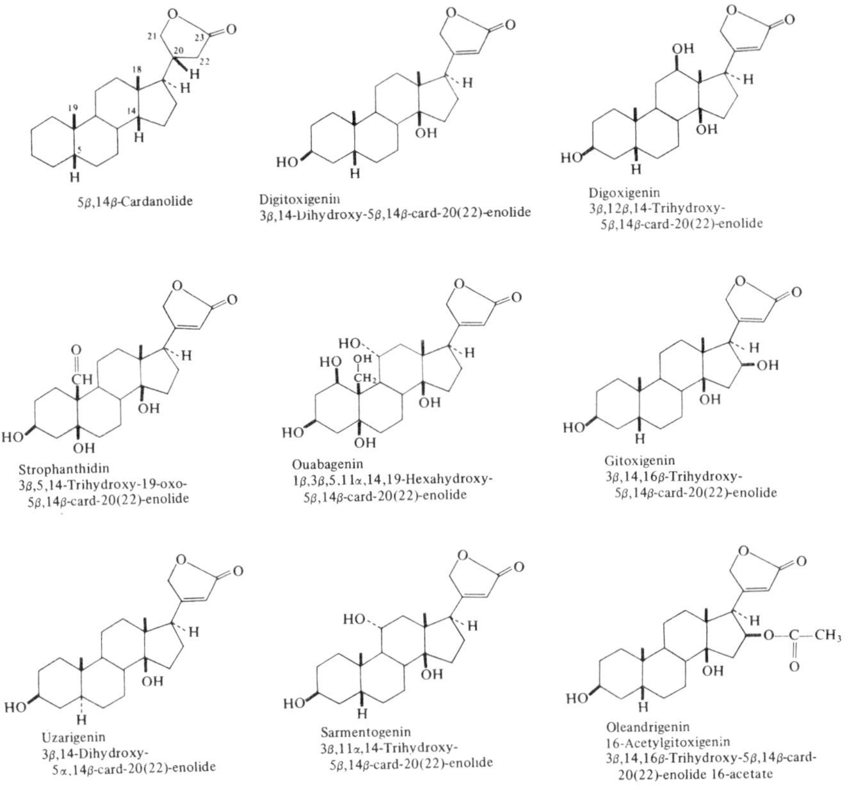

5β,14β-Cardanolide

Digitoxigenin
3β,14-Dihydroxy-5β,14β-card-20(22)-enolide

Digoxigenin
3β,12β,14-Trihydroxy-
5β,14β-card-20(22)-enolide

Strophanthidin
3β,5,14-Trihydroxy-19-oxo-
5β,14β-card-20(22)-enolide

Ouabagenin
1β,3β,5,11α,14,19-Hexahydroxy-
5β,14β-card-20(22)-enolide

Gitoxigenin
3β,14,16β-Trihydroxy-
5β,14β-card-20(22)-enolide

Uzarigenin
3β,14-Dihydroxy-
5α,14β-card-20(22)-enolide

Sarmentogenin
3β,11α-Trihydroxy-
5β,14β-card-20(22)-enolide

Oleandrigenin
16-Acetylgitoxigenin
3β,14,16β-Trihydroxy-5β,14β-card-
20(22)-enolide 16-acetate

Fig. 10.9. Some genins of the cardiac glycosides.

methanolic HCl. Seeds and leaves containing native glycosides also contain enzymes capable of hydrolysing glucose units, but enzymes capable of cleaving linkages bridging rare sugars to one another or to the aglycone appear to be absent. Extraction methods do not usually inhibit these enzymes.

The nomenclature of the cardiac glycosides is based on the fully saturated 5β-cardanolide whose Fischer projection is shown in Fig. 10.9. The configuration at C-20 is the same as in cholesterol, i.e. 20R. Since the highest number is at the top, the usual Fischer projection has been rotated in the plane of the paper through 180°. Names such as "20 (22)-cardenolide" are used for the naturally occurring unsaturated lactones. The names "14,21-" and "16,21-epoxy-cardanolide" are used for the compounds containing a 14,21- or a 16,21-oxygen bridge respectively. The configuration at C-14 should always be stated. As far as is known all the aglycones produce the same type of cardiac effect. The formulae of the most important genins are shown in Fig. 10.9. Hydroxyl groups at 3β and 14β are essential for action. Saturation of the lactone ring reduces activity by at least ten-fold and increases the speed of development of cardiac actions. Uzarigenin glycosides have a very weak action, probably due to the *trans* A/B ring junction which makes the ring system flat as in the allo series of corticosteroids. Digitalis preparations are the ones used medically most often. Strophanthin-K is sometimes used in emergencies as it is absorbed more rapidly than digitalis and is less cumulative. It is usually given intravenously when it acts in 5-15 min and the effect lasts for about 12 h. Semi-synthetic genins are now available and are often preferred because of their uniform potency, e.g. acetyl-digitoxin, acetyl-strophanthidin.

Sarmentogenin is a rare cardenolide in that it has a hydroxyl group at C-11 and at one time there were great hopes that this compound would become a commercially important precursor of cortisone drugs but the identity of the plant source was not clear. Large expeditions were dispatched to Africa by the major drug companies to obtain specimens of as many *Strophanthus* species as possible. It is now apparent that *S. sarmentous* is a polymorphic species showing some morphological differences and striking variations in the glycoside content. It has not yet been possible to obtain this cardenolide on a commercial scale.

B. PHARMACOLOGY

The main action of the cardiac aglycones is to increase the force of systolic myocardial contraction which results in increased cardiac output, decreased heart size, decreased venous blood pressure, decreased blood volume and diuresis which relieves edema. They are used chiefly in congestive heart failure and the best results are obtained in hypertensive or arteriosclerotic heart disease. The rate at which tension or force is developed is increased and the maximum force or tension generated is increased in spite of abbreviation of all phases of systole. The contractile process is not prolonged. In the normal heart the force of systolic contraction is under adrenergic neural control, in addition to a mechanism by which the heart adapts its work output to the load imposed upon it. At any given level of adrenergic influence, an increased end-diastolic pressure is accompanied by an increased work capacity of the muscle. In a failing heart, the work capacity of the ventricle at any given end-diastolic pressure is decreased. The resulting reduction of systolic ejection leads to an increased residual blood volume within the ventricles at the end of systole. If blood continues to enter the ventricle during diastole at the same rate, the end-diastolic pressure increases and the ventricles dilate. The heart compensates for diminished work capacity by progressive dilation. The cardiac aglycones reverse these changes. There is no significant alteration of cardiac output in people without latent or overt heart failure. They do not slow the cardiac rate in normal man but it commonly occurs in the treatment of congestive heart failure which is a secondary effect resulting from improved cardiac output. Cardiac aglycones have a pronounced effect on ventricular rate in atrial fibrillation and are indicated in most cases. Doses should be adjusted to maintain the ventricular rate in a range of 60-80/min at rest.

In congestive heart failure, there are two major causes of edema, namely the increase in hydrostatic pressure in the capillaries, which retards the reabsorption of extracellular fluid, and the reduction in renal blood flood and glomeruler filtration rate. In the latter, the reabsorption of sodium and water is increased. It is thought that decreased renal blood flow causes increased renin production, which causes increased angiotensin formation which stimulates aldosterone production and hence the increased reabsorption of sodium.

All preparations of cardiac glycosides cause toxic systems in too large doses, e.g. sickness, vomiting, giddiness, slow pulse, cold sweating leading to convulsions and death. Dosage must be carefully adjusted on an individual basis. The potency of plant extracts has to be biologically assayed to obtain reliable preparations of uniform action. The official USP assay method is by the fractional, intermittent, intravenous injection of suitable preparations into pigeons. The end point of the assay is death of the animals within an allotted time. It is designed to ensure uniformity in potency of different lots of the same kind of preparation and not for equalizing potency of the various purified glycosides because these have widely differing intestinal absorption rates, speeds of action and duration of effect. One "International Digitalis Unit" represents the potency of 0.1 g of the "International Digitalis Standard Powder". The BP assay method uses guinea pigs.

Many different preparations, mainly of digitalis, are available. The official tincture and powdered leaf forms were the preparations of choice for many years but acceptable purified products are now available. They are given orally whenever possible and absorption is sufficiently rapid to ensure beneficial cardiac effects in 2-6 h. With digitoxin, action starts in 0.5-2 h, reaches a maximum in 4-12 h and regresses for 2-3 days, all action being gone in 2-3 weeks. Digitalis tincture and powdered leaf behave similarly. The fastest action is achieved with intravenous oubain when the action starts in 3-10 min, reaches a maximum in 0.5-2 h, regresses for 8-12 h and is finished in 1-3 days. The initial dose in patients not having received a digitalis preparation is about 12 USP units given in divided doses every 6-8 h for 12-24 h and represents about 1.0-1.5 mg digitoxin USP given orally. Thenceforth the oral daily maintenancy dose is 0.05-0.2 mg.

C. DIGITENOLIDES

The digitenolides occur in *Digitalis purpurea* and *D. lanata* and contain one or more of the rare sugars characteristic of the cardenolides. They are physiologically inactive. Some of the aglycones are shown in Fig. 10.10 and it is possible that these compounds are precursors of the cardenolides.

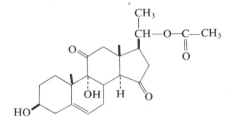

Diginigenin
12α.20α-Epoxy-11,15-dioxo-14β,17α-
pregn-5-en-3β-ol
5,(14β,17α)-Pregnen-3β-ol-11,15-
dione 12α,20α-epoxide

Digacetigenin
11,15-Dioxopregn-5-en-3β,9α,20α-triol
20-acetate
5-Pregnen-3β,9α,20α-triol-11,15
dione 20-acetate

Purprogenin
5-Pregnen-3β,14β,15α-triol-12,20-dione

Fig. 10.10. Some digitenolides.

IV. BUFADIENOLIDES, SCILLADIENOLIDES

A. OF PLANT ORIGIN

The bufadienolides (Table 10.4) are products of synthesis in both plants and animals. Their structure is based on 5β-bufanolide, where the configuration at C-20 is the same as in cholesterol. The configuration at C-14 must always be stated as an affix to the names of these compounds. Scillaren A is the glycoside

10*

of the white Squill or sea onion *Urginea maritima* bulb. It is extracted as the glycoside, scillaridin A, as a terminal glucose is removed by an enzyme present in the plant, leaving rhamnose attached at the 3β position to the genin. Isolation of the true genin, scillarenin (Fig. 10.11), requires the use of a rhamnosidase as mild acid hydrolysis produces the $\Delta^{3,5}$-diene, scillaridin A. Squill glycosides

Table 10.4. *Scilladienolide aglycones*

Derivatives of $3\beta,14$-dihydroxy-$5\beta,14\beta$-bufa-20,22-dienolide

Bufalin				
Bufotalin			16β-acetoxy	
Resibufogenin				14β,15β-epoxide
Cinobufagenin			16β-acetoxy	14β,15β-epoxide
Gammobufogenin	11α-ol			
Arenobufagin	11α-ol	12-one		
Scillarenin	4-ene			
Scillirosidin	4-ene		6β-ace-toxy	8β-ol
Scilliglaucosidin	4-ene			19-one
Telocinobufagin	5β-ol			
Hellebrigenin (Bufotalidin)	5β-ol			19-one
Marinobufagin	5β-ol			14β,15β-epoxide
Bufotalinin	5β-ol		19-one	14β,15β-epoxide
Cinobufotalin	5β-ol		16β-acetoxy	14β,15β-epoxide

Derivatives of $3\beta,14$-dihydroxy-$5\alpha,14\beta$-bufa-20,22-dienolide

Bovogenin A	19-one

have a digitalis-like action on the human heart but are rarely used as they are poorly absorbed from the gastro-intestinal tract. Squill has been used as an expectorant in chronic bronchitis. The white and red varieties of Squill differ so little in morphology that they are not distinguished in botanical classification but they differ markedly in the nature and physiological action of the native principles. Red squill possesses a high specific toxicity for rats and a powder prepared from dried red squills is widely used as a rat poison. Scillaroside is the chief glycoside and the median lethal dose for rats is 0.4-0.7 mg/kg whereas scillaren A from the white Squill is almost inactive. The genin is scillirosidin. Hellebrigenin is the aglycone of hellebrin which occurs as some 2% in the roots of the Christmas rose *Helleborus atrorubeus*.

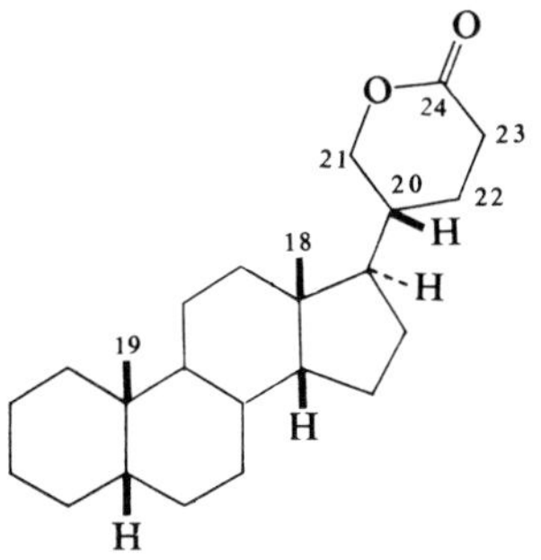

5β,14β-Bufanolide

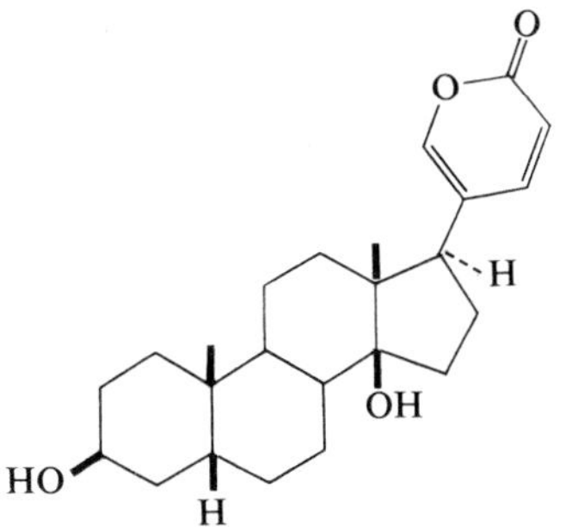

Bufalin
3β,14-Dihydroxy-5β,14β-bufa-20,22-
dienolide

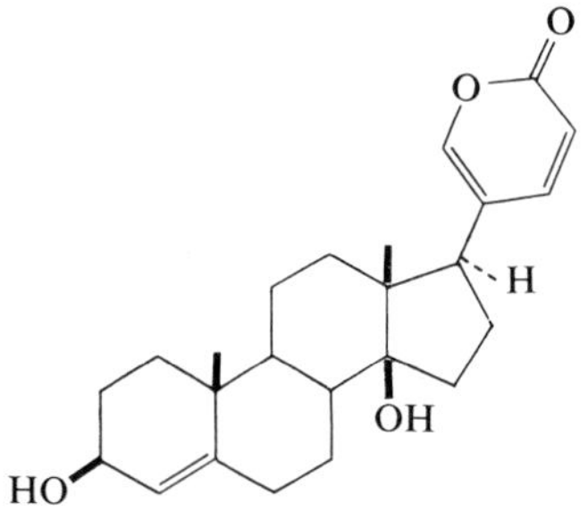

Scillarenin
3β,14-Dihydroxy-14β-bufa-4,20,22-
trienolide

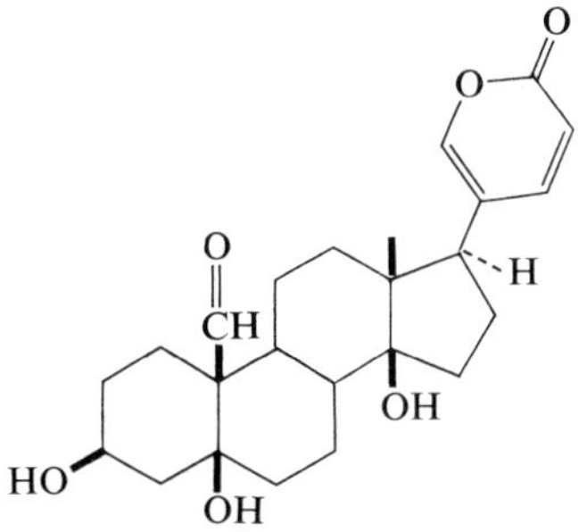

Hellebrigenin
Bufotalidin
3β,5,14-Trihydroxy-19-oxo-5β,14β-bufa-
20,22-dienolide

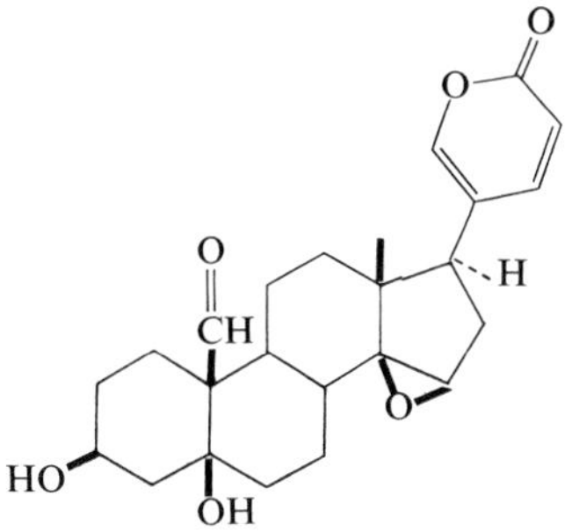

Bufotalinin
3β,5-Dihydroxy-19-oxo-14,15β-epoxy-
5β,14β-bufa-20,22-dienolide

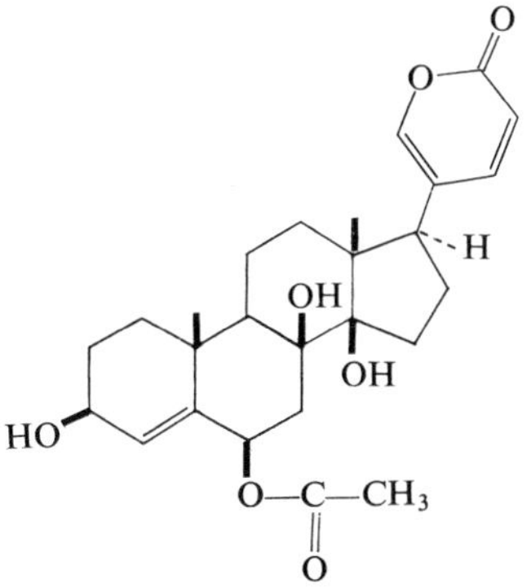

Scillirosidin
3β,6β,8β,14-Tetrahydroxy-5β,14β-bufa-
4,20,22-trienolide 6-acetate

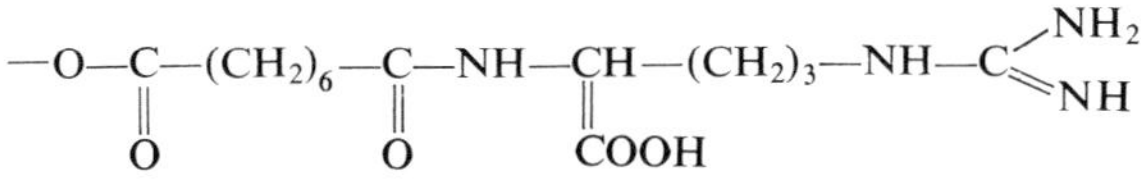

Suberylarginine

Fig. 10.11. Some bufadienolides (scilladienolides).

B. TOAD TOXINS

The venom of the toad has been known from antiquity. For centuries the Chinese have used a preparation from the local toad *Bufo bufo gargarizans* known as "Ch'an Su" as an external drug for the treatment of toothache, sinusitis, and haemorrhages of the gums. Toad venom has a digitalis-like action on the human heart and is highly lethal to mammals and frogs. The venom is located in skin glands, mostly in the parotid glands behind the eyes, whence it can be expressed without damage to the toad. The skin secretions of toads contain bufotoxins, which are the conjugated genins, the free steroid genins, cholesterol, sitosterols and occasionally ergosterol. Adrenalin is not always present but has sometimes been found in very large amounts. Bufotoxin is the principle toxin of the European toad *Bufo vulgaris* and is the 14β-suberyl-arginine ester of the genin bufotalin. The genin of the Chinese toad is bufogenin B which is desacetyl-bufotalin. The processing of dried toad skins usually takes several months of soaking in dilute alcohol and evaporating the extract. When water is added, the genin and the bufotoxin precipitate while the basic constituents remain in solution as salts. A single dried toad skin weighs about 15 g and yields 7-10 mg of genin. Bufotalin is the major constituent (6%) of the dried secretion of *B. vulgaris* but other bufotoxins are present, e.g. bufotalidin (which is identical with hellibrigenin). Garmabufotalin has been isolated from the skin of the Japanese toad.

V. STEROID SAPONINS, SPIROSTANOLS

A. HISTORY

Saponins are plant glycosides characterized by foaming in aqueous solution. The cardiac glycosides also have this property but are separated because of their distinct physiological activity. The saponins are haemolytic when injected into the blood stream of animals and are lethal. The plants have a bitter taste but are practically non-toxic to man when taken orally. They are lethal to fish when introduced into the water and have been used for this purpose by the natives of South America. They form oil-in-water emulsions and act as protective colloids. They have been used as detergents and foaming agents in fire extinguishers. Saponins occur as a combination of a sapogenin (the aglycone) and a glycoside. The aglycone may be either a steroid or a triterpene.

B. STRUCTURE

The structure of the steroid saponins is based on spirostanes of which there are several possible isomers. The name "spirostan" specifies the configurations for all the asymmetric centres except C-5 and C-25. In both the 5α- and

5β-spirostanes the configurations at C-17 and at C-20 are the same as in cholesterol, i.e. the H at C-17 and the CH_3 at C-20 are both α (i.e. 20R). This means that the furan ring, E, sticks up above the plane of the A, B, C, D ring structure and that the two bonds at C-22 are above and below the E ring, i.e. turned through 180° from the plane of the A, B, C, D ring system. If the configurations at C-16 and C-17 are different from those in cholesterol, they are designated as 16β (H) and 17β (H). The configuration at C-22 is implied as 22R unless otherwise stated and means that the C-23 carbon atom is joined to the C-22 carbon atom via that bond at C-22 which is below the E ring. When viewed in three dimensions from above the E ring, the spirostanes are seen as in Fig. 10.12. In the pyran F ring the oxygen atoms, C-26, C-24 and C-23, lie in one plane that is perpendicular to the plane of the paper. The broken line from C-22 to oxygen denotes that the oxygen atom and C-26 lie behind the plane of the paper. Whatever the conformation of ring F, C-27 and the 25-hydrogen atom both lie in the plane of the paper and so cannot be denoted by broken or thickened lines or designated α or β. All the furan E rings of the natural spirostanes have the 20S configuration and most are also (22R,25R)-5α-spirostanes, when the methyl group at C-25 is equatorial to the general plane of the F ring. A few natural spirostanes, e.g. sarsapogenin, are (20S,22R, 25S)-5β-spirostanes, when the methyl group at C-25 is axial to the general plane of the F ring. (The designations α_F, β_F or a, b or a_F, b_F referred to the Fischer convention and have now been superseded by the R and S designations.) The structures of some of the naturally occurring steroid sapogenins are shown in Fig. 10.13 and in Table 10.5.

Cleavage of the F ring of the spirostanes produces the corresponding furostanols, some of which occur naturally. Their nomenclature is based on (22R)-5β-furostan (16β,22-epoxycholestane) which specifies the configurations at all the asymmetric centres except positions 5, 22 and (if position 26 is substituted) also 25. The (20S, 22R, 25R)-spirostanes produce (20S, 22R, 25R)-furostan-26-ols and the (20S, 22R, 25S)-spirostanes produce (20S, 22R, 25S)-furostan-26-ols (Fig. 10.12).

C. DIGITONIN

Digitonin is the steroid saponin present in Digitalis leaves together with the cardiac glycosides and is usually obtained from the seeds of *Digitalis purpurea*. The commercial product usually contains 70-80% digitonin, 10-20% tigonin and gitonin (gitogenin is 15-deoxydigitogenin) and 5-15% minor saponins.

> digitonin = digitogenin + 2 galactose + 2 glucose + 1 xylose
> tigonin   = tigogenin   + 2 galactose + 2 glucose + 1 xylose
> gitonin   = gitogenin   + 3 galactose + 1 xylose

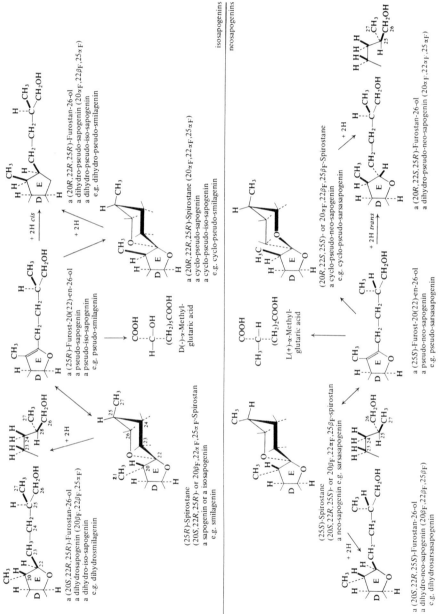

Fig. 10.12. Configurations of the spirostanes and furostanes.

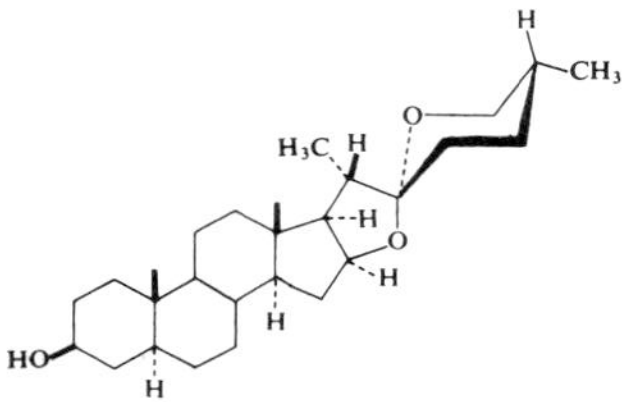

Fig. 10.13. Some naturally occurring steroid sapogenins.

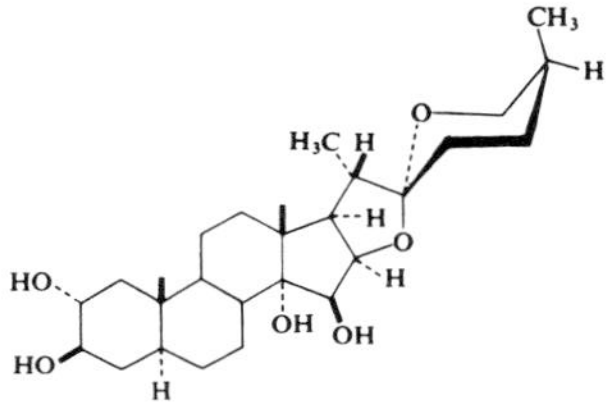

Neodigitogenin
(25S)-5α-Spirostan-2α,3β,15β-triol

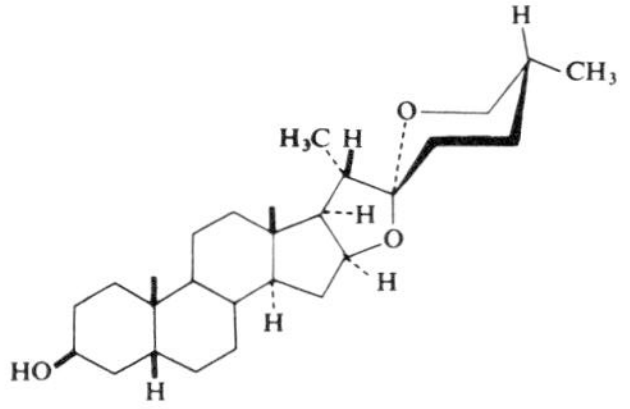

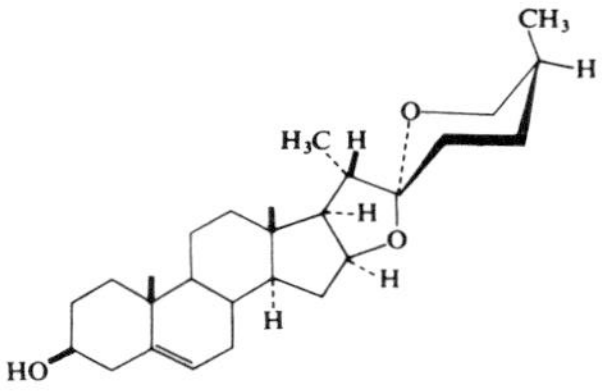

Yamogenin
(25S)-5-Spirosten-3β-ol

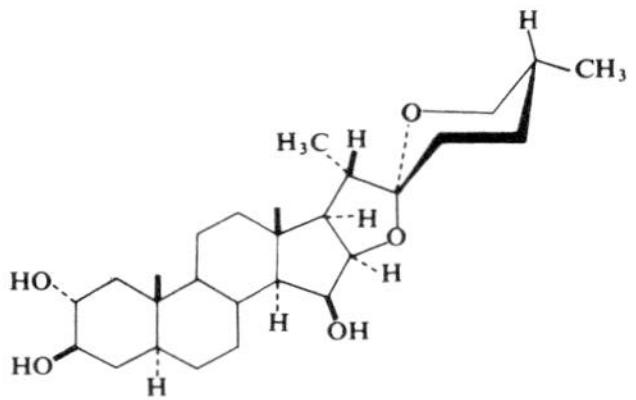

Digitogenin
(25R)-5α-Spirostan-2α,3β,15β-triol

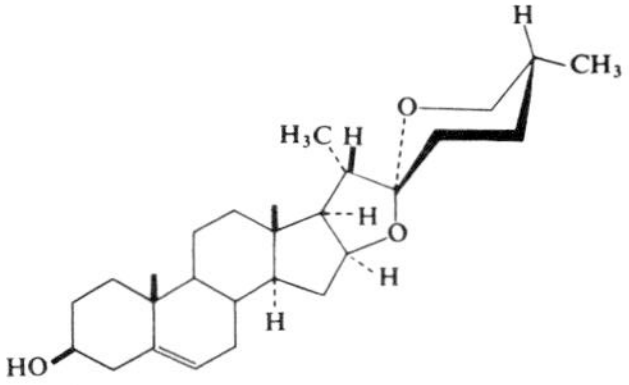

Diosgenin
(25R)-5-Spirosten-3β-ol

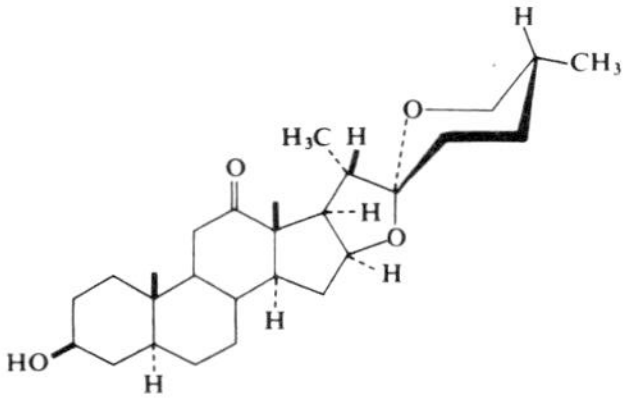

Hecogenin
(25R)-5α-Spirostan-3β-ol-12-one

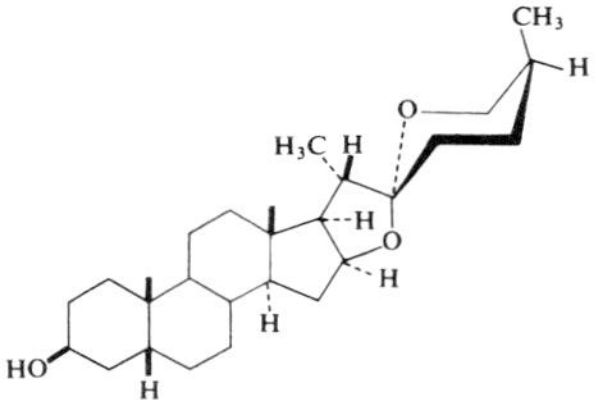

Sarsapogenin
(25S)-5β-Spirostan-3β-ol
5β,20α,22β,25L-Spirostan-3β-ol
5β,22βF,25βF-Spirostan-3β-ol

Tigogenin
(25R)-5α-Spirostan-3β-ol
(20S,22R,25R)-5α-Spirostan-3β-ol
5α,20α,22α,25D-Spirostan-3β-ol
5α,22αF,25αF-Spirostan-3β-ol

Smilagenin
(25R)-5β-Spirostan-3β-ol

Table 10.5. *Naturally occurring steroid sapogenins*

Ring substituent	(25R)-5α-Spirostan-	(25S)-5α-Spirostan-
3β-ol	Tigogenin	Neotigogenin
2α,3β-diol	Gitogenin	Neogitogenin
3β,6α-diol	Chlorogenin	Neochlorogenin
3β,12β-diol	Rockogenin	
2α,3β,5α-triol	Agapanthagenin	
2α,3β,12β-triol	Agavogenin	
2α,3β,15β-triol	Digitogenin	Neodigitogenin
3β-ol-12-one	Hecogenin	Sisalagenin (Neohecogenin)
2α,3β-diol-12-one	Manogenin	

	(25R)-5β-Spirostan-	(25S)-5β-Spirostan-
3β-ol	Smilagenin	Sarsapogenin
1β,3β-diol	Isorhodeasapogenin	Rhodeasapogenin
2β,3β-diol	Samogenin	Markogenin
2β,3α-diol	Yonogenin	
3β,11α-diol	Nogiragenin	
1β,2β,3α-triol	Tokorogenin	
2β,3β,11α-triol	Metagenin	
1β,2β,3α,5β-tetrol	Kogagenin	
2β,3β-diol-12-one	Mexogenin	
3β-ol-12-one		Willagenin

	(25R)-5-Spirosten	(25S)-5-Spirosten-
3β-ol	Diosgenin	Yamogenin
1β,3β-diol	Ruscogenin	Neoruscogenin
2α,3β-diol	Yuccagenin	Lilagenin
3β-ol-12-one	Botogenin (Gentrogenin)	Correlogenin (Neobotogenin)
2α,3β-diol-12-one	Kammogenin	
3β,12β-diol	Isochiapagenin	Chiapagenin

Digitonin is a valuable analytical reagent as it forms an insoluble equimolecular complex with cholesterol, but not with its esters. It is used to precipitate 3β-hydroxy-steroids. This precipitation does not take place if the methyl substituent at C-10 is in the epi configuration. It is also used as a detergent for breaking the membranes of cells, e.g. in the counting of blood white cells after lysis of anuclear erythrocytes.

D. DIOSGENIN

The plants which produce the most important sapogenins are species of *Yucca* and *Agave* (cacti) and *Dioscorea* (yams), as follows:

Source	Saponin	Sapogenin	Sugars
Dioscorea tokoro	Dioscin	Diosgenin	2 rhamnose, 1 glucose
Agave sisila (sisal plant)		Hecogenin	
Radix sarsaparillae		Sarsasapogenin	2 glucose, 1 rhamnose
Yucca schottii			

In *Agave* and *Dioscorea* species there is a reciprocal association between the sterols and sapogenins concentrations. Young *Agave* and *Yucca* plants contain fewer and more oxygenated sapogenins than older ones. During the winter the complexity of the sapogenin mixture increases while the number of oxygen functions and double bonds decreases. Flowering is accompanied by a burst of biosynthetic activity and flowers and stalks have a different sapogenin composition from the rest of the plant. In *Yucca* the highest sapogenin concentration appears in the seeds which may contain up to 18% tigogenin. It is possible the sapogenins stimulate the growth of shoots and roots. Sarsasparilla is an ancient drug and was described in 1568. It became a standard syphilis treatment among pirate surgeons and was popular for rheumatism. In the 1880's in the USA it enjoyed great vogue as a tonic.

The starting materials of about 70-75% of the steroid hormones sold today, mostly as oral contraceptives, are obtained from *Dioscorea* species, the Mexican yam. Other plants, e.g. agaves (sisal) and soya beans, contribute a small amount to the total and the rest comes from animal sources, e.g. ox adrenal glands, wool fat, especially for cholesterol. The principal sapogenins are diosgenin from the yam and hecogenin from the sisal. There are only five synthetic steps from diosgenin to progesterone. There are some 600 species of yams and edible varieties have been cultivated for thousands of years, while the poisonous varieties have been used in the treatment of snake bites, rheumatism and skin diseases. The species of yam most rich in diosgenin has been found in Mexico and in 1944 was the starting point of a vast industry, today worth some fifty million dollars. A satisfactory way of mass cultivation of the special yams has not been achieved as yet and the industry consists mainly of collecting the yams and extracting the saponin for processing elsewhere. The average yam rhizome weighs about 4 lb and about thirty million are collected each year. About 65 lb of dry root yield about 1 lb diosgenin. At the present rate of collection there are enough yams in Mexico to last about 60 years. The saponins are stored in the cytoplasm of the plant not in the juices. Yams are washed and chopped up, then put into shallow concrete fermentation tanks to enable natural bacteria and enzymes to release the diosgenin. The stew is then dried and dispatched to the factory for synthesis into hormones.

VI. STEROID ANTIBIOTICS

Helvolic acid (Fig. 10.14) was first obtained from *Aspergillus fumigatus* in 1943 and in 1965 was prepared from *Cephalosporium mycophyllum*. Cephalo-

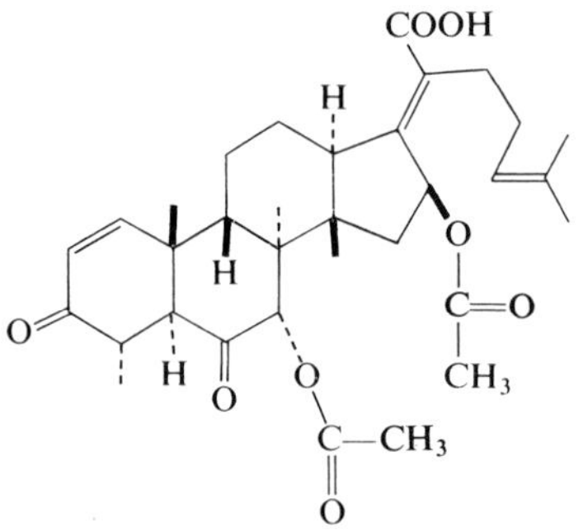

Helvolic acid 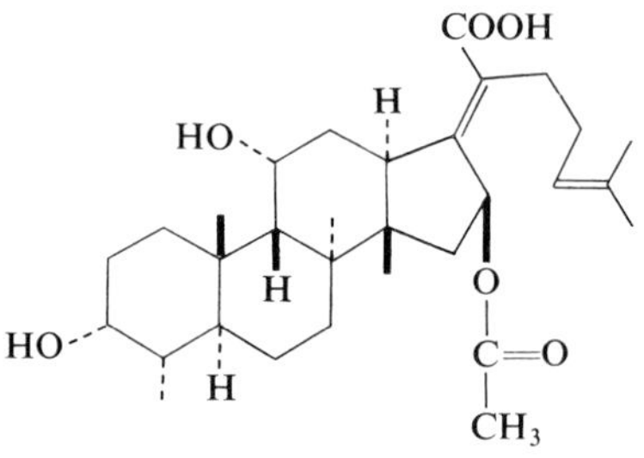   Fusidic acid

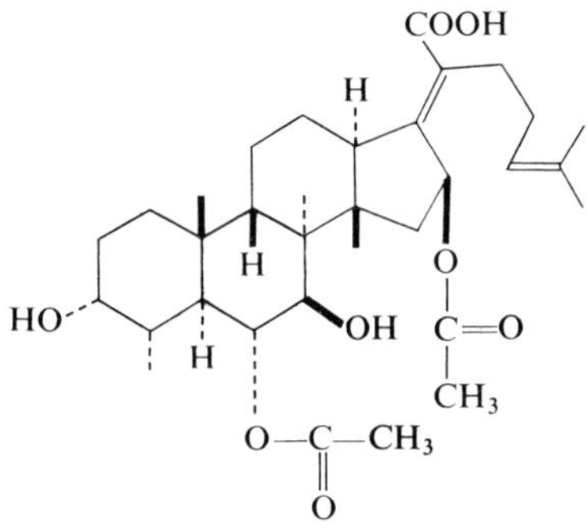

Cephalosporin P_1

Fig. 10.14. Steroid antibiotics.

sporin P_1 was isolated in 1952 from *Cephalosporium brotzu*. Fusidic acid has been known as a metabolite of *Fusidium coccineum* and *Cephalosporium lamelloecola* for many years, but its structure was not determined until 1964. At present it seems to be the steroid antibiotic with the greatest therapeutic potential. It is active against gramme-positive bacteria but not against most gramme-negative bacteria and fungi. It is very insoluble in water but the sodium and potassium salts are soluble and the sodium salt has been marketed as "Fucidin". It is known to inhibit microbial protein synthesis. Although the three antibiotics have similar structures and antibacterial spectra, there is a quantitative difference in activity, cephalosporin P_1 being about sixteen times more active than helvolic acid against *Staphylococcus aureus*. Fusidic acid is more active against a number of gramme-positive bacteria than cephalosporin P_1. Sensitive organisms include some strains of *Staph. aureus* which are resistant to penicillins and other antibiotics. It is active against *Neisseria gonorrheae, Corynebacterium diptheriae, Mycobacterium tuberculosis* and some strains of *Clostridia*. It delays the inactivation of penicillin due to the production of penicillinase by resistant strains and is well absorbed when given by mouth and slowly excreted. It also becomes widely distributed in body tissues but does not reach the spinal cord.

VII. ECDYSONES

The development of insects is accomplished through several larval stages, which are separated from one another by ecdyses. The normal larval ecdysis is started by hormones produced by neurosecretory cells of the brain which stimulate the prothoracic glands. These produce the moulting hormones, the ecdysones, and simultaneously the juvenile hormone is secreted by the corpora allata. Ecdysones control all of the processes which are connected with the ecdyses and are growth and differentiation hormones similar to the estrogens and androgens of mammals.

The best biological assay is the *Calliphora* (blue-bottle) test in which the test object is the isolated abdomen of fully grown maggots. One unit is defined as the amount which after injection evokes the formation of a puaparium in 50-70% of the animals and has now been made equivalent to 0.01 μg crystalline hormone. The cuticle hardens and darkens, i.e. sclerotizes, which depends on the incorporation of quinones. Relative potencies are shown in Table 10.6.

Ecdysone was the first insect steroid hormone isolated in 1954 from *Bombyx mon* pupae and its structure was elucidated in 1965 (Fig. 10.15). Its biological precursor is cholesterol and it belongs to the 5β-series with a *cis* A/B ring junction. The keto group at C-6 is essential for action. This produces appreciable strain in ring B which seems to make the structure fairly labile, even more so in combination with the hydroxyl at C-14. "Ecdysones" is now used as a generic name and the original hormone is distinguished as α-ecdysone. Other ecdysones isolated are 20-hydroxyecdysone from insects and crustacea and 20,26-dihydroxyecdysone from the tobacco hornworm pupa, *Manduca sexta* (Fig. 10.15). Insects are unable to synthesize cholesterol or other sterols from mevalonate and obtain cholesterol as a nutritional factor.

Substances which are either active in inducing puparium formation in Diptera (*Calliphora* and *Musca*) or have chemical structures similar to those of the insect ecdysones have now been isolated from plants. Ecdysone, 20-hydroxyecdysone and other related materials are present in the pinnae of bracken, *Pteridium aquilinum*, and at greater concentrations than in the best insect sources. Other plants, e.g. the fir (*Podocarpus nakaii*), are even richer in these compounds. It is not known whether these phytoecdysones are end products of sterol metabolism, the plant analogues of bile acids, or have a physiological or biochemical function in plant growth and development. It is possible that they protect the plant from insect attack. When 20-hydroxyecdysone is fed to insects, it inhibits ovarian maturation and egg production.

Table 10.6. *Relative potencies of ecdysones*

α-Ecdysone	1
β-Ecdysone	1.9
Cyasterone	2.2
Inokosterone	0.5
Ponasterone A	3.2

VIII. STEROIDAL ALKALOIDS, AZA STEROIDS

Steroidal alkaloids occur in only a few genera of plants, notably *Solanum, Veratrum* and *Holarrhena*. Alkaloids impart a bitter taste to the plant and may act as protection for the plant from insects and other predators. The Colorado beetle avidly devours potato plants but soon dies of alkaloid poisoning. The alkaloid content of potato plants (*Solanum tuberosum*) depends on genetic factors, age, climatic and ecological conditions. During the growing season, the alkaloid content of the leaves rises and that of the tubers declines. Dormant potatoes show the highest concentration in the periphery. Young tomatoes, *Lycopersicon* species, are very rich in tomatine but this gradually disappears and the ripe fruits are the only alkaloid-free organs. The alkaloids occur as glycosides. Solanine consists of the alkylamine, solanidine and one molecule of glucose, galactose and rhamnose. Tomatine consists of tomatidine with two molecules of glucose and one molecule of galactose and xylose. Some of the solanum alkaloids may form sources for the manufacture of steroid hormones in the future.

Connessine is the most abundant and most important of the Kurchi alkaloids and is obtained from the seeds or bark of Indian and African shrubs of *Holarrhena* species. The alkaloids have been used in India for treatment of amoebic dysentry. Holarrhimine is another alkaloid isolated from these species.

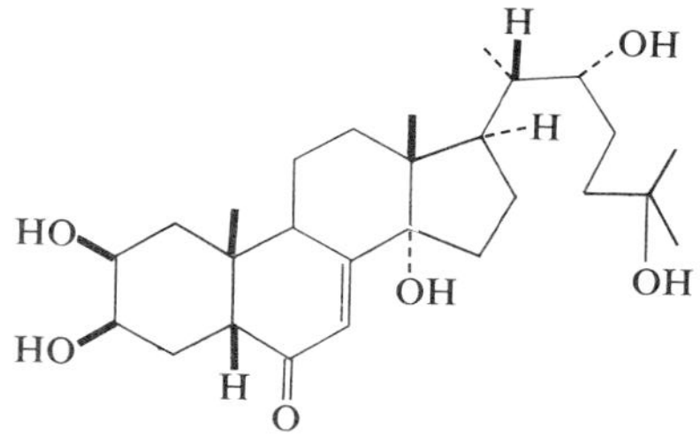

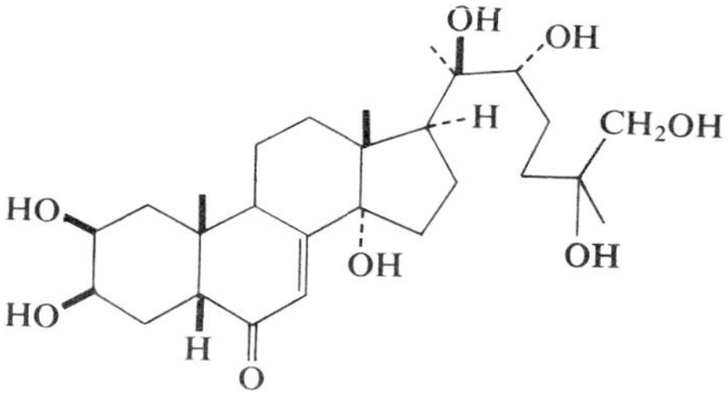

20,26-Dihydroxy-α-ecdysone

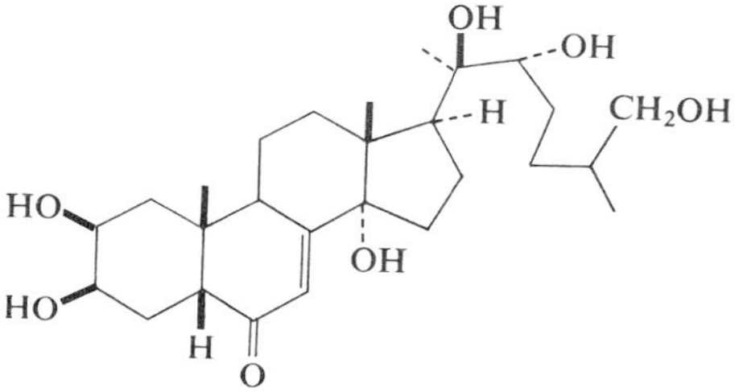

Cyasterone

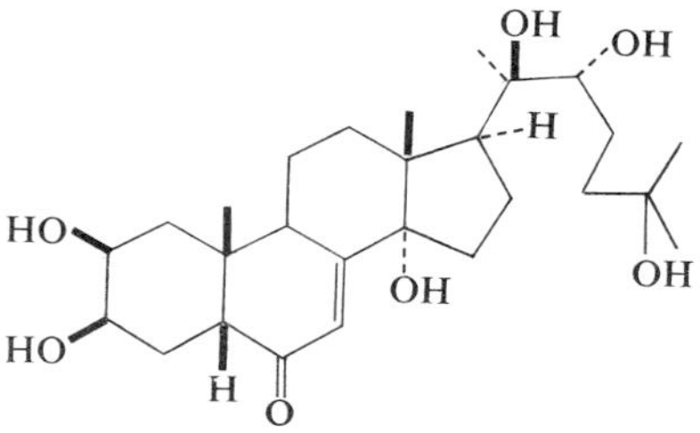

β-Ecdysone
Ecdysterone
20-Hydroxy-α-ecdysone
20R-Hydroxy-ecdysone
Crustecdysone

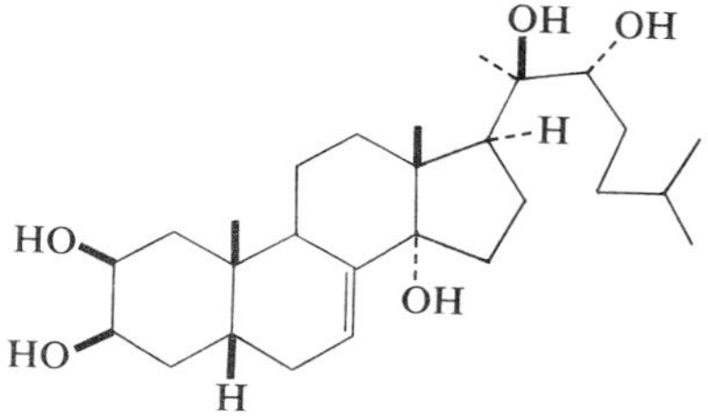

Ponasterone A
(22R)-2β,3β,14,20,22-Pentahydroxy-
5β,14α-cholest-7-en-6-one

α-Ecdysone, Ecdysone
(22R)-2β,3β,14,22,25-Pentahydroxy-
5β,14α-cholest-7-en-6-one
7,(5β)-Cholesten-2β,3β,14α,22βF,25-
pentol-6-one

Inokosterone
(22R)-2β,3β,14,20,22,26-Hexahydroxy-
5β,14α-cholest-7-en-6-one

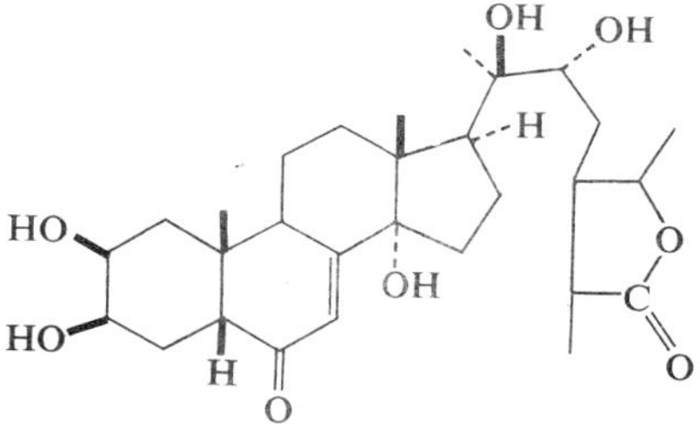

Fig. 10.15. Insect steroid hormones.

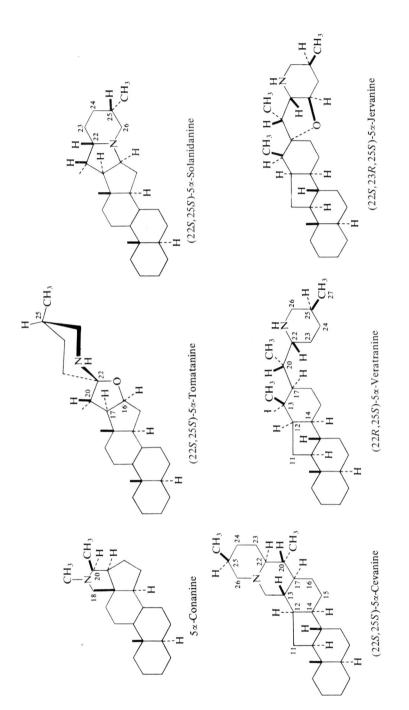

Fig. 10.16. Parent hydrocarbons of the steroid alkaloids.

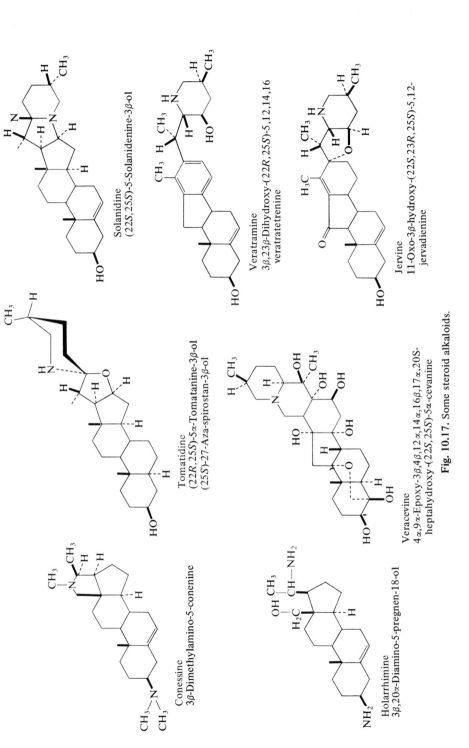

Fig. 10.17. Some steroid alkaloids.

The steroid alkaloids which are obtained from *Veratrum* species fall into two distinct chemical groups—the jerveratrum alkaloids and the ceveratrum alkaloids. The jerveratrum alkaloids are found in unhydrolyzed plant extracts, partly free and partly in conjugation with one molecule of glucose. They contain two or three atoms of oxygen while the ceveratrum alkaloids contain seven to nine atoms of oxygen and usually occur esterified with various acids. The *Veratrum* alkaloids have high hypotensive activity. The species *Veratrum* belongs to the *Liliaceae* family and roots and rhizomes of *V. viride* of the USA and Canada (the American hellebore) are used for many of the extracts. Veratramine contains the unusual C-nor-D-homo ring system but it is commonly considered as a 14(13 → 12) *abeo* structure and numbered as such.

A systematic nomenclature has recently been introduced and the parent saturated alkaloids given specific names for their stereochemistry (Table 10.7 and Fig. 10.16). The structure of some of the alkaloids derived from these parent compounds is shown in Fig. 10.17.

Table 10.7. *Parent names for groups of steroid alkaloids*

Parent name	Stereochemistry implied in the name	Stereochemistry to be indicated by sequence rule prefixes
Conanine	17αH, 20S	—
Tomatanine	16αH, 17αH, 20S	22, 25
Solanidanine	16αH, 17αH, 20S	22, 25
Cevanine	17αH, 17aβH, 20R	22, 25
Veratranine	17αH, 20S	22, 25
Jervanine	17αO, 20R	22, 23, 25

11

INDUSTRIAL PRODUCTION OF
THE STEROIDS

I. INTRODUCTION

Basic organic chemistry has played a fundamental part in steroid bio-chemistry and pharmacology, from the recognition of physiological effects, to the isolation and identification of active compounds, to the synthesis of these compounds and their modifications in pharmaceutical amounts and to their chemical estimation. Raw materials have progressed from human extracts, to plant sterols (e.g. stigmasterol, zymosterol, ergosterol), to bile acids, to plant sapogenins (e.g. diosgenin, hecogenin, sarsasapogenin). These now constitute the major sources of steroids today, though total synthesis from much simpler compounds is fast developing.

II. ISOLATION FROM HUMAN EXTRACTS

A. ESTROGENS

The Allen-Doisy estrogen assay was developed in 1923, but little progress was made in isolation from the follicular fluid of the ovary and from the mammalian placenta until Aschheim and Zondek discovered in 1927 that estrogens were excreted in considerable quantities in the urine of pregnant women. Pure crystalline estrone was isolated in 1929 by Allen and Doisy at St. Louis and by Butenandt of Göttingen and Schering. Improved yields were obtained with Girard's reagent in 1934. Urine is acidified, drastically hydrolysed to break up the water-soluble, ether-insoluble conjugates, extracted with ether and the extract concentrated to a dark oil. This is refluxed for an hour with Girard's reagent T (trimethylaminoacetohydrazide hydrochloride $[(CH_3)_3N^+CH_2CO\,NH\,NH_2]Cl^-$) in alcohol containing 10% acetic acid. The reaction mixture is diluted with water, shaken with ether and the aqueous solution containing the Girard derivative (Fig. 11.1) is clarified, acidified with HCl and warmed to hydrolyse. The regenerated ketonic materials containing estrone are recovered by ether extraction.

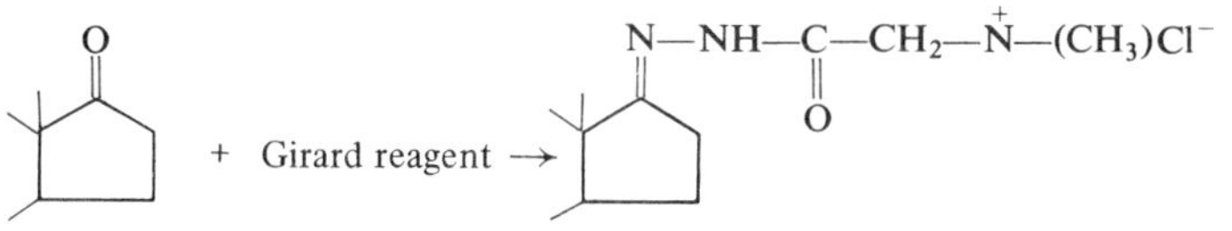

$$N—NH—\underset{\underset{O}{\|}}{C}—CH_2—\overset{+}{N}—(CH_3)Cl^-$$

17-Ketosteroid   + Girard reagent →   Girard derivative

Fig. 11.1. Action of Girard's reagent T.

The average estrogenic activity of human pregnancy urine is about 10,000 mouse units/litre whereas pregnant mares urine contains about ten times this amount. The hormones are more highly conjugated than in human urine and only 10-25% is directly extractable. Processes suitable for the working of human urine required considerable alteration for application to mares urine. Mixed estrogens prepared from pregnant mares urine are still used therapeutically, e.g. "Premarin". Such preparations contain large quantities of equilenin and equilin which are weak estrogens not found in the human.

Estradiol is the most potent estrogen but was not isolated from ovarian tissue until 1935 as the sparingly soluble di-α-naphthoate. Four tons of sow ovaries produce about 12 mg of estradiol. It was later isolated from pregnancy urine.

B. ANDROGENS

The amount of hormone present in genital organs is very small and early attempts at isolation failed. Small amounts occur in blood and urine of normal males and 15,000 litres of male urine were used to produce 15 mg of the first crystalline hormone by Butenandt of Schering in 1931. Its structure as androsterone was determined in 1932. Testosterone was isolated in 1935, 10 mg being obtained from 100 kg of steer testis tissue.

C. PROGESTERONE

By 1932, physiologically active, but very crude, crystalline preparations had been obtained from the corpus luteum of sow ovaries but the degree of purity was not sufficient to enable the active compound(s) to be characterized chemically. In 1934, the independent preparation of the pure corpus luteum hormone was announced from four laboratories, the first being Butenandt's group from the laboratories of Schering, Berlin. The ovaries from a single sow weigh about 12 g and yield about 3 g of corpus luteum tissue and 0.08 mg of crude hormone. In the preparation at the Schering laboratory, about 625 kg of ovaries from 50,000 sows yielded 12.5 g of active extract and 20 mg pure crystalline progesterone.

D. ADRENOCORTICAL STEROIDS

By 1943, twenty-eight steroids had been isolated from the beef and hog adrenal glands in the laboratories of Reichstein (University of Basle), Kendall (The Mayo Clinic) and Wintersteiner (Columbia University). More recently, Wettstein (Ciba, Basle) has isolated a further eighteen compounds and the total number of compounds now known is nearly fifty. About 20,000 cattle are needed to produce 900 g of crude concentrate and about 1000 lb of glands are required to produce 6 mg of cortisone and 6 mg cortisol. Hog adrenals give a considerably higher yield of the more oxygenated components. The full configuration of the compounds was not elucidated until 1948.

III. SYNTHESIS OF PROGESTERONE FROM PLANT STEROIDS

The first synthetic preparation of progesterone (Fig. 11.2) was obtained from 3β-hydroxy-Δ^5-bisnorcholenic acid (II) which had been prepared from stigmasterol (I) by Fernholz at Göttingen in 1933 by ozonolysis of the acetate dibromide, debromination and hydrolysis. This was converted through the ester and the diphenylethylene (III) to pregnenolone. An early German commercial process used this procedure applied to the phytosterol mixture from soya bean oil, which consists mainly of γ-sitosterol but contains 12-25% stigmasterol. Other methods for the degradation of hydroxybisnorcholenic acid were developed. In 1949 the Ciba group converted it to the methyl ketone and carried out a peracid oxidation of the dibromide, debromination, hydrolysis and oxidation to obtain a 40% overall yield of progesterone.

In 1952 the enamine method was developed for the production of progesterone from stigmasterol (Fig. 11.3). Stigmastadienone (I) was prepared by Oppenauer oxidation (aluminium t-butoxide and cyclohexanone in toluene) of

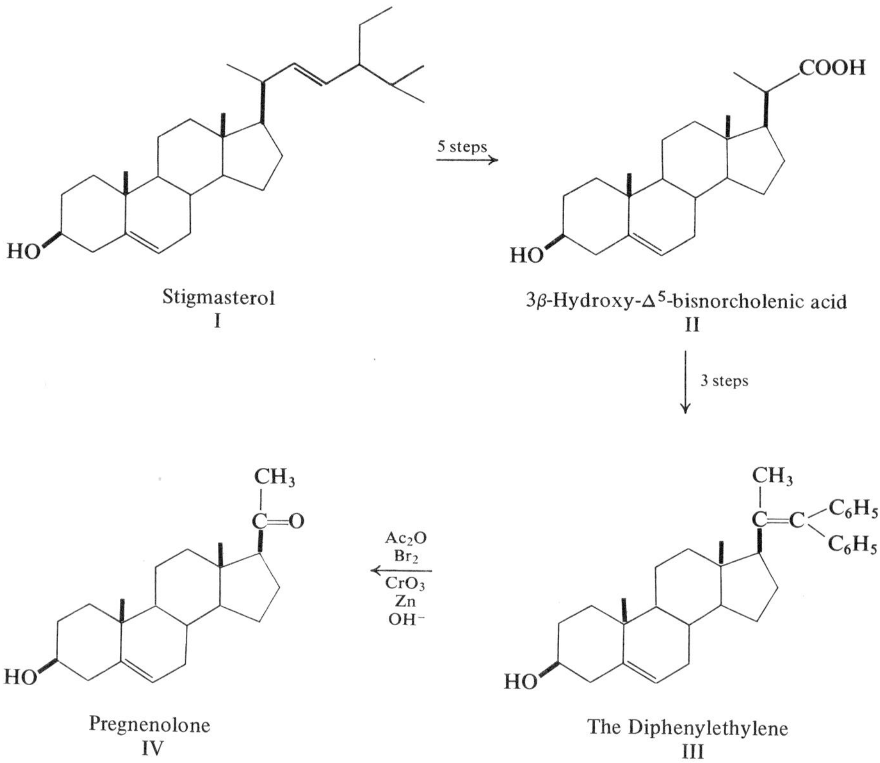

Fig. 11.2. Early preparation of pregnenolone from the stigmasterol of soya bean oil.

stigmasterol and then ozonized directly to produce the ketobisnoraldehyde (II) from which the enamine (III) was prepared by azeotropic distillation with piperidine in benzene. A trace of p-toluene sulphonic acid is added to catalyse enamine formation. Oxidation with sodium dichromate in anhydrous acetic acid-benzene gives progesterone. The yield of progesterone from stigmasterol is about 60% by this method and has forced the price of progesterone down to about 0.2 dollar per gramme.

Ergosterol from yeast has also been extensively investigated as a source of progesterone (Fig. 11.4). Oppenauer oxidation yields ergosterone (I) which on

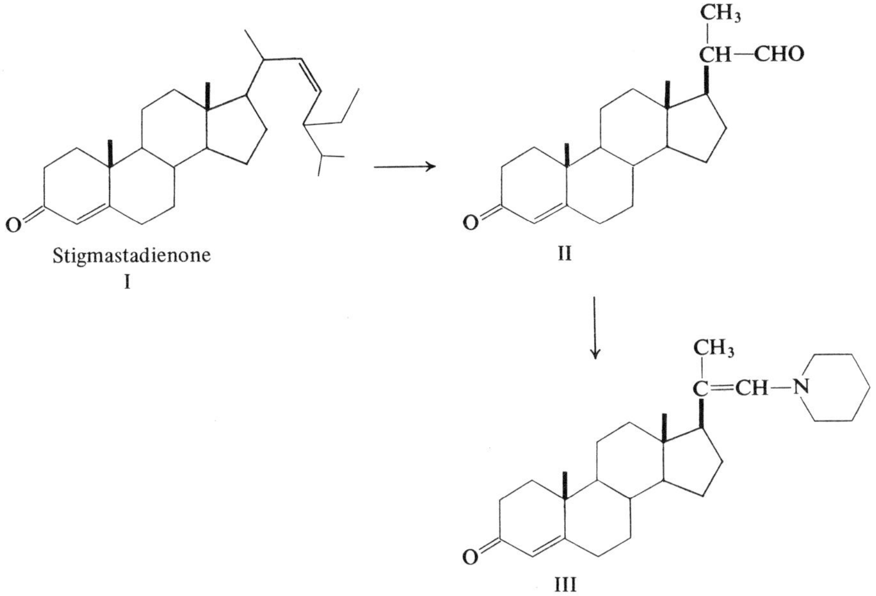

Fig. 11.3. Progesterone from stigmasterol by the enamine method.

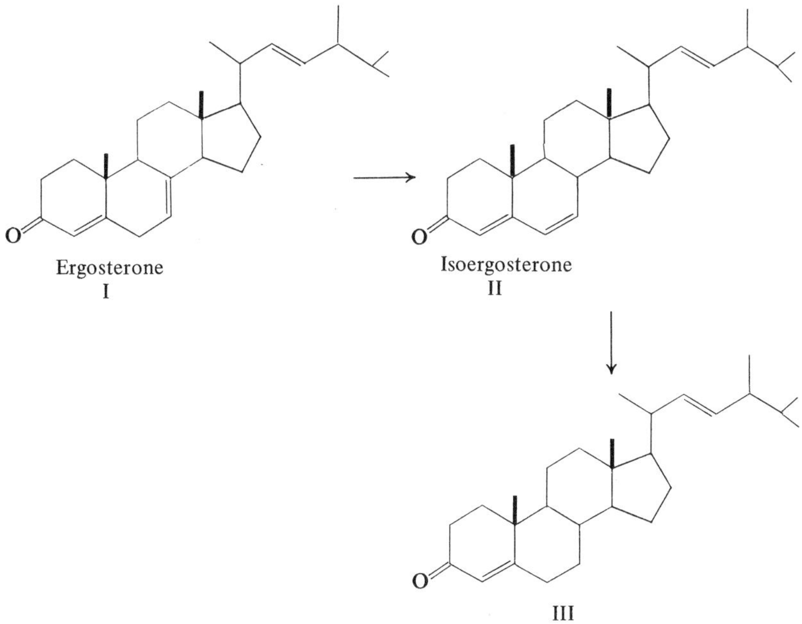

Fig. 11.4. Progesterone from ergosterol.

isomerization with HCl in methanol gives isoergosterone. Selective hydro-genation of the 6,7-double bond is achieved with palladium charcoal in 0.005N alcoholic KOH and the dienone (III) is ozonized to the same ketobisnoraldehyde that is an intermediate in the pathway from stigmasterol. Yields of progesterone are about 80% but this method has not been commercially successful.

IV. SYNTHESIS FROM BILE ACIDS

A. PROGESTERONE

In 1946 a new, highly efficient method (Fig. 11.5) for degrading the bile acid side chain was reported together with the partial synthesis of progesterone from 3β-hydroxy-Δ^5-cholenic acid. This is a by-product in the production of andro-stenolone from cholesterol for which no previous use had been found. The methyl ester (I) was converted to the diphenylethylene derivative at C-24 (II) with phenyl-magnesium-bromide and then dehydrated in acetic anhydride. The more reactive nuclear double bond was protected by the addition of hydrogen

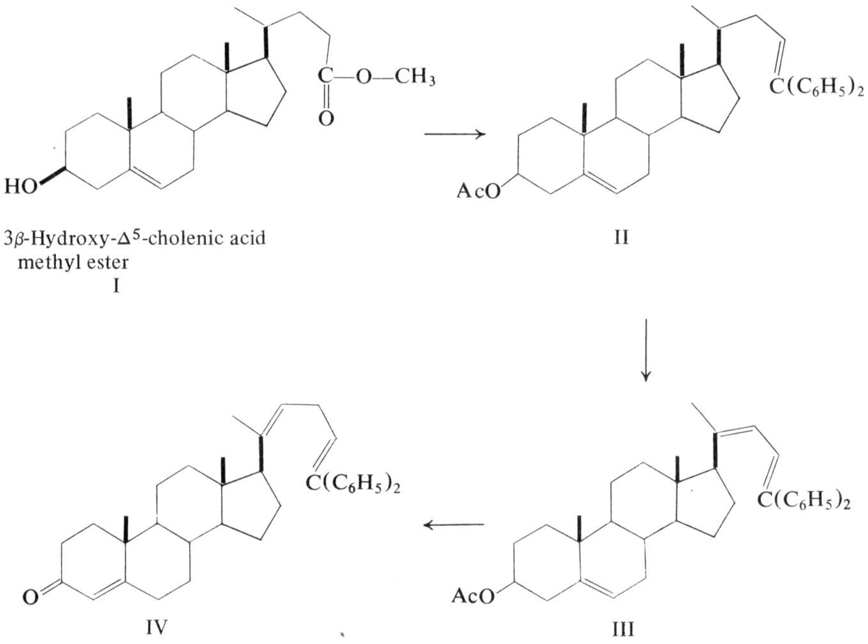

Fig. 11.5. Preparation of progesterone from bile acids.

chloride and bromine was introduced adjacent to the double bond in the side chain with N-bromosuccinimide. The action of dimethylaniline removed both HBr and HCl to give (III). Hydrolysis and Oppenauer oxidation produced (IV) and controlled chromic acid oxidation of the side chain formed progesterone in an overall yield of 33%.

B. CORTISONE

In 1942 research on the synthesis of cortisone (Kendall's compound E) was undertaken by a group of collaborating laboratories in the USA under the sponsorship of the National Research Council in order to obtain sufficient quantities for clinical evaluation. Parallel work was carried out in Switzerland by the Reichstein group. The starting material was cholic acid from ox bile and the first step was the conversion to deoxycholic acid by selective oxidation of the 7α-hydroxyl group to the 7-keto compound and then Wolff-Kishner reduction. About 100 kg of ox bile yields 5-6 kg cholic acid and 600-800 g deoxycholic acid. Initial separation is unnecessary and the total crude bile acid mixture can be oxidized directly with excess reagent. Oxidation was carried out with sodium dichromate or better hypobromous acid generated from N-bromosuccinimide in aqueous medium. The first synthesis of cortisone was achieved by Sarrett in 1945 while 11-dehydrocorticosterone had been synthesized by Reichstein and the Merck group in 1943 in a yield of 0.009%. On the basis of procedures so far known, Merck & Co. initiated work on the large scale production of cortisone in 1946 and were successful in producing about 938 g of cortisone acetate from 1270 lb of starting material.

In the preferred route from deoxycholic acid (I) to cortisone (Fig. 11.6) methyl deoxycholate is converted to the 3-benzoate and oxidized with chromium trioxide to the 12-ketone (II). Dehydrogenation with selenium dioxide in chlorobenzene-acetic acid forms the $\Delta^{9(11)}$-12-ketone (III) and saponification followed by methylation gives the 3-hydroxy-methyl-ester (IV). This is reduced by platinum to the 12-allyl-alcohol and reaction with methanol in the presence of acid gives the 12-methoxy-derivative (V), which yields the 12-chloro-compound after displacement with HCl in chloroform. Bicarbonate forms the $3\alpha,9\alpha$-oxide (VI) which on bromination forms the 11,12-dibromide (VII). This is converted by oxidative hydrolysis with silver chromate-chromic acid to the 12-bromo-11-ketone. Reaction with phenylmagnesium bromide reduces the 12-bromide and forms the diphenylcarbinol which is dehydrated with hot acetic acid to (VIII). This represents the successful incorporation of the 11-keto group. The oxide bridge is cleaved with HBr which inserts a 12β-bromo group which is reduced with zinc, the 3-hydroxyl group is esterified and the side chain converted to the diene (IX) with N-bromosuccinimide followed by

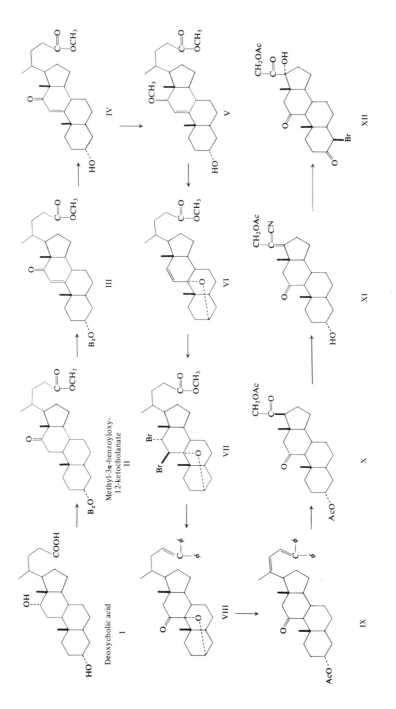

Fig. 11.6. Some steps in the synthesis of cortisone from bile acids.

dehydrobromination. Reaction again with N-bromosuccinimide gives the 21-bromo compound which is displaced by potassium acetate to the 21-acetate. Cleavage of the diene 21-acetate with chromic acid produces pregnane-3α-21-diol-11,20-dione diacetate (X). HCN is then added across the C-20 ketone and dehydration carried out with phosphorus oxychloride-pyridine to give the unsaturated nitrile. The 3- and 21-ester groups are hydrolysed and the primary 21-hydroxyl group selectively acetylated to give (XI). This is hydroxylated with $KMnO_4$ in acetone-piperidine solution with careful pH control to produce the 21-ol-3-ketone, which is acetylated, brominated at C-4 to give the bromo-ketone (XII) which is dehydrobrominated preferably via the 2,4-dinitrophenylhydrasone followed by hydrolysis of the carbonyl derivative with pyruvic acid to give cortisone acetate.

The first compound E was produced in 1948 and sent to the Mayo Clinic where Hench and Kendall investigated its effects in the treatment of rheumatoid arthritis. The results were extremely dramatic and caused formerly bedridden patients to walk again. A sensation was caused in the scientific world and demands were made for more cortisone. Synthesis from bile acids in some thirty steps could not possibly satisfy the demand and an intensive search was made for vegetable starting materials. Possible approaches were to utilize hecogenin, then a rare sapogenin having a keto group at C-12, or to use sarmentogenin, a cardiac aglycone with a hydroxyl group at C-11. Large expeditions were sent to South Africa to identify the plant producing sarmentogenin, but commercial success was finally achieved by the wholly unexpected discovery of microbiological methods for the efficient introduction of oxygen at C-11.

V. SYNTHESIS FROM SAPOGENINS

A. MARKER DEGRADATION OF SAPOGENINS

The three commercially important sapogenins, diosgenin, tigogenin and sarsasapogenin, may be directly degraded to pregnane derivatives. Diosgenin was isolated in 1936 from the root of a Japanese *Dioscorea* and its structure had been elucidated by 1940 when Marker at Pennsylvania State College had developed an efficient process for its degradation to progesterone. In the hope of discovering a practical source of diosgenin, Marker launched a series of extensive botanical collection trips in the southern United States and Mexico when over 400 species of plants were examined. The isolation of twelve new sapogenins and their degradation was not published until 1947. In 1944 Marker set up on his own in Mexico producing progesterone which then cost about 80 dollars per gramme. He joined the owners of the Mexican company "Hormona Laboratories" and established the firm "Syntex" which is now one of the largest companies manufacturing steroids, largely due to the efforts of the Djerrassi group. The price of progesterone eventually fell to 0.48 dollar per gramme and the way was open for the synthesis of hormonal steroids on a massive scale.

1. Production of ψ-sapogenins from sapogenins

Both $25\beta_F$-(neo)-sapogenins (25S-spirostanes), e.g. sarsasapogenin, and $25\alpha_F$-(iso)-sapogenins (25R-spirostanes), e.g. diosgenin (Fig. 11.7, I), undergo a general reaction with neat acetic anhydride at 200°C to give after alkaline hydrolysis, ψ-sapogenins (II) or furost-20(22)-en-27-ols, ($\psi \equiv$ pseudo). The reaction mixture corrodes stainless steel and special apparatus is needed for large scale work. Alternative reagents are n-butyric anhydride, octanoic anhydride and acetic acid at 270°C. The reaction is promoted by zinc acetate, trichloroacetic acid, aluminium chloride, pyridine hydrochloride and ammonium chloride. The best yield (87%) of free furostadiene from diosgenin is obtained by refluxing in n-octanoic acid (B.P. 237°C) containing a little acetic anhydride, distilling off low boiling fractions until the temperature reaches 240°C, refluxing for 2 h and then saponifying.

2. Production of cyclo-ψ-sapogenins and dihydro-ψ-sapogenins

Sapogenins (II) by a very brief treatment with 0.5N ethanolic hydrochloric acid at 0-25°C, or better with ethanolic acetic acid at 100°C, give cyclo-ψ-sapogenins (20R,22R,25-spirostanes) (III). These are saturated but very reactive, probably as a consequence of the strong 13β-methyl:20α_F-methyl steric repulsions. In acidic media an equilibrium exists between:

$$\text{sapogenin} \rightleftharpoons \psi\text{-sapogenin} \rightleftharpoons \text{cyclo-}\psi\text{-sapogenin}$$
e.g. 20S,22R,25S-spirostane $\rightleftharpoons$ a psuedoisogenin $\rightleftharpoons$ 20R,22R,25R-spirostane
(a cyclopseudoneogenin)
20S,22R,25R-spirostane $\rightleftharpoons$ a pseudoisogenin $\rightleftharpoons$ 20R,22R,25R-spirostane
(a cyclopseudoisogenin)

Consequently, hydrogenation with platinum in acetic acid of cyclo-ψ-sapogenins may involve hydrogenation of the ψ-sapogenin, e.g. cyclo-ψ-sarsasapogenin gives dihydro-ψ-sarsasapogenin.

3. Oxidation of ψ-sapogenins, cyclo-ψ-sapogenins and dihydro-ψ-sapogenins

Cyclo-ψ-sapogenins and dihydro-ψ-sapogenins are readily oxidized by chromium trioxide whereas sapogenins and dihydro-sapogenins are not. ψ-Sapogenins of both the 25R and 25S series are oxidized by chromium trioxide

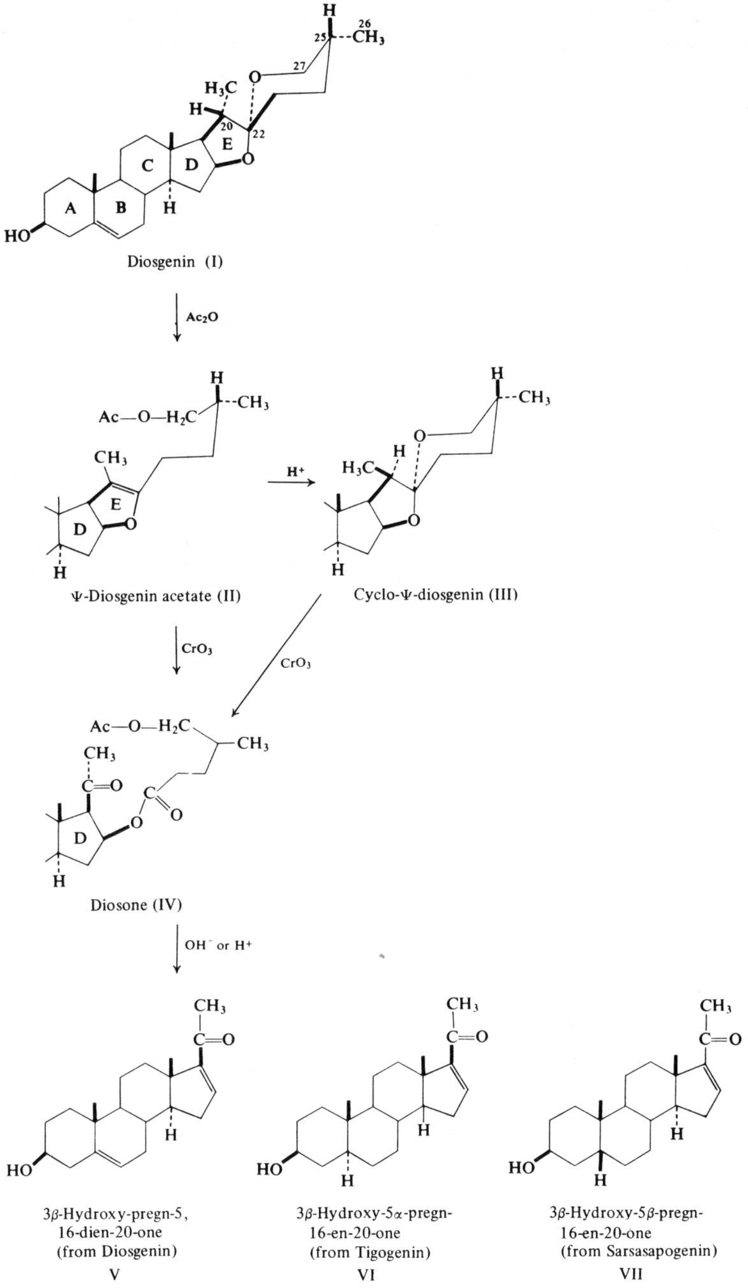

Diosgenin (I)

Ac₂O

Ψ-Diosgenin acetate (II)

H⁺

Cyclo-Ψ-diosgenin (III)

CrO₃

CrO₃

Diosone (IV)

OH⁻ or H⁺

3β-Hydroxy-pregn-5,
16-dien-20-one
(from Diosgenin)
V

3β-Hydroxy-5α-pregn-
16-en-20-one
(from Tigogenin)
VI

3β-Hydroxy-5β-pregn-
16-en-20-one
(from Sarsasapogenin)
VII

Fig. 11.7. Marker degradation of sapogenins.

to β-acyl ketones. ψ-Sapogenin acetates with chromium trioxide at 30°C give crystalline ester acetates. ψ-Diosgenin as the 3,27-diacetate (II) is oxidized so rapidly at the 20(22)-position that protection of the nuclear double bond is unnecessary and 3β-hydroxypregna-5,16-dien-20-one is produced (V). This is the most commercially important method and omits the formation of a cyclo-ψ-sapogenin or a dihydro-ψ-sapogenin.

4. Hydrolysis

Hydrolysis with either alkali or acid, e.g. potassium hydroxide in t-butanol or boiling acetic acid of the β-acyl ketones of ψ-sapogenins, yields L(+)- or D(−)-α-methylglutaric acid and 5ξ-pregn-16-en-20-ones, or hydrogenation and subsequent hydrolysis yields 5ξ-pregnane-16β,20β-diols. ψ-Sapogenin ester-acetates also give 16-en-20-ones and 16β,20β-diols. Similar treatment of 22R- or 22S-cyclo-ψ-sapogenins or of dihydro-ψ-sapogenins gives 5-pregn-16-en-20-ones. When the cyclo-ψ-sapogenins are of the "iso" series *only*, the usual pregn-16-en-20-ones are accompanied by tertiary 20-alcohols, e.g. cyclo-ψ-tigogenin acetate yields about 45% of the 20S-ol. Similarly, cyclo-ψ-hecogenin gives some of the 3,12,-dioxo-20S-ol.

By the Marker degradation process diosgenin yields mainly 3β-hydroxypregn-5,16-dien-20-one (V), tigogenin yields 3β-hydroxy-5α-pregn-16-en-20-one (VI) and sarsasapogenin yields 3β-hydroxy-5β-pregn-16-en-20-one (VII). The industrial yield of 16-dehydropregnenolone from diosgenin is about 60%.

5. Hydrogenation of 16-enes

Selective hydrogenation is carried out with palladium, e.g. 3β-hydroxypregn-5,16-diene-20-one produces 3β-hydroxypregn-5-en-20-one (pregnenalone). An important alternative pathway is via the 16α,17α-epoxide which readily gives 17α-hydroxypregnenolone which is an important starting material.

6. Conversion of pregnenolone to progesterone

Originally this was accomplished by direct oxidation with chromium trioxide or copper oxide but later by the addition of bromine, oxidation and debromination, and by dehydrogenation with aluminium isopropoxide or platinum black.

B. CORTISONE

There does not appear to be a naturally occurring sapogenin in any quantity with an oxygen function at C-11 and considerable ingenuity has been exerted in order to insert such a group. It has been found easier to accomplish this before the Marker degradation.

Oxidation of diosgenin with sodium dichromate, perbenzoic or performic acids yields $\Delta^{7,9(11)}$-tigogenin acetate (Fig. 11.8, IV). Treatment of the diene with sodium dichromate in acetic acid-benzene gives a $\Delta^{8(9)}$-7,11-dione (V) which is converted to 11-oxotigogenin (III) by zinc reduction and removal of the 7-ketone through the cycloethylene thioketal. Alternatively, the 1,4-addition of hypobromous acid to the diene produces the 11-bromo-$\Delta^{8(9)}$-7-ketone and reaction with silver nitrate replaces the halogen by a hydroxyl group. Oxidation then gives the $\Delta^{8(9)}$-7,11-dione.

Performic acid oxidation of a $\Delta^{7,9(11)}$-diene yields a 7-keto-9α,11α-oxide which under mild alkaline treatment with potassium *tert.*-butoxide isomerizes to the saturated 7,11-diketone. The 7-ketone can be removed through desulphurization of the 7-thioketal.

Hecogenin (12-oxotigogenin) can be used to prepare C-11 oxygenated compounds (Fig. 11.8). Transfer of the oxygen from C-12 to C-11 can be accomplished by conversion of hecogenin acetate to the 11α,23ξ-dibromide, which by substitution and inversion at C-11 by alkali and debromination with zinc at C-23 gives a 60% yield of 3β,12β-dihydroxy-5α25R-spirostan-11-one (II). Oxidation with bismuth oxide to the 11,12-diketone and Wolff-Kishner reduction gives 11-oxotigogenin (III) with some 11β-hydroxytigogenin and tigogenin. Reduction of the diketone by the thioketal-Raney nickel procedure gives 11-oxotigogenin only. The best yields (80%) of 11-oxotigogenin are now given by direct reduction of 3β,12-dihydroxy-5α-25R-spirostan-11-one with calcium in liquid ammonia. The overall yield of 11-oxotigogenin by this three-step procedure from hecogenin is 55%. Although hecogenin can be isolated from *Agave* species, the chief commercial source is now the waste liquors from sisal manufacture. The sisal plant, *Agave sisalana*, is widely cultivated in East Africa yielding over 100,000 tons per year of sisal, a strong white fibre 3-5 ft long derived from the leaf. Expressed waste material on fermentation deposits a sediment which contains 4-12% of the saponin as glycoside. Probably more hecogenin is now produced from Yucatan sisal which contains more admixed tigogenin.

Botogenin is Δ^5-hecogenin and occurs together with neobotogenin as 15-25% in a *Dioscorea* species. As the 5α,6β,11α,23ξ-tetrabromide-3-acetate, botogenin is converted by the same reaction sequences as hecogenin into 11-oxodiosgenin. If a proton donor, e.g. ethanol, is added at the calcium in liquid ammonia stage, the product is 11α-hydroxydiosgenin.

The Marker degradation of 11-oxotigogenin and 11-oxodiosgenin yields 3β-hydroxy-5α-pregn-16-en-11,20-dione and 3β-hydroxy-pregn-5,16-diene-11,20-dione respectively.

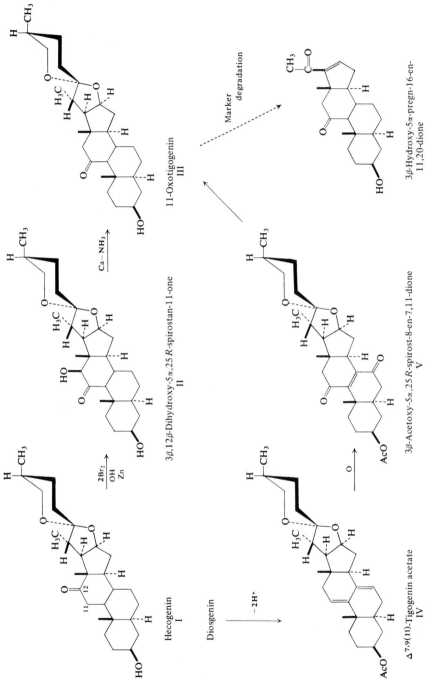

Fig. 11.8. Insertion of oxygen at C-11 into the sapogenins

VI. MICROBIOLOGICAL CONVERSIONS USED
IN SYNTHESES

The steroid industry was revolutionized in 1953 when the Upjohn Group discovered that progesterone may be 11α-hydroxylated by molds of the *Rhizopus* family, so making 11-hydroxy steroids available in unlimited quantities. That yeasts could dehydrogenate and hydrogenate steroids had been known since 1937. The substrates are foreign to the micro-organisms and natural sterols, e.g. ergosterol, are resistant to microbiological transformations. A given micro-organism reduces a 3-keto group to either the 3α- or the 3β-alcohol and the 17-ketones are reduced in all cases to the 17β-alcohols. The Upjohn Group deliberately set out to find a soil micro-organism capable of hydroxylating a steroid at C-11 and found this in a culture of *Rhizopus arrhizus* isolated from Kalamazoo air on exposure of an agar plate on a window sill. Better yields were obtained with *Rhizopus nigricans* which caused 80-90% yields of 11α-hydroxy-progesterone from progesterone, with minor amounts of 6α,11α-dihydroxy-progesterone and 11α-hydroxy-5α-pregnane-3,20-dione.

11α-Hydroxy progesterone (Fig. 11.9, II) is catalytically hydrogenated giving primarily the 5β-derivative (III) and chromic acid oxidation gives pregnane-3,11,20-trione (IV). Selective reduction with borohydride gives pregnan-3α-ol-11-dione (V) and this may be converted to cortisone via the Gallagher enol acetate method. This involves forming the dienol acetate by treatment with acetic anhydride-*p*-toluenesulphonic acid. Selective reduction with peracid of the 17,20 double bond forms the 17α,20α-oxide which is hydrolysed by mild alkali treatment to give the 17α-hydroxy-ketone (VI). Bromination yields the 21-bromide and this is converted to the 21-hydroxy compound by mild alkaline hydrolysis. Oxidation at C-3, then bromination and dehydrobromination yields cortisone.

Shortly afterwards the Squibb Group reported 11α-hydroxylations carried out by *Aspergillus niger*, e.g. of cortexolone to 11-epicortisol (Fig. 11.10) in 25% yields. The 11-epicortisol is converted to its monoacetate and oxidized with chromic acid to yield cortisone acetate. 11β-Hydroxylation by fungi is much rarer than 11α-hydroxylation and yields are not so high. Nevertheless, the direct conversion of cortexolone to cortisol by *Streptomyces fradiae*, or *Cunninghamella blakesleeana* (in 35% yield) or by *Curvularia lunata* (in 40% yield) are now important commercial processes. Variation of the culture medium has produced yields of over 80%. Many organisms have now been found which can hydroxylate at almost any position of the steroid nucleus. It has been established that microbiological enzymatic transformation does not proceed through the $\Delta^{9(11)}$-intermediate but involves the direct displacement with retention of configuration of a hydrogen by atmospheric oxygen.

Since microbiological oxidation of cortexolone affords an effective route to cortical hormones, the synthesis of this intermediate has been the subject of

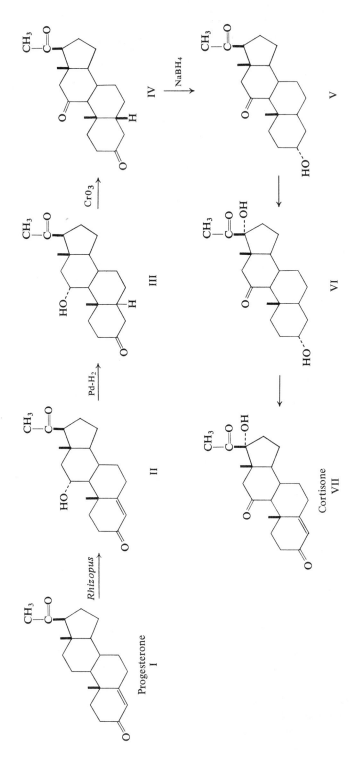

Fig. 11.9. Cortisone from progesterone using *Rhizopus nigricans*.

considerable investigation. The best process uses 16-dehydropregnenolone oxide (Fig. 11.11, I) as the starting material. This is prepared by the action of alkaline hydrogen peroxide on 16-dehydropregnenolone which is readily available from diosgenin. The oxide is reacted in methylene chloride solution with HBr in acetic acid and produces the bromohydrin (II). Bromine is removed by hydrogenation in methanol in the presence of ammonium acetate to react with the HBr formed and so prevent reduction of the 5,6-double bond. The debrominated product (III) is formylated at C-3 giving a 76% yield of (IV). (The production of 17α-acetoxyprogesterone, an oral progestogen, is produced in 53% yield by

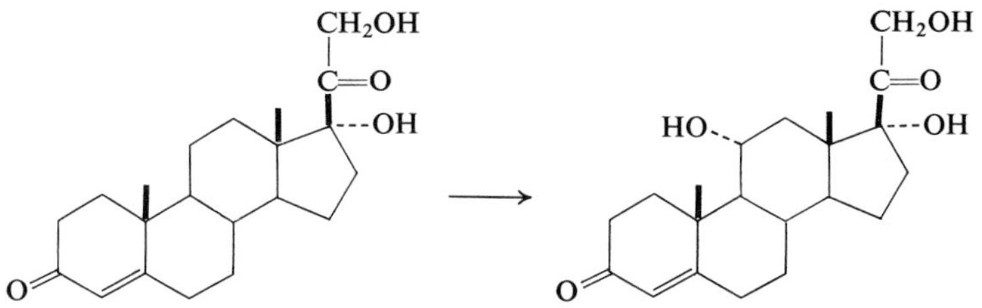

Cortexolone
Reichstein substance S

11-Epicortisol

Fig. 11.10. 11α-Hydroxylation with *Aspergillus niger*.

Oppenauer oxidation of the 17-acetate of (IV).) For the synthesis of cortexolone diacetate, the formate is treated with bromine to produce the 5,6,21-tribromoderivative (V) which is debrominated at C-5 and C-6 by treatment with sodium iodide in acetone, producing the 21-iodide. Reaction with potassium acetate then gives the 3-formate-21-acetate. To prevent formation of a D-homo derivative in the next step, the 17α-hydroxyl group is first acetylated and then an Oppenauer oxidation of the 3-formate-17,21-diacetate produces cortexolone diacetate (VII). Saponification to cortexolone is carried out by a brief reaction in methanol at 0-5°C with 1.15 equivalents of potassium hydroxide. The overall yield is 48%.

VII. TOTAL SYNTHESIS

Although it is possible to degrade the pregnane derivatives produced from sapogenins and bile acids to androstane and estrane derivatives, these compounds are increasingly made by total synthesis. The pioneer in this field was Sir Robert Robinson who developed many of the key reactions and with Cornforth was responsible for one of the first syntheses of a non-aromatic steroid, epiandrosterone.

11*

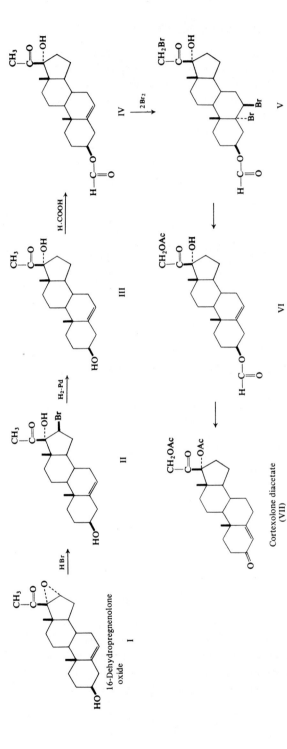

Fig. 11.11. 16-Dehydropregnenolone to cortexolone.

A. EPIANDROSTERONE

1,6-Dimethoxynaphthalene (Fig. 11.12, I) is reduced with sodium and alcohol to 5-methoxytetralone-2 and methylation gives (II). Ring A was then added by condensation with methyl vinyl ketone as its diethylaminobutanone methiodide, the ether being hydrolysed to the free phenol (IV). Catalytic hydrogenation produces selectively a 5β A/B ring junction and a 3α-hydroxyl group which is then acetylated. Further hydrogenation reduces the aromatic ring and gives two B/C cis and two B/C *trans* DL-monoacetates (IV). The two *trans* forms were separated by oxidation of the ring C hydroxyl groups, equilibration of the ketone with alcoholic alkali, inversion at C-8 and formation of the brucine succinates. C-methylation was accomplished by the condensation of the ketone (V) with ethyl formate and sodium methoxide to give the formyl derivative, reaction of the enolate with methyl iodide and cleavage with potassium carbonate to give (VI). One of the optically active hydroxy-ketones on oxidation gives the diketone. Bromination and dehydrobromination gives the unsaturated diketone (VII). Transformation to (VIII) is accomplished by ammonolysis of the enol acetate with potassium amide in liquid ammonia, followed by the addition of ammonium chloride. Reduction of both ketone groups and selective alkylation gives the monotrityl derivative (IX) which on oxidation and hydrolysis gives the ketone (X). Carbonation of the benzoate with triphenylmethylsodium and then carbon dioxide, and esterification gives the keto ester (XI). This has three asymmetric centres and hence four racemic forms are possible. The correct isomer is then subjected to a Reformatsky reaction to give (XII). Dehydration and hydrogenation gives (XIII) which gives epiandrosterone in five steps.

B. ESTRONE

A number of syntheses of estrone have been developed, the first being in 1942 when a stereoisomer was produced. One of the more important recent (1957) routes is known as "Johnson's second synthesis" (Fig. 11.13). The starting material is ethyl-γ-anisoylbutyrate (I) readily available by Friedel-Crafts acylation of anisole with glutaric acid anhydride. A Stobbe condensation with diethylsuccinate gives (II) and hydrogenation and esterification gives the triester (III). On Dieckmann cyclization with sodium hydride and methylation of the resulting sodio derivative of the resulting β-ketoester, the ketoester (IV) of the correct configuration crystallizes directly from the reaction mixture in 36% yield. A Reformatsky condensation gives (V) and ring B is closed by intramolecular Friedel-Crafts condensation to give (VI). Acid catalysed hydrogenation removes the 6-keto group and saturates the double bond, the product being the dimethyl ester of DL-marrianolic acid methyl ether (VII). D-ring closure is carried out by acyloin condensation to (VIII) which may be converted to estradiol, estrone or estriol.

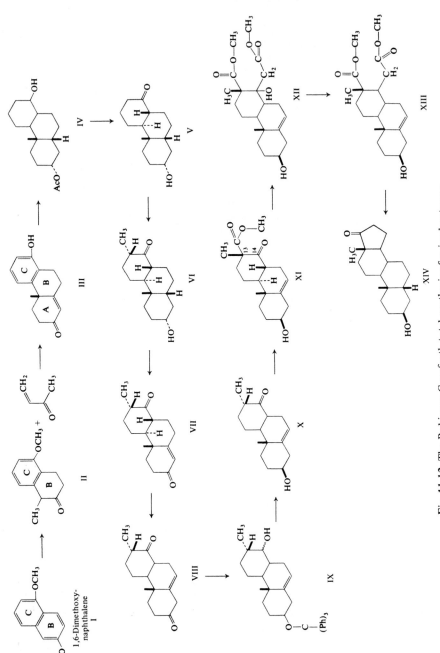

Fig. 11.12. The Robinson-Cornforth total synthesis of epiandrosterone.

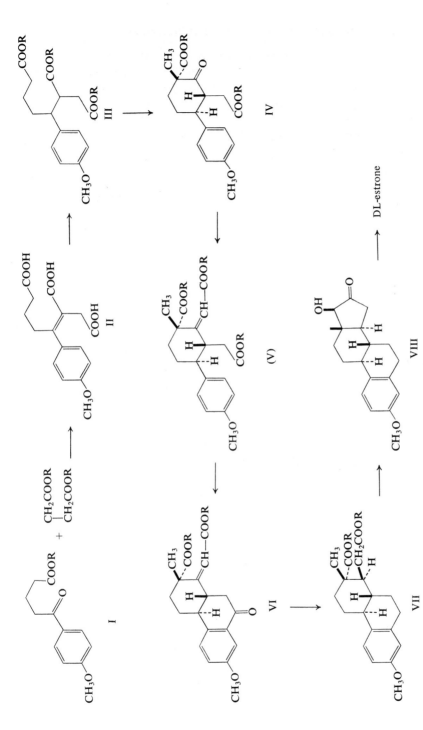

Fig. 11.13. Johnson's second synthesis of estrone.

More recently commercial syntheses have been starting with anisole derivatives. The vinyl ketone (Fig. 11.14, I) is reacted under mildly basic conditions
with 2-methylcyclopentane-1,3-dione to form the trione (II) which is subjected
to cyclodehydration with polyphosphoric acid to form (III). By catalytic and
then lithium aniline-liquid ammonia reduction this is converted to ±-estrone. The
overall yield from 3-*m*-methoxyphenylpropyl bromide, which is used to make
the vinyl ketone, is 18%.

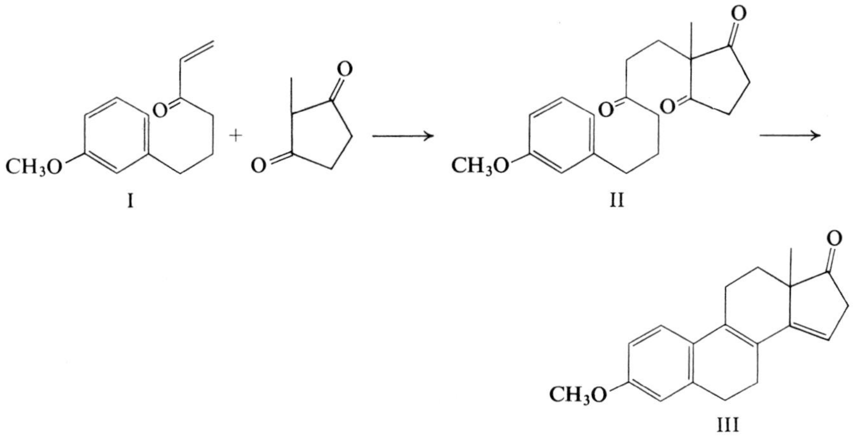

Fig. 11.14. Short synthesis of estrone.

VIII. MODIFICATIONS OF THE NATURAL STEROIDS

A. RING DEHYDROGENATION

In 1953 it was believed that modification of the naturally occurring
hormones could only result in loss of activity but this was dispelled when it was
shown that 9α-chlorohydrocortisone was a more potent anti-inflammatory
agent than hydrocortisone. A major achievement was the synthesis in 1954 of
prednisone and prednisolone, the Δ^1-analogues of cortisone and hydrocortisone,
by the Schering group. An efficient synthesis due to the Upjohn Group is shown
in Fig. 11.15, the starting material being 11-ketoprogesterone (I) which is
condensed with two molecules of diethyl oxalate in the presence of sodium
ethoxide in t-butyl alcohol to form the salt (II). This is neutralized with acetic
acid and on treatment with bromine in the presence of sodium acetate gives the
2,21,21-tribromo derivative (III). Treatment with sodium methoxide in
methanol produces the 2-bromo-*cis*-$\Delta^{17(20)}$-ene-21-oate (IV) which is dehydro-
genated with lithium chloride in dimethyl formamide and converted to predni-

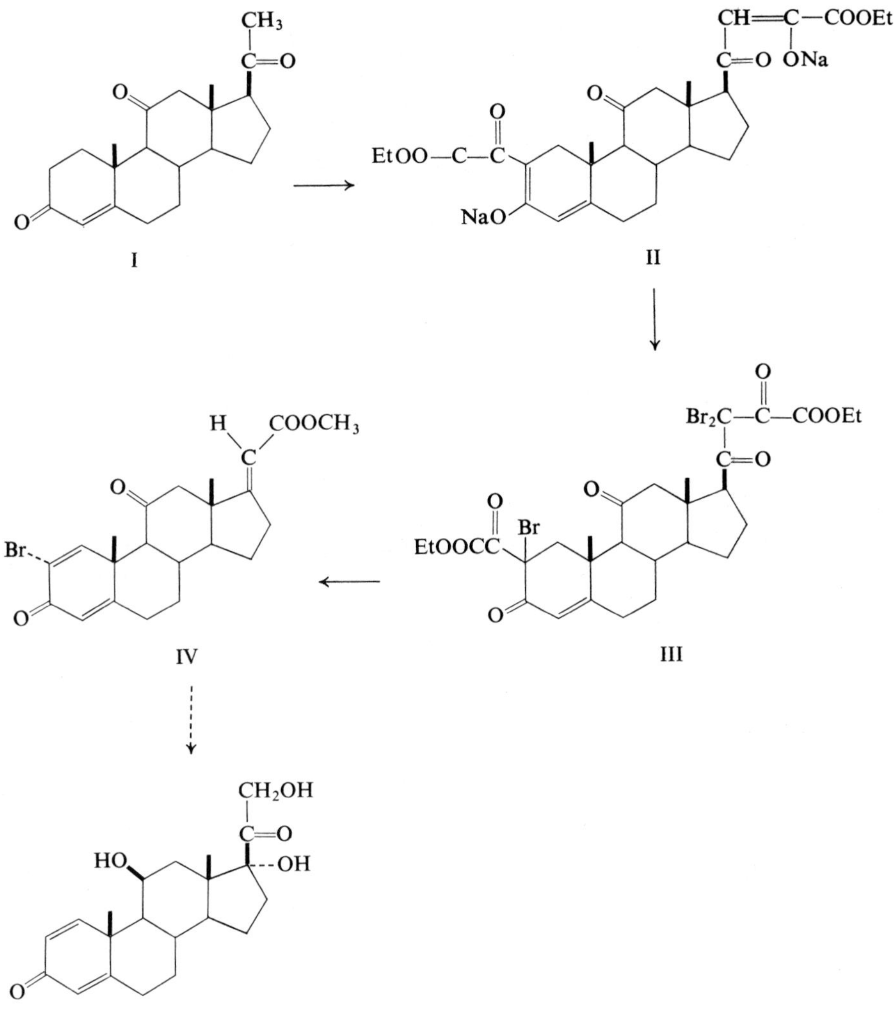

Fig. 11.15. Chemical synthesis of prednisolone.

solone (V). Prednisolone is now more often prepared by microbial dehydrogenation with *Corynebacterium simplex*. Dehydrogenation can be effected either before or after microbiological oxidation at C-11 and is also applicable to 9α-fluoro and 16α-hydroxy derivatives. Yields are about 60-90% and the most common by-products are 20β-hydroxy-steroids.

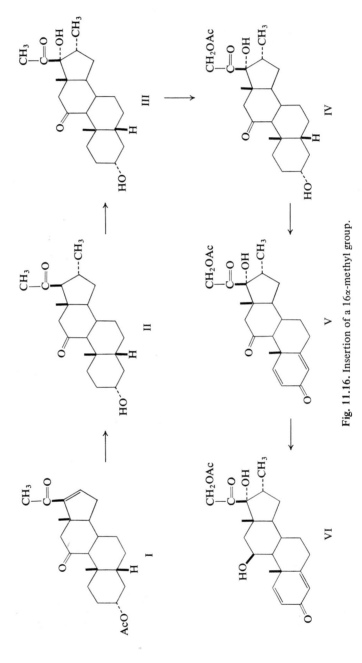

Fig. 11.16. Insertion of a 16α-methyl group.

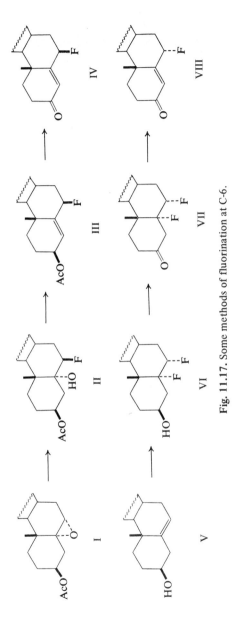

Fig. 11.17. Some methods of fluorination at C-6.

B. METHYLATION

Methyl groups have been introduced into cortisone, hydrocortisone and their Δ^1-analogues at eleven different positions throughout the steroid nucleus. The most important are the 6α- and 16α-positions. The starting material for a 16α substitution is 5β-Δ^{16}-pregnen-3α-ol-11,20-dione acetate (I) (Fig. 11.16) which is treated with methyl Grignard reagent in the presence of cuprous chloride to

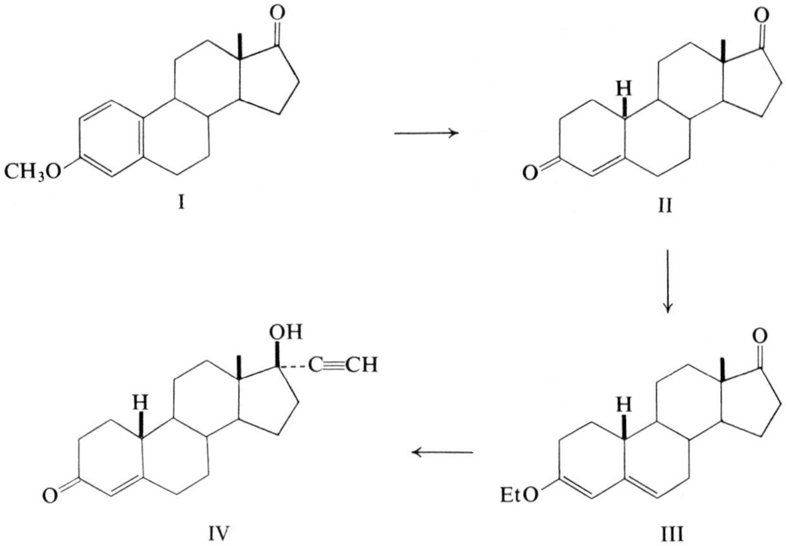

Fig. 11.18. Insertion of a 17α-ethinyl group.

obtain the 16α-methyl-20-ketone (II). Introduction of the 17α-hydroxyl is carried out by the Gallagher procedure to give (III). Bromination at C-21 followed by acetate displacement produces (III) and oxidation at C-3, bromination and dehydrobromination of the 2,4-dibromide gives 16α-methyl-prednisone (V). Sodium borohydride reduction of the 3,20-bissemicarbazone and acid hydrolysis gives 16α-methylprednisolone (VI).

C. FLUORINATION

Fluoro derivatives have now been prepared at many positions of the steroid nucleus of testosterone, progesterone and cortisone series. To achieve fluorination at the C-6 position, the 3β-acetoxy-5α,6α-epoxide (Fig. 11.17, I) of the cholestane, androstane and pregnane series is treated with boron trifluoride etherate in benzene solution and gives the fluorohydrin (II). Dehydration of the 5α-hydroxyl group with thionyl chloride gives the allylic acetate (III) and removal of the acetate group with lithium aluminium hydride followed by oxidation with chromium trioxide gives the 6β-fluoro-Δ^4-3-ketone (IV). Acid treatment produces the more stable 6α (equatorial) fluoro compound. The 6α-fluoro-Δ^4-3-ketones can be prepared directly by the *cis* addition of fluorine from lead tetrafluoride to a Δ^5-3β-alcohol (V). The resulting 5α,6α-difluoride (VI) is oxidized to the 3-ketone (VII) and treated with sodium acetate in methanol to give the 6α-fluoro-Δ^4-3-ketone (VIII).

D. INSERTION OF AN ETHINYL GROUP

The synthesis of 19-nor-ethisterone (Fig. 11.18) illustrates the process of inserting an ethinyl group. Estrone methyl ether (I) undergoes a Birch reduction with lithium in liquid ammonia and mild acid hydrolysis to give 19-nor-testosterone which is oxidized to the 3,17-dione (II) and further converted with ethyl orthoformate to its 3-enol ether (III). This is then treated with acetylene in the presence of potassium t-amylate and after hydrolysis of the protective enol ether function, 19-nor-ethisterone (IV) is produced.

BIBLIOGRAPHY

Chapter 1

Barton, D. H. R. and Cookson, R. C. (1956). Principles of conformation analysis. *Q. Rev. chem. Soc.* **10**, 44-82.

Cahn, R. S. and Ingold, C. K. (1951). Specification of configuration about quadrivalent asymmetric carbon atoms. *J. chem. Soc.* 612-22.

Cahn, R. S., Ingold, C. K. and Prelog, V. (1956). The specification of asymmetric configuration in organic chemistry. *Experientia* **12**, 81-124.

Cahn, R. S., Ingold, C. K. and Prelog, V. (1966). Specification of molecular chirality. *Angew. Chem.* (International Edition in English) **5**, 385-415.

Dorfman, R. I. and Ungar, F. (1965). "Metabolism of Steroid Hormones". Academic Press, London and New York.

Fieser, L. F. and Fieser, M. (1959). "Steroids". Reinhold, New York.

Fieser, L.F. and Fieser, M. (1960). Steroid nomenclature. *Tetrahedron* **8**, 360-65.

Florkin, M. and Stotz, E. H. (eds.) (1963). "Sterols, Bile Acids and Steroids", Comprehensive Biochemistry, Vol. 10. Elsevier, Amsterdam.

IUPAC (1958). "Nomenclature of Organic Chemistry", pp. 73-82. Butterworths, London.

IUPAC (1960). Definitive rules for nomenclature of steroids. *J. Am. chem. Soc.* **82**, 5577-81.

IUPAC (1968). IUPAC/IUB 1967 Revised tentative rules for nomenclature of steroids. *Pure appl. Chem.* 23-65; and *Biochim. biophys. Acta,* **164**, 453-86.

Klyne, W. (1965). "The Chemistry of the Steroids". Methuen, London.

Mueller, C. P. and Pettit, G. R. (1962). Nomenclature of the steroidal sapogenins. *Experientia* **18**, 404-5.

Shoppee, C. W. (1964). "Chemistry of the Steroids", 2nd Edn. Butterworths, London.

Chapter 2

Assali, N. S. (ed.) (1968). "Biology of Gestation", Vol. 1. Academic Press, London and New York.

Bell, E. T. and Loraine, J. A. (1967). "Recent Research in Gonadrotrophic Hormones". E. & S. Livingstone, Edinburgh.

Brown-Grant, K. and Cross, B. A. (eds.) (1966). Recent studies on the hypothalamus. *Br. med. Bull.* **22**, 195-277.

Butt, W. R. (1967). "Hormone Chemistry". Van Nostrand, London.

Cameron, C. B. (1963). *In* "The Liver—Morphology, Biochemistry, Physiology", Vol. 2, pp. 91-132 (edited by C. Rouiller). Academic Press, London and New York.

Davies, D. V. and Davies, F. (eds.) (1962). "Gray's Anatomy", 33rd Ed. Longmans, London.

Fraschini, F., Mess, B. and Martini, L. (1968). Pineal gland, melatonin and the control of luteinising hormone secretion. *Endocrinology* **82**, 919-24.

Grant, J. K. (1968). The biosynthesis of adrenocortical steroids. *J. Endocr.* **41**, 111-35.

Ham, A. W. and Leeson, T. S. (1965). "Histology", 2nd Edn. Pitman Medical Publishing Co., Ltd., London and J. B. Lippincott Company, Philadelphia.

Harris, G. W. and Donovan, B. T. (eds.) (1966). "The Pituitary Gland", 3 Vols. Butterworths, London.

Harris, G. W., Reed, M. and Fawcett, C. P. (1966). Hypothalamic releasing factors and the control of the anterior pituitary function. *Br. med. Bull.* **22**, 266-72.

Kandutsch, A. A. (1964). *In* "The Epidermis", pp. 493-510 (edited by W. Montagna and W. C. Lobitz). Academic Press, London and New York.

Lever, W. F. (1967). "Histopathology of the Skin". Pitman Medical Publishing Co., Ltd., London and J. B. Lippincott Company, Philadelphia.

Loomis, W. F. (1967). Skin pigment regulation of vitamin-D biosynthesis in man. *Science, N.Y.* **157**, 501-6.

Martini, L. and Ganong, W. F. (1966 and 1967). "Neuroendocrinology", 2 Vols. Academic Press, London and New York.

Martini, L., Fraschini, F. and Motta, M. (1968). Neural control of anterior pituitary functions. *Recent Prog. Horm. Res.* **24**, 439-96.

Maximow, A. A. and Bloom, W. (1952). "A Textbook of Histology", 6th Edn. W. B. Saunders Company, Philadelphia.

Peart, W. S. (1965). The renin-angiotensin system. *Pharmac. Rev.* **17**, 143-82.

Reichert, L. E., Kathan, R. H. and Ryan, R. J. (1968). Studies on the composition and properties of immunological grade human pituitary follicle stimulating hormone (FSH): comparison with luteinising hormone (LH). *Endocrinology* **82**, 109-14.

Sloper, J. C. (1966). Hypothalamic neurosecretion. *Br. med. Bull.* **22**, 208-15.

Szentagothai, J., Flerkó, B., Mess, B. and Halász, B. (1968). "Hypothalamic Control of the Anterior Pituitary", 3rd Edn. Akad. Kiado, Budapest.

Turner, C. D. (1966). "General Endocrinology", 4th Edn. W. B. Saunders Company, Philadelphia.

Chapter 3

Akhtari, M., Watkinson, I. A., Rahimtula, A. D., Wilton, D. C. and Munday, K. A. (1969). The role of a cholesta-8,14-dien-3-ol system in cholesterol biosynthesis. *Biochem. J.* **111**, 757-61.

Bergström, S., Danielsson, H. and Samuelsson, B. (1960). *In* "Lipid Metabolism" (edited by K. Bloch). John Wiley, New York.

Bloch, K. (1965). The biological synthesis of cholesterol. *Science, N.Y.* **150**, 19-28.

Clayton, R. B. (1965). Biosynthesis of sterols, steroids and terpenoids. I. Biogenesis of cholesterol and the functional steps in terpenoid biosynthesis. II. Phytosterols, terpenes and the physiologically active steroids. *Q. Rev. chem. Soc.* **19**, 168.

Cornforth, J. W. (1968). Terpenoid biosynthesis. *Chem. in Britain* 102-6.

Dorfman, R. I. and Ungar, F. (1965). "Metabolism of Steroid Hormones". Academic Press, London and New York.

Frantz, I. D. and Schroepfer, G. J. (1967). Sterol biosynthesis. *A. Rev. Biochem.* **36**, 691-726.

Goodwin, T. W. (ed.) (1963). "The Biosynthesis of Vitamins and Related Compounds". Academic Press, London and New York.

Grant, J. K. (1962). Biogenesis of the adrenal steroids. *Br. med. Bull.* **18**, 99-105.

Grant, J. K. (1968). The biosynthesis of adrenocortical steroids. *J. Endocr,* **41**, 111-35.

Greengard, P., Psychoyos, S., Tallan, H. H., Cooper, D. Y., Rosenthal, O. and Estabrook, R. W. (1967). Aldosterone synthesis by adrenal mitochondria. *Archs Biochem. Biophys.* **121**, 298-303.

György, P. and Pearson, W. N. (eds.) (1967). "The Vitamins", 2nd Edn., Vol 6. Academic Press, London and New York.

Hall, P. F. and Young, D. G. (1968). Site of action of trophic hormones upon the biosynthetic pathways to steroid hormones. *Endocrinology* **82**, 559-68.

Haslewood, G. A. D. (1967). "Bile Salts". Methuen, London.

Hayaishi, O. (ed.) (1962). "Oxygenases". Academic Press, London and New York.

Kandutsch, A. A. (1964). *In* "The Epidermis" (edited by W. Montagna and W. C. Labitz). Academic Press, London and New York.

Pasqualini, J. R. and Jayle, M. F. (eds.) (1964). "The Structure and Metabolism of Corticosteroids". Academic Press, London and New York.

Sebrell, Jr., W. H. and Harris, R. S. (eds.) (1969). "The Vitamins", 2nd Edn., Vol 3. Academic Press, London and New York.

Wilson, L. D., Oldham, S. B. and Harding, B. W. (1968). Cytochrome P450 and steroid 11β-hydroxylation in mitochondria from human adrenal cortex. *J. clin. Endocr. Metab.* **28**, 1143-52.

Chapter 4

Alexander, P. (1967). Hormone cosmetics. *Am. Perfumer Cosmet.* **82**, 31.

Applezweig, N. (1962). "Steroid Drugs". McGraw-Hill, New York.

Applezweig, N. (1964). "Index of Biologically Active Steroids". Holden-Day Inc., San Francisco.

Biggers, J. D. (1959). *In* "The Pharmacology of Plant Phenolics" (edited by J. W. Fairbairn). Academic Press, London and New York.

Bishop, P. M. F. (1968). Oral contraceptives. *Practitioner* **200**, 121-28.

Dickey, R. P. and Dorr, C. H. (1969). Oral contraceptives: selection of the proper pill. *Obstet. Gynec., N.Y.* **33**, 273-87.

Diczfalusy, E. (1968). Mode of action of contraceptive drugs. *Am. J. Obstet. Gynec.* **100**, 136-63.

Dorfman, R. I. (ed.) (1964). "Steroid Activity in Experimental Animals and Man (Part A)", Methods in Hormone Research, Vol. 3. Academic Press, London and New York.

Dorfman, R. I. (ed.) (1965). "Steroidal Activity in Experimental Animals and Man (Part B)", Methods in Hormone Research, Vol. 4. Academic Press, London and New York.

Dorfman, R. I. (ed.) (1968). "Chemical Determinations", 2nd Edn., Methods in Hormone Research, Vol. 1. Academic Press, London and New York.

Dorfman, R. I. (ed.) (1969). "Bioassay (Part A)", 2nd Edn., Methods in Hormone Research, Vol 2. Academic Press, London and New York.

Dorfman, R. I. (ed.) (1969). "Bioassay (Part B)", 2nd Edn., Methods in Hormone Research, Vol. 2. Academic Press, London and New York.

Dukes, H. H. (1965). "The Physiology of Domestic Animals", 7th Edn. Balliere, Tindall & Cox, London.

Duncan, G. W. (1968). Current research on new contraceptives. *Adv. Planned Parenthood* 3, 69-74. Excerpta Medica Foundation, Amsterdam.

Goodman, L. S. and Gilman, A. (eds.) (1965). "The Pharmacological Basis of Therapeutics", 3rd Edn. Macmillan, London.

Hamilton, T. H. (1968). Control by estrogen of genetic transcription and translation. *Science, N.Y.* 161, 649-61.

Jacobs, A. and Butler, E. B. (1965). Menstrual blood-loss in iron-deficiency anaemia. *Lancet* i, 407-9.

Karlson, P. (1968). Regulation of gene activity by hormones. *Human genetik* 6, 99-109.

Leavitt, W. W. and Meismer, D. M. (1968). Sexual development altered by non-steroidal estrogens. *Nature, Lond.* 218, 181-82.

Loraine, J. A. and Bell, E. T. (1966). "Hormone Assays and their Clinical Application". E. & S. Livingstone, Edinburgh.

MacDonald, R. R. (1967). Cervical mucus. *Post-grad. med. J.* (Dec.) Suppl. pp. 28-33.

Martindale (1967). "Extra Pharmacopoeia", 25 Edn. (edited by R. G. Todd). The Pharmaceutical Press, London.

Morgan, C. F. (1963). A comparison of topical and subcutaneous methods of administration of sixteen estrogens. *J. Endocr,* 26, 317-29.

Segal, S. J. (1967). Regulatory action of estrogenic hormones. *Develop. Biol. Supplement* 1, 264-80.

Turner, C. D. (1966). "General Endocrinology", 4th Edn. W. B. Saunders Company, Philadelphia.

Ufer, J. (1969). "The Principles and Practice of Hormone Therapy in Gynaecology and Obstetrics", (Schering Handbook). Walter de Gruyter & Co., Berlin.

Velardo, J. T. (ed.) (1958). "The Endocrinology of Reproduction". Oxford University Press, New York.

Vickery, B. H. and Bennett, J. P. (1968). The cervix and its secretion in mammals. *Physiol. Rev.* 48, 135-54.

Wynn, R. M. (ed.) (1967). "Cellular Biology of the Uterus". North Holland Publishing Co., Amsterdam.

Chapter 5

Alexander, P. (1967). Hormone cosmetics. *Am. Perfumer Cosmet.* 82, 31.

Bobroff, A. (1964). "Acne and Related Disorders of Complexion and Scalp". Charles C. Thomas, Springfield.

Briggs, M. H., Caldwell, A. D. S. and Pitchford, A. G. (1967). Treatment of cancer by progestogens. *Hosp. Med.* 63-9.

Diczfalusy, E. (1968). Mode of action of contraceptive drugs. *Am. J. Obstet. Gynec.* 100, 136-63.

Dorfman, R. I. (1963). *In* "The Biology of the Prostate and Related Tissues", Monograph 12. National Cancer Institute, U.S.A.

Duncan, G. W. (1968). Current research on new contraceptives. *Adv. Planned Parenthood* 3, 69-74. Excerpta Medica Foundation, Amsterdam.

Fox, B. W. and Fox, M. (1967). Biochemical aspects of the action of drugs on spermatogenesis. *Pharmac. Rev.* **19**, 21-57.

Goodman, L. S. and Gilman, A. (eds.) (1965). "The Pharmacological Basis of Therapeutics", 3rd Edn. Macmillan, London.

Hamilton, J. B. (1951). Patterned loss of hair in man: types and incidence. *Ann. N.Y. Acad. Sci.* **53**, 708-28.

Idson, B. (1966). Hormones and the skin. *Drug Cosmet. Ind.* **98** (3), 30 and (4), 45.

Kihlman, B. A. (1966). "Action of Chemicals on Dividing Cells". Prentice-Hall Inc., Englewood Cliffs, N.J.

Kruskemper, H. L. (1968). "Anabolic Steroids", translation by C. H. Doering. Academic Press, London and New York.

Levine, R. and Luft, R. (1965). Nitrogen-retaining steroids and their application in disease. *Adv. Metabolic Disorders* **2**, 79-111.

Loraine, J. A. and Bell, E. T. (1966). "Hormone Assays and their Clinical Application". E. & S. Livingstone, Edinburgh.

Martindale (1967). "Extra Pharmacopoeia", 25th Edn. (edited by R. G. Todd). The Pharmaceutical Press, London.

Mercantini, E. S. (1965). Hair and physiological baldness. *Can. med. Ass. J.* **92**, 1345-48.

Montagu, A. (1960). "Human Heredity". World Publishing Co., New York.

Owens, D. W. and Knox, J. M. (1967). The effect of hormones on the sebaceous glands. *Acta derm.-vener., Stockh.* **47**, 363-68.

Strauss, J. S. and Pochi P. E. (1963). The human sebaceous gland: its regulation by steroidal hormones and its use as an end organ for assaying androgenicity *in vivo. Recent Prog. Horm. Res.* **19**, 385-444.

Tata, J. R. (1968). Hormonal regulation of growth and protein synthesis. *Nature, Lond.* **219**, 331-37.

Turner, C. D. (1966). "General Endocrinology", 4th Edn. W. B. Saunders Company, Philadelphia.

Velardo, J. T. (ed.) (1958). "The Endocrinology of Reproduction". Oxford University Press, New York.

Wynn, V. (1968). The anabolic steroids. *Practitioner,* **200**, 509-18.

Chapter 6

Anderson, W. A. D. (1961). "Pathology", 4th Edn. C. V. Mosby Company, St. Louis.

Berliner, D. L. and Nabors, C. J. (1968). *In* "Topics in Pharmaceutical Sciences", Vol. 1, pp. 99-124 (edited by D. Perlman). H. K. Lewis & Co. Ltd., London.

Black, D. A. K. (ed.) (1967). "Renal Disease", 2nd Edn. Blackwell, Oxford.

Cooper, M. D., Gabrielson, A. F. and Good, R. A. (1967). Role of the thymus and other central lymphoid tissues in immunological disease. *A. Rev. Med.* **18**, 113-38.

Criep, L. H. (1967). "Dermatologic Allergy: Immunology, Diagnosis, Management". W. B. Saunders Company, Philadelphia.

Dorfman, R. I. (1969). *In* "Methods in Hormone Research", 2nd Edn., Vol. 2, p. 325 (edited by R. I. Dorfman). Academic Press, London and New York.

Ehrlich, E. N. (1968). Aldosterone, the adrenal cortex and hypertension. *A. Rev. Med.* **19**, 373-98.

Eisenstein, A. B. (ed.) (1967). "The Adrenal Cortex". J. & A. Churchill Ltd., London.

Frangione, B., Milstein, G. and Pink, J. R. L. (1969). Immunoglobulins. *Nature, Lond.* **221**, 145-54.

Gell, P. G. H. and Coombs, R. R. A. (eds.) (1968) "Clinical Aspects of Immunology", 2nd Edn. Blackwell, Oxford.

Hadgraft, J. W. (1967). The influence of formulation on skin absorption. *J. Mond. Pharm.* **3**, 309-21.

Hirsch, J. G. and Fedorko, M. E. (1968). Ultrastructure of human leukocytes. *J. Cell Biol.* **38**, 615.

Houck, J. C. and Forscher, B. K. (eds.) (1968). "Chemical Biology of Inflammation". Pergamon Press, Oxford.

Lerner, L. J., Bianchi, A., Turkheimer, A. R., Singer, F. M. and Borman, A. (1964). Anti-inflammatory steroids: potency, duration and modification of activities. *Ann. N.Y. Acad. Sci.* **116**, 1071-77.

Macaulay, D. B. (1967). Allergic diseases and associated conditions. *Br. J. Clin. Pract.* **21**, 157-62.

Mills, L. C. and Moyer, J. H. (eds.) (1961). "Inflammation and Diseases of Connective Tissue". W. B. Saunders Company, Philadelphia.

Nossal, G. T. V. (1967). Mechanisms of antibody production. *A. Rev. Med.* **18**, 81-96.

Peart, W. S. (1965). The renin-angiotensin system. *Pharmac. Rev.* **17**, 143.

Ringler, I. (1964). Activities of adrenocorticosteroids in experimental animals and man. *Meth. Hormone Res.* **3A**, 227-349.

Robson, J. S. (1968). Current concepts in renal physiology. *Practitioner* **201**, 413-26.

Ross, E. J. (1965). Aldosterone and its antagonists. *Clin. Pharmac. Ther* **6**, 65.

Schlagel, C. A. (1965). Comparative efficacy of topical anti-inflammatory steroids. *J. pharm. Sci.* **54**, 335-54.

Schur, P. H. and Austen, K. F. (1968). Complement in human disease. *A. Rev. Med.* **19**, 1-24.

Sibler, R. H. and Arcese, P. S. (1964). *In* "Animal and Clinical Pharmacologic Techniques in Drug Evaluation", p.542 (edited by J. H. Nodine and P. E. Siegler). Year Book Medical Publishing Company, Chicago.

Spector, W. G. and Willoughby, D. A. (1968). "The Pharmacology of Inflammation". The English Universities Press, London.

Turk, J. L. (1967). "Delayed Hypersensitivity". North Holland Publishing Co., Amsterdam.

Wardener, H. E. de (1967). "The Kidney: An Outline of Normal and Abnormal Structure and Function", 3rd Edn. J. & A. Churchill Ltd., London.

Wilson, D. B. and Billingham, R. E. (1967). Lymphocytes and transplantation immunity. *Adv. Immunology* **7**, 189-273.

Yoffey, J. M. (ed.) (1967). "The Lymphocyte in Immunology and Haemopoiesis". Edward Arnold, London.

Chapter 7

Bolis, L. and Pethica, B. A. (eds.) (1968). "Membrane Models and the Formation of Biological Membranes". North Holland Publishing Co., Amsterdam.

Chapman, D. (ed.) (1968). "Biological Membranes". Academic Press, London and New York.

Constantinides, P. (1965). "Experimental Atherosclerosis". Elsevier, Amsterdam.

Cook, R. P. (ed.) (1958). "Cholesterol-Chemistry, Biochemistry and Pathology". Academic Press, London and New York.

Copp, D. H. (1969). Endocrine control of calcium homeostasis. *J. Endocr.* **43**, 137-61.

Danielsson, H. (1963). Present status of research on catabolism and excretion of cholesterol. *Adv. Lipid Res.* **1**, 335-85.

De Luca, H. F. (1967). Mechanism of action and metabolic fate of vitamin D. *Vitams Horm.* **25**, 315-367.

Dietschy, J. M. (1968). Mechanism for the intestinal absorption of bile acids. *J. Lipid Res.* **9**, 297-309.

Hofmann, A. F. and Small, D. M. (1967). Detergent properties of the bile salts: correlation with physiological function. *A. Rev. Med.* **18**, 333-76.

Northcote, N. H. (ed.) (1968). Structure and function of membranes. *Br. med. Bull.* **24**, 99-184.

Popper, H. (1968). Cholestasis. *A. Rev. Med.* **19**, 39-56.

Roberts, J. C. and Straus, R. (1965). "Comparative Atherosclerosis". Harper and Row, New York.

Schettler, F. G. and Boyd G. S. (eds.) (1969). "Atherosclerosis: Pathology, Physiology, Aetiology, Diagnosis and Clinical Management". Elsevier, Amsterdam.

Seeman, P. M. (1966). Membrane stabilisation by drugs: tranquilisers, steroids and anaesthetics. *Int. Rev. Neurobiol.* **9**, 145-221.

Sperry, W. M. and Webb, M. (1950). Revision of the Schoenheimer-Sperry method for cholesterol determination. *J. biol. Chem.* **187**, 97.

Stein, W. D. and Danielli, J. F. (1956). *Discuss. Faraday Soc.* **21**, 238.

Taylor, S. F. (ed.) (1968). "Calcitonin". William Heinemann Medical Books Ltd., London.

Weissman, G. (1968). The role of lysosomes in inflammation and disease. *A. Rev. Med.* **18**, 97-112.

Wiseman, G. (1964). "Absorption from the Intestine". Academic Press, London and New York.

Zemplenyi, T. (1968). "Enzyme Biochemistry of the Arterial Wall as Related to Atherosclerosis". Lloyd-Luke (Medical), London.

Chapter 8

Bongiovanni, A. F., Eberlein, W. R., Goldman, A. S. and New, M. (1967). Disorders of adrenal biogenesis. *Recent Prog. Horm. Res.* **23**, 375-449.

Bransome, E. D. (1968). The adrenal cortex. *A. Rev. Physiol.* **30**, 171-212.

Brown, J. and Pearson, C. M. (eds.) (1962). "Clinical Uses of Adrenal Steroids". McGraw-Hill, New York.

Cope, C. L. (1964). "Adrenal Steroids and Disease". Pitman Medical Publishing Co. Ltd., London.

Gaunt, R., Steinetz, B. G. and Chart, J. J. (1968). Pharmacologic alteration of steroid hormone functions. *Clin. Pharmac. Ther.* **9**, 657-81.

Gray, C. H. and Bacharach, A. L. (1967). "Hormones in Blood", 2nd. Edn. 2 Vols. Academic Press, London and New York.

Gray, C. H., Baron, D. N., Brooks, R. V. and James, V. H. T. (1969). A critical appraisal of a method of estimating urinary 17-oxosteroids and total 17-oxogenic steroids. *Lancet* **i**, 124-27.

Gray, M. S. Strausfeld, K. S., Watanabe, M., Sims, E. A. H. and Solomon, S. (1968). Aldosterone secretory rates in the normal menstrual cycle. *J. clin. Endocr. Metab.* **28**, 1269-75.

Holt, K. S. and Raine, D. N. (eds.) (1966). "Basic Concepts of Inborn Errors and Defects of Steroid Biosynthesis". E. & S. Livingstone, Edinburgh.

James, V. H. T. and Landon, J. (1968). "The Investigation of the Hypothalamic-Pituitary-Adrenal Function". Cambridge University Press, London.

Laragh, J. H. and Kelly, W. G. (1964). Aldosterone: its biochemistry and physiology. *Adv. Metab. Disorders* **1**, 217-62.

Loraine, J. A. and Bell, E. T. (1966). "Hormone Assays and their Clinical Application". E. & S. Livingstone, Edinburgh.

McKerns, K. W. (ed.) (1968). "Functions of the Adrenal Cortex". 2 Vols. North Holland Publishing Co., Amsterdam.

Nichols, C. T. and Tyler, F. H. (1967). Diurnal variation in adrenal function. *A. Rev. Med.* **18**, 313-24.

Thomas, P. (1968). "Guide to Steroid Therapy". Lloyd-Luke (Medical), London.

Chapter 9

Assali, N. S. (ed.) (1968). "Biology of Gestation", Vol. 1. Academic Press, London and New York.

Baird, D., Horton, R., Longcope, C. D. and Tait, J. F. (1968). Steroid prehormones. *Perspect. Biol. Med.* **11**, 384-421.

Briggs, M. H., Caldwell, A. D. S. and Pitchford, A. G. (1967). The treatment of cancer by progestogens. *Hosp. Med.* 63-9.

Curstensen, H. (ed.) (1967). "Steroid Hormone Analysis". Edward Arnold, London.

Dale, S. L. (1967). "Principles of Steroid Analysis". Henry Kempton, London.

Gandy, H. M. and Peterson, R. E. (1968). Measurement of testosterone and 17-ketosteroids in plasma by the double isotope dilution derivative technique. *J. clin. Endocr. Metab.* **28**, 949-77.

Gray, C. H. and Bacharach, A. L. (1967). "Hormones in Blood", 2nd Edn. 2 Vols. Academic Press, London and New York.

Hobson, B. M (1967). Pregnancy diagnosis. *J. Reprod. Fert.* **12**, 33-48.

Hytten, F. E. and Leitch, I. (1964). "The Physiology of Human Pregnancy". Blackwell, Oxford.

Israel, S. L. (1967). "Diagnosis and Treatment of Menstrual Disorders and Sterility", 5th Edn. Hoeber Medical Division, Harper and Row, New York.

Jensen, V., Deshpande, N., Bulbrook, R. D. and Doouss, T. W. (1968). Adrenal function in breast cancer. *J. Endocr.* **42**, 425-39.

Jones, B. M. and Kemp, R. B. (1969). Self-isolation of the foetal trophoblast. *Nature, Lond.* **221**, 829-31.

Loraine, J. A. and Bell, E. T. (1966). "Hormone Assays and their Clinical Application". E. & S. Livingstone, Edinburgh.

Peterson, N. T., Midgley, A. R. and Jaffe R. B. (1968). Regulation of human gonadotrophins, III Luteinising hormone and follicle stimulating hormone in sera from adult males. *J. clin. Endocr. Metab.* **28**, 1473.

Riondel, A., Tait, J. F., Gut, M., Tait, S. A. S., Joachim, E. and Little, B. (1963). Estimation of testosterone in human peripheral blood using S^{35}-thiosemicarbazide. *J. clin. Endocr. Metab.* **23**, 620-28.

Saxena, B. B., Demura, H., Gandy, H. M. and Peterson, R. E. (1968). Radioimmunoassay of human follicle stimulating and luteinising hormones in plasma. *J. clin. Endocr. Metab.* **28**, 519-34.

Selenkow, H. A., Wool, M. S. and Refetoff, S. (1967). Radioimmunoassay of anterior pituitary hormones. *Radiol. Clin. N. Amer.* **5**, 317-31.

Southren, A. L. (1965). The syndrome of testicular feminisation. *Adv. Metabolic Disorders* **2**, 227-55.

Stirrat, G. M. (1968). Suppression of lactation by stilboestrol. *J. Obstet. Gynaec. Br. Commonw.* **75**, 313.

Tanner, J. M. and Gupta, D. (1968). A longitudinal study of the urinary excretion of individual steroids in children from 8 to 12 years old. *J. Endocr.* **41**, 139-56.

Vande Wels, R. L., Macdonald, P. C., Grupide, E. and Lieberman, S. (1963). Studies on the secretion and interconversion of the androgens. *Recent Prog. Horm. Res.* **19**, 275-310.

Wallach, E. E. and Touchstone, J. C. (1967). Comparison of methods for pregnanediol determination. *Clin. Chem.* **13**, 976-84.

Wang, D. Y. and Bulbrook, R. D. (1968). Steroid sulphates in foetal-placental endocrinology. *Adv. Reprod. Physiol.* **3**, 113-46.

Zuppinger, K., Engel, E., Forbes, A. P., Mantooth, L. and Claffey, J. (1967). Klinefelter's syndrome, a clinical and cytogenic study in twenty-four cases. *Acta endocr., Copenh.* **54**, suppl. 113.

Chapter 10

Bates, R. B. (1967). *In* "Antibiotics", Vol. 2, pp. 134-51 (edited by D. Gottlieb and P. D. Shaw). Springer-Verlag, Berlin.

Boiteau, P., Pasich, B. and Ratsimamanga, R. (1964). "Les Triterpenoids en Physiologie Vegetale et Animale". Gauthier-Villars, Paris.

Bonner, J. and Varner, J. E. (eds.) (1965). "Plant Biochemistry". Academic Press, London and New York.

IUPAC (1968). IUPAC/IUB (1967). Revised tentative rules for nomenclature of steroids. *Pure appl. Chem.* 23-65; and *Biochim. biophys. Acta* **164**, 453-86.

Karlson, P. and Sekeris, C. E. (1966). Ecdysone, an insect steroid hormone and its mode of action. *Recent Prog. Horm. Res.* **22**, 473-502.

Kreig, M. B. (1965). "Green Medicine". George G. Harrap & Co., London.

Manske, R. H. F. and Holmes, H. L. (eds.) (1953). "The Alkaloids: Chemistry and Physiology", Vol. 3. Academic Press, London and New York.

Ohtaki, T., Milkman, R. D. and Williams, C. M. (1967). Ecdysone and ecdysone analogues: their assay on the fleshfly *Sarcophaga peregrina. Proc. natn. Acad. Sci. U.S.A.* **58**, 981-84.

Pridham, J. B. (ed.) (1967). "Terpenoids in Plants". Academic Press, London and New York.

Schreiber, K., Adam, G., Aurich, O., Horstmann, C., Ripperger H. and Ronsch, H. (1967). "Recent Advances in the Preparation of Hormone Steroids from Solanum Alkaloids". Proc. 2nd Internat. Congress Hormonal Steroids (edited by L. Martini, F. Fraschini and M. Motta), pp. 334-53. Excerpta Medica Foundation, Amsterdam.

Shoppee, C. W. (1964). "Chemistry of the Steroids", 2nd Edn. Butterworths, London.

Chapter 11

Charney, W. and Herzog, H. L. (1967). "Microbial Transformation of Steroids". Academic Press, London and New York.
Djerassi, C. (1963). "Steroid Reactions". Holden-Day Inc., San Francisco.
Fieser, L. F. and Fieser, M. (1959). "Steroids". Reinhold, New York.
Florkin, M. and Stotz, E. H. (1963). "Sterols, Bile Acids and Steroids", Comprehensive Biochemistry, Vol. 10. Elsevier, Amsterdam.
Hanson, J. R. (1968). "Introduction to Steroid Chemistry". Pergamon Press, Oxford.
Iizuka, H. and Atsushi, N. (1966). "Microbial Transformation of Steroids and Alkaloids". University Park Press, Manchester.
Klyne, W. (1965). "The Chemistry of the Steroids". Methuen, London.
Shoppee, C. W. (1964). "Chemistry of the Steroids", 2nd Edn. Butterworths, London.

APPENDIX I

TRIVIAL AND SYSTEMATIC NAMES OF STEROIDS

Trivial name	IUPAC (1968) Systematic Name	Alternative systematic name
A		
Acovenosigenin	1β,3β,14-Trihydroxy-5β,14β-card-20(22)-enolide	20(22),(5β,14β)-Cardenolide-1β,3β,14-triol
Adenosterone	4-Androstene-3,11,17-trione	4-Androsten-3,11,17-trione
Adynerigenin	3β,16β-Dihydroxy-5β-card-8(14),20(22)-dienolide	8(14),20(22),(5β)-Cardadienolide-3β,16β-diol
Aetio–	*see* Etio–	
Agapanthagenin	(25R)-5α-Spirostane-2α,3β,5-triol	(25R)-5α-Spirostan-2α,3β,5-triol
Agavogenin	(25R)-5α-Spirostane-2α,3β,12β-triol	(25R)-5α-Spirostan-2α,3β,12β-triol
Agnosterol	5α-Lanosta-7,9(11),24-trien-3β-ol	7,9(11),24,(5α)-Lanostatrien-3β-ol
Aldactone	3-(3-Oxo-7α-acetvlthio-17β-hydroxy-4-androsten-17α-yl) propionic acid α-lactone	4-Androsten-17β-ol-3-one-17α-propionic acid 17α,17β-lactone,7α-acetylmercaptide
Aldosterone	{11β,21-Dihydroxy-3,20-dioxo-4-pregn-ene-18-al(11→18)-lactol / 3,20-Dioxo-11β,18-oxido-4-pregnene-18,21-diol	4-Pregnen-18-al-11β,21-diol-3,20-dione (11→18)-lactol
Allocholanes	*see* 5α-Cholanes	
Allocholesterol	4-Cholesten-3β-ol	4-Cholesten-3β-ol
Allocholic acid	3α,7α,12α-Trihydroxy-5α-cholan-24-oic acid	24,(5α)-Cholanic acid-3α,7α,12α-triol
Allocortol	5α-Pregnane-3α,11β,17,20α,21-pentol	5α-Pregnan-3α,11β,17α,20α,21-pentol
β-Allocortol	5α-Pregnane-3α,11β,17,20β,21-pentol	5α-Pregnan-3α,11β,17α,20β,21-pentol
Allocortolone	3α,17,20α,21-Tetrahydroxy-5α-pregnan-11-one	5α-Pregnan-3α,17α,20α,21-tetrol-11-one
β-Allocortolone	3α,17,20β,21-Tetrahydroxy-5α-pregnan-11-one	5α-Pregnan-3α,17α,20β,21-tetrol-11-one
Allodihydrocortisol	11β,17,21-Trihydroxy-5α-pregnane-3,20-dione	5α-Pregnan-11β,17α,21-triol-3,20-dione
Allodihydrocortisone	17α,21-Dihydroxy-5α-pregnane-3,11,20-trione	5α-Pregnan-17α,21-diol-3,11,20-trione
Allodihydrotestosterone	17β-Hydroxy-5α-androstan-3-one	5α-Androstan-17β-ol-3-one
Allopregnanolone	3β-Hydroxy-5α-pregnan-20-one	5α-Pregnan-3β-ol-20-one
Allopregnanes	*see* 5α-Pregnanes	
Allotetrahydrocortisol	3α,11β,17,21-Tetrahydroxy-5α-pregnan-20-one	5α-Pregnan-3α,11β,17α,21-tetrol-20-one
Androisoxazole	17β-Hydroxy-17-methyl-5α-androstan-[3,2-c]-isoxazole	17α-Methyl-5α-androstan-17β-ol[3,2-c]-isoxazole
Androstadienedione	1,4-Androstadiene-3,17-dione	1,4-Androstadien-3,17-dione
Androstadienolone	17β-Hydroxy-1,4-androstadien-3-one	1,4-Androstadien-17β-ol-3-one
Androstanazole	17β-Hydroxy-17-methyl-5α-androstane[3,2-c]-pyrazole	17α-Methyl-5α-androstan-17β-ol[3,2-c]-pyrazole
Androstanediol	5α-Androstane-3β,17β-diol	5α-Androstan-3β,17β-diol
Androstane	5α-Androstane	5α-Androstane
Androstanedione	5α-Androstane-3,17-dione	5α-Androstan-3,17-dione
Androstanolone	17β-Hydroxy-5α-androstan-3-one	5α-Androstan-17β-ol-3-one
Androstenediol	5-Androstene-3β,17β-diol	5-Androsten-3β,17β-diol
Androstenedione	4-Androstene-3,17-dione	4-Androsten-3,17-dione
Androstenolone	3β-Hydroxy-5-androsten-17-one	5-Androsten-3β-ol-17-one
Androsterone	3α-Hydroxy-5α-androstan-17-one	5α-Androstan-3α-ol-17-one
Anhydrohydroxyprogesterone	17α-Ethinyl-17-hydroxy-4-androsten-3-one	17α-Ethinyl-4-androsten-17β-ol-3-one

Name		
Antiarigenin	3β,5,12β,14-Tetrohydroxy-19-oxo-5β,14β-card-20(22)-enolide	20(22),(5β,14β)-Cardenolide-3β,5,12β,14-tetrol-19-one
Apocholic acid	3α,12α-Dihydroxy-5β-chol-8(14)-enic acid	8(14),(5β)-Cholenic acid-3α,12α-diol
Arenobufagin	3β,11α,14-Trihydroxy-12-oxo-5β,14β-bufa-20,22-dienolide	20,22,(5β,14β)-Bufadienolide-3β,11α,14-triol-12-one
Ascosterol	24-Methyl-5α-cholesta-8,23-dien-3β-ol	24-Methyl-8,23,(5α)-cholestadien-3β-ol
B		
Basseol	5α-Eupha-7,24-dien-3β-ol	7,24,(5α)-Euphadien-3β-ol
Beclomethasone dipropionate	9α-Chloro-11β,17,21-trihydroxy-16β-methyl-1,4-pregnadiene-3,20-dione 17,21-dipropionate	9α-Chloro-16β-methyl-1,4-pregnadien-11β,17α,21-triol-3,20-dione 17,21-dipropionate
Betamethasone valerate	9α-Fluoro-11β,17,21-trihydroxy-16β-methyl-1,4-pregnadiene-3,20-dione 17-n-valerate	9α-Fluoro-16β-methyl-1,4-pregnadien-11β,17α-21-triol-3,20-dione 17-n-valerate
Bipindogenin	3β,5,11α,14-Tetrahydroxy-5β,14β-card-20(22)-enolide	20(22),(5β,14β)-Cardenolide-3β,5,11α,14-tetrol
22,23-Bisnorallocholanic acid-3β-ol	3β-Hydroxy-5α-pregnane-21-carboxylic acid	5α-Pregnan-3β-ol-21-carboxylic acid
Botogenin	(25R)-3β-Hydroxy-5-spirosten-12-one	(25R)-5-Spirosten-3β-ol-12-one
Bovogenin A	3β,5,14-Trihydroxy-19-oxo-5β,14β-bufa-20,22-dienolide	20,22,(5β,14β)-Bufadienolide-3β,5,14-triol-19-one
Brassicasterol	(24S)-24-Methylcholest-5,22-dien-3β-ol	5,22-Ergostadien-3β-ol
Bufalin	3β,14-Dihydroxy-5β,14β-bufa-20,22-dienolide	20,22,(5β,14β)-Bufadienolide-3β,14-diol
Bufotalin	16β-Acetoxy-3β,14-dihydroxy-5β,14β-bufa-20,22-dienolide	20,22,(5β,14β)-Bufadienolide-3β,14,16β-triol 16-acetate
Bufotalidin	3β,5,14-Trihydroxy-19-oxo-5β,14β-bufa-20,22-dienolide	20,22,(5β,14β)-Bufadienolide-3β,5,14-triol-19-one
Bufotalinin	14,15β-Epoxy-3β,5-dihydroxy-19-oxo-5β,14β-bufa-20,22-dienolide	20,22,(5β,14β)-Bufadienolide-3β,5-diol-19-one 14,15β-epoxide
Butyrospermol	5α-Eupha-7,24-dien-3β-ol	7,24,(5α)-Euphadien-3β-ol
C		
Calciferol	9,10-Secocholesta-5,7,10(19)-trien-3β-ol	9,10-Seco-5,7,10(19)-cholestatrien-3β-ol
Campestanol	(24R)-24-Methyl-5α-cholestan-3β-ol	(24R)-Methyl-5α-cholestan-3β-ol
Campesterol	(24R)-24-Methyl-5-cholesten-3β-ol	(24R)-24-Methyl-5-cholesten-3β-ol
Cannogenin	3β,14-Dihydroxy-19-oxo-5β,14β-card-20(22)-enolide	20(22),(5β,14β)-Cardenolide-3β,14-diol-19-one
Carbenoxolone	3β-(3-Carboxypropionyloxy)-11-oxo-12,(18β)-olean-en-30-oic acid	12,(18β)-Oleanen-3β-ol-11-one-30-oic acid 3-hemisuccinate
Caudogenin	3β,12α,14-Trihydroxy-11-oxo-5β,14β-card-20(22)-enolide	20(22),(5β,14β)-Cardenolide-3β,12α,14-triol-11-one
Chalinasterol	24-Methylene-5-cholesten-3β-ol	24-Methylene-5-cholesten-3β-ol
Chenodeoxycholic acid	3α,7α-Dihydroxy-5β-cholan-24-oic acid	24,(5β)-Cholanic acid-3α,7α-diol
Chiapagenin	(25S)-5-Spirostene-3β,12β-diol	(25S)-5-Spirosten-3β,12β-diol
Chlocortolone	9α-Chloro-6α-fluoro-11β,21-dihydroxy-16α-methyl-1,4-pregnadiene-3,20-dione	9α-Chloro-6α-fluoro-16α-methyl-1,4-pregnadien-11β,21-diol-3,20-dione
Chlormadinone acetate	17-Acetoxy-6-chloro-4,6-pregnadiene-3,20-dione	6-Chloro-4,6-pregnadien-17α-ol-3,20-dione 17-acetate
Chlorogenin	(25R)-5α-Spirostane-3β,6α-diol	(25R)-5α-Spirostan-3β,6α-diol
Cholaic acid	3α,7α,12α-Trihydroxy-5β-cholan-24-oic acid N-(2-sulphoethyl)-amide	24,(5β)-Cholanic acid-3α,7α,12α-triol N-(2-sulphoethyl)-amide
Cholecalciferol	9,10-Secocholesta-5,7,10(19)-trien-3β-ol	9,10-Seco-5,7,10(19)-cholestatrien-3β-ol
α-Cholestanol (Epicholestanol)	5α-Cholestan-3α-ol	5α-Cholestan-3α-ol
β-Cholestanol (Cholestanol)	5α-Cholestan-3β-ol	5α-Cholestan-3β-ol
Cholestanone	5α-Cholestan-3-one	5α-Cholestan-3-one
Cholestene	5-Cholestene	5-Cholestene
Cholestenone	4-Cholesten-3-one	4-Cholesten-3-one

APPENDIX I—*continued*

Trivial Name	IUPAC (1968) Systematic Name	Alternative systematic name
Cholesterol	5-Cholesten-3β-ol	5-Cholesten-3β-ol
Cholesteryl chloride	3β-Chloro-5-cholestene; 5-cholesten-3β-yl chloride	5-Cholesten-3β-yl chloride
Cholesterylene	3,5-Cholestadiene	3,5-Cholestadiene
Cholic acid	3α,7α,12α-Trihydroxy-5β-cholan-24-oic acid	24,(5β)-Cholanic acid-3α,7α,12α-triol
Chondrillasterol	(24S)-24-Ethyl-5α-cholesta-7,22-dien-3β-ol	(24S)-24-Ethyl-7,22,(5α)-cholestadien-3β-ol
Chryseogenin	7α,15α-Epoxy-3β,14-dihydroxy-11,12-dioxo-5β,14β-card-20(22)-enolide	20(22),(5β,14β)-Cardenolide-3β,14-diol-11,12-dione 7α,15α-epoxide
Cinchol	(24R)-24-Ethyl-5-cholesten-3β-ol	5-Stigmasten-3β-ol
Cinobufagenin	14,15β-Epoxy-3β-hydroxy-5β,14β-bufa-20,22-dienolide	20,22,(5β,14β)-Bufadienolide-3β-ol 14,15β-epoxide
Cinobufotalin	6β-Acetoxy-14,15β-epoxy-3β,5-dihydroxy-5β,14β-bufa-20,22-dienolide	20,22,(5β,14β)-Bufadienolide-3β,5,6β-triol 6-acetate, 14,15β-epoxide
Cis-testosterone	17α-Hydroxy-4-androsten-3-one	4-Androsten-17α-ol-3-one
Clionasterol	(24S)-24-Ethyl-5-cholesten-3β-ol	(24S)24-Ethyl-5-cholesten-3β-ol
Coprostane	5β-Cholestane	5β-Cholestane
Coprostanol (Coprosterol)	5β-Cholestan-3β-ol	5β-Cholestan-3β-ol
Coprostenol	4-Cholesten-3β-ol	4-Cholesten-3β-ol
Coroglaucigenin	3β,14,19-Trihydroxy-5α,14β-card-20(22)-enolide	20,(22),(5α,14β)-Cardenolide-3β,14,19-triol
Corotoxigenin	3β,14-Dihydroxy-19-oxo-5α,14β-card-20(22)-enolide	20,(22),(5α,14β)-Cardenolide-3β,14-diol-19-one
Correlogenin	(25S)-3β-Hydroxy-5-spirosten-12-one	(25S)-5-Spirosten-3β-ol-12-one
Cortexolone	17,21-Dihydroxy-4-pregnene-3,20-dione	4-Pregnen-17α,21-diol-3,20-dione
Cortexone	21-Hydroxy-4-pregnene-3,20-dione	4-Pregnen-21-ol-3,20-dione
Corticosterone	11β,21-Dihydroxy-4-pregnene-3,20-dione	4-Pregnen-11β,21-diol-3,20 dione
Cortisol	11β,17,21-Trihydroxy-4-pregnene-3,20-dione	4-Pregnen-11β,17α,21-triol-3,20-dione
Cortisone	17,21-Dihydroxy-4-pregnene-3,11,20-trione	4-Pregnen-17α,21-diol-3,11,20-trione
Δ-Cortisone	17,21-Dihydroxy-1,4-pregnadiene-3,11,20-trione	1,4-Pregnadien-17α,21-diol-3,11,20-trione
Cortol (α-Cortol)	5β-Pregnane-3α,11β,17,20α,21-pentol	5β-Pregnan-3α,11β,17α,20α,21-pentol
β-Cortol	5β-Pregnane-3α,11β,17,20β,21-pentol	5β-Pregnan-3α,11β,17α,20β,21-pentol
Cortolone (α-Cortolone)	3α,17,20α,21-Tetrahydroxy-5β-pregnan-11-one	5β-Pregnan-3α,17α,20α,21-tetrol-11-one
β-Cortolone	3α,17,20β,21-Tetrahydroxy-5β-pregnan-11-one	5β-Pregnan-3α,17α,20β,21-tetrol-11-one
Cronolone	17-Acetoxy-9α-fluoro-11β-hydroxy-4-pregnene-3,20-dione	9α-Fluoro-4-pregnen-11β,17α-diol-3,20-dione 17-acetate
Cycloartenol	9β,19-Cyclo-24-lanosten-3β-ol	24-Cycloarten-3β-ol
Cycloeucalenol	{ 24-Methylene-9β,19-cyclo-31-nor-5α-lanostan-3β-ol / 4α,14α-Dimethyl-24-methylene-9β,19-cyclo-5α-cholestan-3β-ol }	24-Methylene-31-nor-5α-cycloartan-3β-ol
Cyclolaudenol	{ (24S)-24-Methyl-9β,19-cyclo-5α-lanost-25(26)-en-3β-ol / 4,4,14α-Trimethyl-9β,19-cyclo-25(26),(5α)-ergosten-3β-ol }	(24S)-24-Methyl-25(26),(5α)-cycloarten-3β-ol
Cyproterone acetate	17-Acetoxy-6-chloro-1α,2α-methylene-1α,2α-methylene-4,6-pregnadiene-3,20-dione	6-Chloro-1α,2α-methylene-4,6-pregnadien-17α-ol-3,20-dione 17-acetate
5α-Cucurbitane	19(10→9β)-abeo-5α-Lanostane	5α-Cucurbitane
D		
5α-Dammarane	8-Methyl-18-nor-5α-lanostane	5α-Dammarane
Decogenin	3β,14-Dihydroxy-11,12-dioxo-5β,14β-card-20(22)-enolide	20(22),(5β,14β)-Cardenolide-3β,14-diol-11,12-dione
7-Dehydroandrostenolone	3β-Hydroxy-5,7-androstadien-17-one	5,7-Androstadien-3β-ol-17-one

Name	Systematic name	Systematic name
24-Dehydrocholesterol	5,24-Cholestadien-3β-ol	5,24-Cholestadien-3β-ol
Dehydrocholic acid	3,7,12-Trioxo-5β-cholan-24-oic acid	24,(5β)-Cholanic acid-3,7,12-trione
Dehydrocortisol	11β,17,21-Trihydroxy-1,4-pregnadiene-3,20-dione	1,4-Pregnadien-11β,17α,21-triol-3,20-dione
Dehydrocortisone	17,21-Dihydroxy-1,4-pregnadiene-3,11,20-trione	1,4-Pregnadien-17α,21-diol-3,11,20-trione
Dehydroepiandrosterone	3β-Hydroxy-5-androsten-17-one	5-Androsten-3β-ol-17-one
Dehydrohydrocortisone	11β,17,21-Trihydroxy-1,4-pregnadiene-3,20-dione	1,4-Pregnadien-11β,17α,21-triol-3,20-dione
1-Dehydromethyltestosterone	17β-Hydroxy-17-methyl-1,4-androstadien-3-one	17α-Methyl-1,4-androstadien-17β-ol-3-one
1-Dehydrotestosterone	17β-Hydroxy-1,4-androstadien-3-one	1,4-Androstadien-17β-ol-3-one
Deoxycholic acid	3α,12α-Dihydroxy-5β-cholan-24-oic acid	24,(5β)-Cholanic acid-3α,12α-diol
Deoxycorticosterone	21-Hydroxy-4-pregnene-3,20-dione	4-Pregnen-21-ol-3,20-dione
21-Deoxycortisone	17α-Hydroxy-4-pregnene-3,11,20-trione	4-Pregnen-17α-ol-3,11,20-trione
Deoxyequilenin	1,3,5(10),6,8-Estrapentaen-17-one	1,3,5(10),6,8-Estrapenten-17-one
Desfluocortolone	9α-Chloro-11β,21-dihydroxy-16α-methyl-1,4-pregnadiene-3,20-dione	9α-Chloro-16α-methyl-1,4-pregnadien-11β,21-diol-3,20-dione
Desmosterol	5,24-Cholestadien-3β-ol	5,24-Cholestadien-3β-ol
Desoxy—	see Deoxy—	—
Dexamethasone	9α-Fluoro-11β,17,21-trihydroxy-16α-methyl-1,4-pregnadiene- 3,20-dione	9α-Fluoro-16α-methyl-1,4-pregnadien-11β,17α-21-triol-3,20-dione
Dichlorisone acetate	21-Acetoxy-9α,11β-dichloro-17,21-hydroxy-1,4-pregnadiene-3,20-dione	9α,11β-Dichloro-1,4-pregnadien-17α,21-diol-3,20-dione acetate
Digacetigenin	20α-Acetoxy-3β,9α-dihydroxy-5-pregnene-11,15-dione	5-Pregnen-3β,9α,20α-triol-11,15-dione 20-acetate
Diginigenin	12α,20α-Epoxy-3β-hydroxy-14β,17α-pregn-5-ene-11,15-dione	5,(14β,17α)-Pregnen-3β-ol-11,15-dione 12α,20α-epoxide
Digitogenin	(25R)-5α-Spirostane-2α,3β,15β-triol	(25R)-5α-Spirostan-2α,3β,15β-triol
Digitoxigenin	3β,14-Dihydroxy-5β,14β-card-20(22)-enolide	20(22),(5β,14β)-Cardenolide-3β,14-diol
Digoxigenin	3β,12β,14-Trihydroxy-5β,14β-card-20(22)-enolide	20(22),(5β,14β)-Cardenolide-3β,12β,14-triol
Dihydroallocortisone	17,21-Dihydroxy-5α-pregnane-3,11,20-trione	5α-Pregnan-17α,21-diol-3,11,20-trione
Dihydroandrosterone	5α-Androstane-3α,17β-diol	5α-Androstan-3α,17β-diol
Dihydroequilenin	1,3,5(10),6,8-Estrapentaene-3,17β-diol	1,3,5(10),6,8-Estrapenten-3,17β-diol
Dihydrocholesterol	5α-Cholestan-3β-ol	5α-Cholestan-3β-ol
Dihydrocorticosterone	11β,21-Dihydroxy-5β-pregnane-3,20-dione	5β-Pregnan-11β,21-diol-3,20-dione
Dihydrocortisol	11β,17,21-Trihydroxy-5β-pregnane-3,20-dione	5β-Pregnan-11β,17α-triol-3,20-dione
Dihydrocortisone	17,21-Dihydroxy-5β-pregnane-3,11,20-trione	5β-Pregnan-17α,21-diol-3,11,20-trione
Dihydrotestosterone	17β-Hydroxy-5α-androstan-3-one	5α-Androstan-17β-ol-3-one
Dimethisterone	17α-Ethinyl-17-hydroxy-6α,21-dimethyl-4-androsten-3-one	17α-Ethinyl-6α,21-dimethyl-4-androsten-17β-ol-3-one
Diosgenin	(25R)-5-Spirosten-3β-ol	(25R),5-Spirosten-3β-ol
Dromostanolone propionate	2α-Methyl-17β-propionyloxy-5α-androstan-3-one	2α-Methyl-5α-androstan-17β-ol-3-one 17-propionate
Drostanolone	17β-Hydroxy-2α-methyl-5α-androstan-17-one	2α-methyl-5α-androstan-17β-ol-3-one

Name	Systematic name	Systematic name
E		
Eburicoic acid	3β-Hydroxy-4,4,14α-trimethyl-5α-ergosta-8,24(28)-dien-21-oic acid	⎰24-Methylene-8,(5α)-lanosten-3β-ol-21-oic acid ⎱4,4,14α-Methyl-8,24(28),(5α)-ergostadien-3β-ol-20β-oic acid
Ecdysone (α-Ecdysone)	(22R)-2β,3β,14,22,25-Pentahydroxy-5β,14α-cholest-7-en-6-one	7,(5β,14α,22R)-Cholesten-2β,3β,14,22,25-pentol-6-one
Ecdysterone	(22R)-2β,3β,14,20,22,25-Hexahydroxy-5β,14α-cholest-7-en-6-one	7,(5β,14α,22R)-Cholesten-2β,3β,14,20,22,25-hexol-6-one
Electrocortin	see Aldosterone	—
Elemolic acid	3β-Hydroxy-5α-tirucalla-8,24-dien-21-oic-acid	8,24,(5α)-Tirucalladien-3β-ol-21-oic acid
Enoxolone	3β-Hydroxy-11-(18β)-oxo,(18β)-olean-12-en-30-oic acid	12-Oleanen-3β-ol-11-one-30-oic acid
Epiandrosterone	3β-Hydroxy-5α-androstan-17-one	5α-Androstan-3β-ol-17-one

APPENDIX 1—*continued*

Trivial Name	IUPAC (1968) Systematic Name	Alternative systematic name
Epicholestanol	5α-Cholestan-3α-ol	5α-Cholestan-3α-ol
Epicoprostanol	5β-Cholestan-3α-ol	5β-Cholestan-3α-ol
Epidihydrocholesterol	5α-Cholestan-3α-ol	5α-Cholestan-3α-ol
16,17-Epiestriol	1,3,5(10)-Estratriene-3,16β,17α-triol	1,3,5(10)-Estratrien-3,16β,17α-triol
17-Epiestriol	1,3,5(10)-Estratriene-3,16α,17α-triol	1,3,5(10)-Estratrien-3,16α,17α-triol
16-Epiestriol	1,3,5(10)-Estratriene-3,16β,17β-triol	1,3,5(10)-Estratrien-3,16β,17β-triol
Epipregnanolone	3α-Hydroxy-5β-pregnan-20-one	5β-Pregnan-3α-ol-20-one
Episterol	24-Methylene-5α-cholest-7-en-3β-ol	24-Methylene-7,(5α)-cholesten-3β-ol
Epitestosterone	17α-Hydroxy-4-androsten-3-one	4-Androsten-17α-ol-3-one
Equilenin	3-Hydroxy-1,3,5(10),6,8-estrapentaen-17-one	1,3,5(10),6,8-Estrapenten-3-ol-17-one
Equilin	3-Hydroxy-1,3,5(10),7-estratetraen-7-one	1,3,5(10),7-Estratetren-3-ol-17-one
Ergocalciferol	9,10-Seco-ergosta-5,7,10(19),22-tetraen-3β-ol	9,10-Seco-5,7,10(19),22-ergostatetren-3β-ol
Ergostanol	(24S)-24-Methyl-5α-cholestan-3β-ol	5α-Ergostan-3β-ol
Ergosterol	(24S)-24-Methyl-5,7,22-cholestatrien-3β-ol	5,7,22-Ergostatrien-3β-ol
Estradiol, Estradiol-17β	1,3,5(10)-Estratriene-3,17β-diol	1,3,5(10)-Estratrien-3,17β-diol
17α-Estradiol	1,3,5(10)-Estratriene-3,17α-diol	1,3,5(10)-Estratrien-3,17α-diol
16α-Estradiol	1,3,5(10)-Estratriene-3,16α-diol	1,3,5(10)-Estratrien-3,16α-diol
Estrenol	4-Estren-17β-ol	4-Estren-17β-ol
Estriol	1,3,5(10)-Estratriene-3,16α,17β-triol	1,3,5(10)-Estratrien-3,16α,17β-triol
Estrone	3-Hydroxy-1,3,5(10)-estratrien-17-one	1,3,5(10)-Estratrien-3-ol-17-one
5β,17(αH)-Etianic acid	5β-Androstane-17β-carboxylic acid	5β-Androstan-17β-carboxylic acid
α-Etianolone	3α-Hydroxy-5β-androstan-17-one	5β-Androstan-3α-ol-17-one
Etioallocholane	5α-Androstane	5α-Androstane
Etiocholane	5β-Androstane	5β-Androstane
Etiocholanic acid	5β-Androstane-17β-carboxylic acid	5β-Androstane-17β-carboxylic acid
Etiocholanolone	3α-Hydroxy-5β-androstan-17-one	5β-Androstan-3α-ol-17-one
Ethisterone (Ethindrone)	17α-Ethinyl-17-hydroxy-4-androsten-3-one	17α-Ethinyl-4-androsten-17β-ol-3-one
Ethylestrenol	17α-Ethyl-4-estren-17-ol	17α-Ethyl-4-estren-17β-ol
Ethyiferone	17α-Chloroethinyl-17-hydroxy-4,9-estradien-3-one	17α-Chloroethinyl-4,9-estradien-17β-ol-3-one
Ethynodiol diacetate	3β,17β-Diacetoxy-17-ethinyl-4-estrene	17α-Ethinyl-4-estren-3β,17β-diol diacetate
5α-Euphane	5α,13α,14β,17α-Lanostane	5α-Euphane
Euphol	5α-Eupha-8,24-dien-3β-ol	8,24,(5α)-Euphadien-3β-ol
Euphorbol	24-Methylene-5α-tirucall-8-en-3β-ol	24-Methylene-8,(5α)-tirucullen-3β-ol

F
Fecosterol	24-Methylene-5α-cholest-8-en-3β-ol	24-Methylene-8,(5α)-cholesten-3β-ol
Fludrocortisone	9α-Fluoro-11β,17α,21-trihydroxy-4-pregnene-3,20-dione	9α-Fluoro-4-pregnen-11β,17α,21-triol-3,20-dione
Flumedroxone acetate	17-Acetoxy-6α-(trifluoromethyl)-4-pregnene-3,20-dione	6α-Trifluoromethyl-4-pregnen-17α-ol-3,20-dione 17-acetate
Flumethasone pivalate	6α,9α-Difluoro-11β,17,21-trihydroxy-16α-methyl-1,4-pregnadiene-3,20-dione 21-pivalate	6α,9α-Difluoro-16α-methyl-1,4-pregnadien-11β,17α,21-triol-3, 20-dione 21-pivalate

Fluocinolone acetonide	6α,9α-Difluoro-16α,17-isopropylidenedioxy-1,4-pregnadiene-3,20-dione 6α,9α-Difluoro-11β,16α,17,21-tetrahydroxy-1,4-pregnadiene-3,20-dione cyclic 16, 17-acetal with acetone	6α,9α-Difluoro-1,4-pregnadien-11β,17α,21-triol-3,20-dione 16α,17-acetonide
Fluocortolone caproate	21-Caproyloxy-6α-fluoro-11β-hydroxy-16α-methyl-1,4-pregnadiene-3,20-dione	6α-Fluoro-16α-methyl-1,4-pregnadien-11β,17α,21-diol-3,20-dione 21-caproate
Fluorohydrocortisone	9α-Fluoro-11β,17,21-trihydroxy-4-pregnene,3,20-dione	9α-Fluoro-4-pregnen-11β,17α,21-triol-3,20-dione
Fluorometholone	9α-Fluoro-11β,17-dihydroxy-6α-methyl-1,4-pregnadiene-3,20-dione	9α-Fluoro-6α-methyl-1,4-pregnadien-11β,17α,diol-3,20-dione
Fluoxymesterone	9α-Fluoro-11β,17β-dihydroxy-17-methyl-4-androsten-3-one	9α-Fluoro-17α-methyl-4-androsten-11β,17β-diol-3-one
Fluperolone acetate	9α-Fluoro-11β,17,21-trihydroxy-21-methyl-1,4-pregnadiene-3,20-dione 21-acetate 17β-[2-Acetoxypropionyl]-9α-fluoro-11β,17-dihydroxy-1,4-androstadien-3-one	9α-Fluoro-21-methyl-1,4-pregnadien-11β,17α,21-triol-3,20-dione 21-acetate 9α-Fluoro-21-hydroxypropyl-1,4-androstadien-11β,17α-diol-3, 20-dione
Fluprednisolone	6α-Fluoro-11β,17,21-trihydroxy-1,4-pregnadiene-3,20-dione	6α-Fluoro-1,4-pregnadien-11β,17α,21-triol-3,20-dione
Flurandrenolone	6α-Fluoro-11β,16α,17,21-tetrahydroxy-4-pregnene-3,20-dione	6α-Fluoro-4-pregnen-11β,16α,17α,21-tetrol-3,20-dione
Flurandrenolone acetonide	6α-Fluoro-16α,17-isopropylidenedioxy-11β,21-dihydroxy-4-pregnene-3, 20-dione	6α-Fluoro-4-pregnen-11β,17α,21-triol-3,20-dione 16α,17-acetonide
Flurogestone acetate	9-Fluoro-11β,17-dihydroxy-4-pregnene-3,20-dione 17-acetate	9α-Fluoro-4-pregnen-11β,17-diol-3,20-dione 17-acetate
Fucosterol	24-Ethylidene-5-cholesten-3β-ol	5,E-24(28)-Stigmastadien-3β-ol
Fungisterol	5α-Ergosta-6,8,22-trien-3β-ol; (24S)-24-Methyl-5α-cholest-6,8,22-trien-3β-ol	6,8,22,(5α)-Ergostatrien-3β-ol
Funtamine	3α-Amino-5α-pregnan-20-one	3α-Amino-5α-pregnan-20-one
Fusidic acid	3,11,16-Trihydroxy-4,8,10,14-tetramethyl-17-(1'-carboxyisohept-4'-enylidene)cyclopentanoperhydrophenanthrene 16-acetate	17(20)[16,21-cis],24-Fusidadien-3α,11α,16β-triol-20-oic acid 16-acetate

G

Gammabufogenin	3β,11α,14-Trihydroxy-5β,14β-bufa-20,22-dienolide	20,22,(5β,14β)-Bufadienolide-3β,11α,14-triol
Gestonorone caproate	17α-Caproyloxy-19-nor-4-pregnene-3,20-dione	19-Nor-4-pregnen-17α-ol-3,20-dione 17-caproate
Gitaloxigenin	16β-Formoyloxy-3β,14-dihydroxy-5β-14β-card-20(22)-enolide	20,(22),(5β,14β)-Cardenolide-3β,14,16β-triol 16-formate
Gitogenin	(25R)-5α-Spirostane-2α,3β-diol	(25R)-5α-Spirostan-2α,3β-diol
Gitoxigenin	3β,14,16β-Trihydroxy-5β,14β-card-20(22)-enolide	20(22),(5β,14β)-Cardenolide-3β,14,16β-triol
Glycochenodeoxycholic acid	3α,7α-Dihydroxy-5β-cholan-24-oic acid N-(carboxymethyl)-amide	24,(5β)-Cholanic acid-3α,7α-diol N-(carboxymethyl)-amide
Glycocholic acid	3α,12α-Dihydroxy-5β-cholan-24-oic acid N-(carboxymethyl)-amide	24,(5β)-Cholanic acid-3α,12α-diol N-(carboxymethyl)-amide
Glycodehydrocholic acid	3,7,12-Trioxo-5β-cholan-24-oic acid N-(carboxymethyl)-amide	24,(5β)-Cholanic acid-3,7,12-trione N-(carboxymethyl)-amide
Glycodeoxycholic acid	3α,7α,12α-Trihydroxy-5β-cholan-24-oic acid N-(carboxymethyl)-amide	24,(5β)-Cholanic acid-3α,7α,12α-triol N-(carboxymethyl)-amide
Glycolithocholic acid	3α-Hydroxy-5β-cholan-24-oic acid N-(carboxymethyl)-amide	24,(5β)-Cholanic acid-3α-ol N-(carboxymethyl)-amide
Glycyrrhet(in)ic acid	3β-Hydroxy-11-oxo-12-oleanen-30-oic acid	12-Oleanen-3β-ol-11-one-30-oic acid

H

Hecogenin	(25R)-3β-Hydroxy-5α-spirostan-12-one	(25R)-5α-Spirostan-3β-ol-12-one
Hellebrigenin	3β,5,14-Trihydroxy-19-oxo-5β,14β-bufa-20,22-dienolide	20,22,(5β,14β)-Bufadienolide-3β,5,14-triol-19-one
Hippulin	3-Hydroxy-1,3,5(10),8-estratetraen-17-one	1,3,5(10),8-Estratetren-3-ol-17-one
Hydrocortisone	11β,17α,21-Trihydroxy-4-pregnene-3,20-dione	4-Pregnen-11β,17α,21-triol-3,20-dione
Hyocholic acid	3α,6α,7α-Trihydroxy-5β-cholan-24-oic acid	24,(5β)-Cholanic acid-3α,6α,7α-triol
Hyodeoxycholic acid	3α,6α-Dihydroxy-5β-cholan-24-oic acid	24,(5β)-Cholanic acid-3α,6α-diol

343

APPENDIX I—*continued*

Trivial Name	IUPAC (1968) Systematic Name	Alternative systematic name
I		
Inertogenin	7α,15α-Epoxy-3β,12α,14-trihydroxy-11-oxo-5β,14β-card-20(22)-enolide	20(22),(5β,14β)-Cardenolide-3β,12α,14-triol-11-one 7α,15α-epoxide
Inokosterone	(22R)-2β,3β,14,20,22,26-Hexahydroxy-5β,14α-cholest-7-en-6-one	7,(5β,14α,22R)-Cholesten-2β,3β,14,20,22,26-hexol-6-one
Iso—	see Epi—	—
Isocholesterol	3α,5-Cyclo-5α-cholestan-6β-ol	3α,5-Cyclo-5α-cholestan-6β-ol
"Isocholesterol"	Lanosterol	—
K		
Kammogenin	(25R)-2α,3β-Dihydroxy-5-spirosten-12-one	(25R)-5-Spirosten-2α,3β-diol-12-one
Keto—	see Oxo—	—
Ketocholanic acid	3,7,12-Trioxo-5β-cholan-24-oic acid	24,(5β)-Cholanic acid-3,7,12-trione
18-Ketocorticosterone	see Aldosterone	—
7-Ketodeoxycholic acid	3α,12α-Dihydroxy-7-oxo-5β-cholan-24-oic acid	24,(5β)-Cholanic acid-3α,12α-diol-7-one
3-Ketoetiocholanic acid methyl ether	17β-Methoxycarbonyl-5β-androstan-3-one	5β-Androstan-3-one-17β-carboxylic acid 17-methyl ether
11-Ketoetiocholanolone	3α-Hydroxy-5β-androstane-11,17-dione	5β-Androstan-3α-ol-11,17-dione
3-Keto-4-etiocholenic acid	17β-Carboxy-4-androsten-3-one	4-Androsten-3-one-17β-carboxylic acid
L		
5α-Lanostane	4,4,14α-Trimethyl-5α-cholestane	5α-Lanostane
Lanosterol	5α-Lanosta-8,24-dien-3β-ol	8,24,(5α)-Lanostadien-3β-ol
Lathosterol	5α-Cholest-7-en-3β-ol	7,(5α)-Cholesten-3β-ol
Leptogenin	7α,15α-Epoxy-3β,12β,14-trihydroxy-11-oxo-5β,14β-card-20(22)-enolide	20(22),(5β,14β)-Cardenolide-3β,12β,14-triol-11-one 7α,15α-epoxide
Lilagenin	(25S)-5-Spirostene-2α,3β-diol	(25S)-5-Spirosten-2α-3β-diol
Lithocholic acid	3α-Hydroxy-5β-cholan-24-oic acid	24,(5β)-Cholanic acid-3α-ol
Lophenol	4α-Methyl-5α-cholest-7-en-3β-ol	4α-Methyl-7,(5α)-Cholesten-3β-ol
Lumisterol₂	9β,10α-Ergosta-5,7,22-trien-3β-ol	5,7,22,(9β,10α)-Ergostatrien-3β-ol
Lutinyl	17α-Acetoxy-6-chloro-4,6-pregnadiene-3,20-dione	6-Chloro-4,6-pregnadien-17α-ol-3,20-dione 17-acetate
Lynestrenol	17α-Ethinyl-4-estren-17β-ol	17α-Ethinyl-4-estren-17β-ol
M		
Manogenin	(25R)-2α,3β-Dihydroxy-5α-spirostan-12-one	(25R)-5α-Spirostan-2α,3β-diol-12-one
Marinobufagin	14,15β-Epoxy-3β,5-dihydroxy-5β,14β-bufa-20,22-dienolide	20,22,(5β,14β)-Bufadienolide-3β,5-diol 14,15β-epoxide
Masticadienoic acid	3-Oxo-5α-tirucalla-7,24-dien-26-oic acid	7,24,(5α)-Tirucalladien-3-one-26-oic acid
Medrogestone	6,17-Dimethyl-4,6-pregnadiene-3,20-dione	6,17α-Dimethyl-4,6-pregnadien-3,20-dione
Medroxyprogesterone acetate	17-Acetoxy-6α-methyl-4-pregnene-3,20-dione	6α-Methyl-4-pregnen-17α-ol-3,20-dione 17-acetate
Medrysone	11β-Hydroxy-6α-methyl-4-pregnene-3,20-dione	6α-Methyl-4-pregnen-11β-ol-3,20-dione
Megestrol acetate	17-Acetoxy-6-methyl-4,6-pregnadiene-3,20-dione	6-Methyl-4,6-pregnadien-17α-ol-3,20-dione 17-acetate

Name		
Melengestrol acetate	17-Acetoxy-6-methyl-16-methylene-4,6-pregnadiene-3,20-dione	6-Methyl-16-methylene-4,6-pregnadien-17α-ol-3,20-dione 17-acetate
Mestanolone	17β-Hydroxy-17-methyl-5α-androstan-3-one	17α-Methyl-5α-androstan-17β-ol-3-one
Mesterolone	17β-Hydroxy-1α-methyl-5α-androstan-3-one	1α-Methyl-5α-androstan-17β-ol-3-one
Mesterone	17β-Hydroxy-17-methyl-4-androsten-3-one	17α-Methyl-4-androsten-17β-ol-3-one
Mestranol	17α-Ethinyl-3-methoxy-1,3,5(10)-estratrien-17β-ol	17α-Ethinyl-1,3,5(10)-estratrien-3,17β-diol-3-methyl ether
Metagenin	(25R)-5β-Spirostane-2β,3β,11α-triol	(25R)-5β-Spirostan-2β,3β,11α-triol
Methalone	17β-Hydroxy-2β,17-dimethyl-5-androstan-3-one	2β,17α-Dimethyl-5-androstan-17β-ol-3-one
Methandienone	17β-Hydroxy-17-methyl-1,4-androstadien-3-one	17α-Methyl-1,4-androstadien-17β-ol-3-one
Methandriol	17α-Methyl-5-androstene-3β,17-diol	17α-Methyl-5-androsten-3β-17β-diol
Methandrostenolone	17β-Hydroxy-17-methyl-1,4-androstadien-3-one	17α-Methyl-1,4-androstadien-17β-ol-3-one
Methenolone	17β-Hydroxy-1-methyl-5α-androst-1-en-3-one	1-Methyl-1,(5α)-androsten-17β-ol-3-one
Methostenol	4α-Methyl-5α-cholest-7-en-3β-ol	4α-Methyl-7,(5α)-Cholesten-3β-ol
Δ⁸-Methostenol	4α-Methyl-5α-cholest-8-en-3β-ol	4α-Methyl-8,(5α)-Cholesten-3β-ol
Methyldiacetoxybisnorcho-lanate	3α,12α-Dihydroxy-5β-pregnane-21-carboxylic acid 3,12-diacetate, 21-methyl ether	5β-Pregnan-3α,12α-diol-21-carboxylic acid 3,12-diacetate,21-methyl ether
Methyldihydrotestosterone	17β-Hydroxy-17-methyl-5α-androstan-3-one	17α-Methyl-5α-androstan-17β-ol-3-one
Methyl-3-ketoetiocholanate	17β-Methoxycarbonyl-5β-androstan-3-one	5β-Androstan-3-one-17β-carboxylic acid
Δ¹-Methyl-testosterone	17β-Hydroxy-17-methyl-1,4-androstadien-3-one	17α-Methyl-1,4-androstadien-17β-ol-3-one
Methyltrienolone	17β-Hydroxy-17-methyl-4,9,11-estratrien-3-one	17α-Methyl-4,9,11-estratrien-17β-ol-3-one
Metrogestone	6,17-Dimethyl-4,6-pregnadiene-3,20-dione	6,17-Dimethyl-4,6-pregnadien-3,20-dione
Mexogenin	(25R)-2β,3β-Dihydroxy-5β-spirostan-12-one	(25R)-5β-Spirostan-2β,3β-diol-12-one
N		
Nandrolone	17β-Hydroxy-4-estren-3-one	4-Estren-17β-ol-3-one
Neoergosterol	19-Nor-5,7,9,22-ergostatetraen-3β-ol	19-Nor-5,7,9,22-ergostatetren-3β-ol
Neochlorogenin	(25S)-5α-Spirostane-3β,6α-diol	(25S)-5α-Spirostan-3β,6α-diol
Neocholestene	5α-Cholest-2-ene	2,(5α)-Cholestene
Neodigitogenin	(25S)-5α-Spirostan-2α,3β,15β-triol	(25S)-5α-Spirostan-2α,3β,15β-triol
Neogitogenin	(25S)-5α-Spirostane-2α,3β-diol	(25S)-5α-Spirostan-2α,3β-diol
Neoruscogenin	(25S)-5-Spirosten-1β,3β-diol	(25S)-5-Spirosten-1β,3β-diol
Neotigogenin	(25S)-5α-Spirostan-3β-ol	(25S)-5α-Spirostan-3β-ol
Neriantogenin	3β,16β-Dihydroxy-5β-card-14,20(22)-dienolide	14,20(22),(5β)-Cardadienolide-3β,16β-diol
Nogiragenin	(25R)-5β-Spirostane-3β,11α-diol	(25R)-5β-Spirostan-3β,11α-diol
19-Nor-androstane	see Estrane	—
Norcholanic acid	23-Nor-5β-cholan-24-oic-acid	23-Nor-24,(5β)-cholanic acid
Norcholic acid	3α,7α,12α-Trihydroxy-23-nor-5β-cholan-24-oic acid	23-Nor-24,(5β)-cholanic acid-3α,7α,12α-triol
Norethandrolone	17α-Ethyl-17-hydroxy-4-estren-3-one	17α-Ethyl-4-estren-17β-ol-3-one
Norethindrone	17α-Ethinyl-17-hydroxy-4-estren-3-one	17α-Ethinyl-4-estren-17β-ol-3-one
Norethisterone	17α-Ethinyl-17-hydroxy-4-estren-3-one	17α-Ethinyl-4-estren-17β-ol-3-one
Norethynodrel	17α-Ethinyl-17-hydroxy-5(10)-estren-3-one	17α-Ethinyl-5(10)-estren-17β-ol-3-one
D-Norgestrel	D-17α-Ethinyl-17-hydroxy-18-methyl-4-estren-3-one	D-17α-Ethinyl-18-methyl-4-estren-17β-ol-3-one
Norlanosterol	4,4-Dimethyl-5α-cholesta-8,24-diene-3β-ol	4,4-Dimethyl-8,24,(5α)-cholestadien-3β-ol
Norlutin	17α-Ethinyl-17-hydroxy-4-estren-3-one	17α-Ethinyl-4-estren-17β-ol-3-one
Normethandrone	17α-Methyl-17-hydroxy-4-estren-3-one	17α-Methyl-4-estren-17β-ol-3-one

345

APPENDIX 1—continued

Trivial Name	IUPAC (1968) Systematic Name	Alternative systematic name
19-Nor-17α-pregnane	see 17β-Hydroxy-17-ethyl-estrane	
19-Nortestosterone	17β-Hydroxy-4-estren-3-one	4-Estren-17β-ol-3-one
O		
Oleandrigenin	16β-Acetoxy-3β,14-dihydroxy-5β,14β-card-20(22)-enolide	20(22),(5β,14β)-Cardenolide-3β,14,16β-triol 16-acetate
Ouabagenin	1β,3β,5,11α,14,19-Hexahydroxy-5β,14β-card-20(22)-enolide	20(22),(5β,14β)-Cardenolide-1β,3β,5,11α,14,19-hexol
Oxandrolone	17β-Hydroxy-17-methyl-2-oxa-5α-androstan-3-one	17α-Methyl-2-oxa-5α-androstan-17β-ol-3-one
Oxymesterone	4,17β-Dihydroxy-17-methyl-4-androsten-3-one	17α-Methyl-4-androsten-4,17β-diol-3-one
Oxymetholone	17β-Hydroxy-2-(hydroxymethylene)-17-methyl-5α-androstan-3-one	2-Hydroxymethylene-17α-methyl-5α-androstan-17β-ol-3-one
P		
Paramethasone acetate	6α-Fluoro-11β,17-21-trihydroxy-16α-methyl-1,4-pregnadiene-3,20-dione 21-acetate	6α-Fluoro-16α-methyl-1,4-pregnadien-11β,17α,21-triol-3,20-dione 21-acetate
Parkeol	5α-Lanosta-9(11),24-dien-3β-ol	9(11),24,(5α)-Lanostadien-3β-ol
Periplogenin	3β,5,14-Trihydroxy-5β,14β-card-20(22)-enolide	20(22),(5β,14β)-Cardenolide-3β,5,14-triol
Phanurane	(17-Hydroxy-3-oxo-17α-pregna-4,6-diene-21-carboxylic acid γ-lactone (17α-(2-Carboxyethyl)-17-hydroxy-4,6-androstadien-3-one lactone	4,6-Androstadien-17β-ol-3-one-17α-carboxylic acid 17α,17β-lactone
Phenesterine	{p-[bis(2-chloroethyl)amino]} phenyl acetic acid cholesterol ester	Cholesteryl p-bis(2-chloroethyl)aminophenylacetate
Pinicolic acid A	4,4,14α-Trimethyl-3-oxo-5α-cholesta-8,24-dien-21-oic acid	8,24,(5α)-Lanostadien-3-one-21-oic acid
Polyporenic acid A	3α,12α-Dihydroxy-24-methylene-5α-lanost-8-en-27-oic acid	24-Methylene-8,(5α)-lanosten-3α,12α-diol-27-oic acid
Polyporenic acid C	16α-Hydroxy-24-methylene-3-oxo-5α-lanosta-7,9(11)-dien-21-oic acid	24-Methylene-7,9(11),(5α)-lanostadien-16α-ol-3-one-21-oic acid
Ponasterone A	(22R)-2β,3β,14,20,22-Pentahydroxy-5β,14α-cholest-7-en-6-one	7,(5β,14α,22R)-Cholesten-2β,3β,14,20,22-pentol-6-one
Poriferasterol	(24S)-24-Ethyl-5,22-cholestadien-3β-ol	24S-(24-Ethyl)-5,22-cholestadien-3β-ol
Prednisolone	11β,17,21-Trihydroxy-1,4-pregnadiene-3,20-dione	1,4-Pregnadien-11β,17α,21-triol-3,20-dione
Prednisone	17,21-Dihydroxy-1,4-pregnadiene-3,11,20-trione	1,4-Pregnadien-17α,21-diol-3,11,20-trione
Prednival	11β,17,21-Trihydroxy-1,4-pregnadiene-3,20-dione 17-valerate	1,4-Pregnadien-11β,17α,21-triol-3,20-dione 17-valerate
Prednylidene	11β,17,21-Trihydroxy-16-methylene-1,4-pregnadiene-3,20-dione	16-Methylene-1,4-pregnadien-11β,17,21-triol-3,20-dione
Pregnanediol	5β-Pregnane-3α,20α-diol	5β-Pregnan-3α,20α-diol
Pregnanedione	5β-Pregnane-3,20-dione	5β-Pregnan-3,20-dione
Pregnanetriol	5α-Pregnane-3α,17,20α-triol	5α-Pregnan-3α,17α,20α-triol
Pregnanolone	3β-Hydroxy-5β-pregnan-20-one	5β-Pregnan-3β-ol-20-one
Pregnenolone	3β-Hydroxy-5-pregnen-20-one	5-Pregnen-3β-ol-20-one
Premarin	Mainly sodium estrone sulphate	
Progesterone	4-Pregnene-3,20-dione	4-Pregnen-3,20-dione
Provera	17-Acetoxy-6α-methyl-4-pregnene-3,20-dione	6α-Methyl-4-pregnen-17α-ol-3,20-dione 17-acetate
Provitamin D₂	see Ergosterol	
Provitamin D₃	see 7-Dehydrocholesterol	
Provitamin D₄	see 22,23-Dihydroergosterol	

Purprogenin	3β,14β,15α-Trihydroxy-5-pregnene-12,20-dione	5-Pregnen-3β,14β,15α-triol-12,20-dione
Pyrocalciferol	10α-Ergosta-5,7,22-trien-3β-ol	(10α)5,7,22-Ergostatrien-3β-ol
Q		
Quinestradiol	3-(Cyclopentyloxy)-1,3,5(10)-estratriene-16α,17β-diol	1,3,5(10)-Estratrien-3,16α,17β-triol 3-cyclopentyl ether
Quingestrone	3-(Cyclopentyloxy)-3,5-pregnadien-20-one	3,5-Pregnadien-3-ol-20-one 3-cyclopentyl ether
R		
Resibufogenin	14,15β-Epoxy-3β-hydroxy-5β,14β-bufa-20,22-dienolide	20,22,(5β,14β)-Bufadienolide-3β-ol-14,15β-epoxide
Retroprogesterone	9β,10α-Pregna-4,6-diene-3,20-dione	4,6,(9β,10α)-Pregnadien-3,20-dione
Rhodeasapogenin	(25S)-5β-Spirostane-1β,3β-diol	(25S)-5β-Spirostan-1β,3β-diol
Rockogenin	(25R)-5α-Spirostane-3β,12β-diol	(25R)-5α-Spirostan-3β,12β-diol
Ruscogenin	(25R)-5-Spirostene-1β,3β-diol	(25R)-5-Spirosten-1β,3β-diol
S		
Samogenin	(25R)-5β-Spirostan-2β,3β-diol	(25R)-5β-Spirostan-2β,3β-diol
Sargasterol	(20S)-24-Ethylidene-5-cholesten-3β-ol	(20S)-24-Ethylidene-5-cholesten-3β-ol
Sarmentogenin	3β,11α,14-Trihydroxy-5β,14β-card-20(22)-enolide	20(22),(5β,14β)-Cardenolide-3β,11α,14-triol
Sarmentologenin	3β,5,11α,14,19-Pentahydroxy-5β,14β-card-20(22)-enolide	20(22),(5β,14β)-Cardenolide-3β,5,11α,14,19-pentol
Sarmutogenin	3β,12β,14-Trihydroxy-11-oxo-5β,14β-card-20(22)-enolide	20(22),(5β,14β)-Cardenolide-3β,12β,14-triol-11-one
Sarsapogenin	(25S)-5β-Spirostan-3β-ol	(25S)-5β-Spirostan-3β-ol
Scillarenin	3β,14-Dihydroxy-5β,14β-bufa-4,20,22-trienolide	4,20,22,(5β,14β)-Bufatrienolide-3β,14-diol
Scilliglaucosidin	3β,14-Dihydroxy-19-oxo-5β,14β-bufa-4,20,22-trienolide	4,20,22,(5β,14β)-Bufatrienolide-3β,14-diol-19-one
Scillirosidin	6β-Acetoxy-3β,8,8β,14-trihydroxy-5β,14β-bufa-4,20,22-trienolide	4,20,22,(5β,14β)-Bufatrienolide-3β,6β,8β,14-tetrol 6-acetate
Sinogenin	3β,11α,14-Trihydroxy-12-oxo-5β,14β-card-20(22)-enolide	20(22),(5β,14β)-Cardenolide-3β,11α,14-triol-12-one
α₁-Sitosterol	4α-Methyl-5α-stigmasta-7,24(28)-dien-3β-ol	4α-Methyl-7,24(28),(5α)-stigmastadien-3β-ol
β-Sitosterol	5-Stigmasten-3β-ol; (24R)-24-Ethyl-5-cholesten-3β-ol	5-Stigmasten-3β-ol
γ-Sitosterol	(24S)-24-Ethyl-5-cholesten-3β-ol	(24S)-24-Ethyl-5-cholesten-3β-ol
Sisalagenin	(25S)-3β-Hydroxy-5α-spirostan-12-one	(25S)-5α-Spirostan-3β-ol-12-one
Smilagenin	(25R)-5β-Spirostan-3β-ol	(25R)-5β-Spirostan-3β-ol
α-Spinasterol	7,22-Stigmastadien-3β-ol	7,22-Stigmastadien-3β-ol
Spironolactone	⎰3-(3-Oxo-7α-acetylthio-17β-hydroxy-4-androsten-17α-yl) propionic acid γ-lactone	4-Androsten-3-one-17α-propionic acid 17α,17β-lactone, 7α-acetylmercaptide
	⎱17β-Hydroxy-7-mercapto-3-oxo-17α-pregn-4-ene-21-carboxylic acid γ-lactone, 7-acetate	—
Spongesterol	(24S)-24-Ethyl-22-cholesten-3β-ol	(24S)-24-Ethyl-22-cholesten-3β-ol
Squalene	2,6,10,15,19,23-Hexamethyl-2,6,10,14,18,22-tetracosahexaene	
Stanolone	17β-Hydroxy-5α-androstan-3-one	5α-Androstan-17β-ol-3-one
Stanozolol	17β-Hydroxy-17-methyl-5α-androstan[3,2-c]-pyrazole	17α-Methyl-5α-androstan-17β-ol[3,2-c]-pyrazole
Stellasterol	(5α,20S,24R)-24-Methyl-7,22-cholestadien-3β-ol	(20S,24R)-24-Methyl-(5α)7,22-cholestadien-3β-ol
Stenbolone	17β-Hydroxy-2-methyl-5α-androst-1-en-3-one	2-Methyl-1-(5α)-androsten-17β-ol-3-one
Stigmastanol	(24R)-24-Ethyl-5α-cholestan-3β-ol; 5α-Stigmastan-3β-ol	5α-Stigmastan-3β-ol
Stigmastadienone	24-Ethyl-4,22-cholestadien-3-one; 4,22-Stigmastadien-3-one	4,22-Stigmastadien-3-one

347

APPENDIX I—*continued*

Trivial Name	IUPAC (1968) Systematic Name	Alternative systematic name
Stigmasterol	5,22-Stigmastadien-3β-ol	5,22-Stigmastadien-3β-ol
Strophanthidin	3β,5,14-Trihydroxy-19-oxo-5β,14β-card-20(22)-enolide	20,22,(5β,14β)-Cardenolide-3β,5,14-triol-19-one
T		
Taurocholanic acid	5β-Cholan-24-oic acid N-(2-sulphoethyl)-amide	24,(5β)-Cholanic acid N-(2-sulphoethyl)-amide
Taurocholic acid	3α,7α,12α-Trihydroxy-5β-cholan-24-oic acid N-(2-sulphoethyl)-amide	24,(5β)-Cholanic acid-3α,7α,12α-triol N-(2-sulphoethyl)-amide
Taurodehydrocholic acid	3,7,12-Trioxo-5β-cholan-24-oic acid N-(2-sulphoethyl)-amide	24,(5β)-Cholanic acid-3,7,12-trione N-(2-sulphoethyl)-amide
Taurodeoxycholic acid	3α,12α-Dihydroxy-5β-cholan-24-oic acid N-(2-sulphoethyl)-amide	24,(5β)-Cholanic acid-3α,12α-diol N-(2-sulphoethyl)-amide
Taurolithocholic acid	3α-Hydroxy-5β-cholan-24-oic acid N-(2-sulphoethyl)-amide	24,(5β)-Cholanic acid-3α-ol N-(2-sulphoethyl)-amide
Tachysterol₂	9,10-Seco-5(10),6,8,22-ergostatetraen-3β-ol	9,10-Seco-5(10),6,8,22-ergostatetren-3β-ol
Tanghinigenin	7α,15α-Epoxy-3β,14-dihydroxy-5β,14β-card-20(22)-enolide	20,(22),(5β,14β)-Cardenolide-3β,14-diol 7α,15α-epoxide
Telocinobufagin	3β,5,14-Trihydroxy-5β,14β-bufa-20,22-dienolide	20,(22),(5β,14β)-Bufadienolide-3β,5,14-triol
Testane	5β-Androstane	5β-Androstane
Testolactone	17α-Oxo-D-homo-1,4-androstadiene-3,17-dione	17α-Oxa-D-homo-1,4-androstadien-3,17-dione
Testosterone	17β-Hydroxy-4-androsten-3-one	4-Androsten-17β-ol-3-one
Δ¹-Testosterone	17β-Hydroxy-1,4-androstadien-3-one	1,4-Androstadien-17β-ol-3-one
Tetrahydrocortisol	3α,11β,17,21-Tetrahydroxy-5β-pregnan-20-one	5β-Pregnan-3α,11β,17α,21-tetrol-20-one
Tetrahydrocortisone	3α,17,21-Trihydroxy-5β-pregnane-11,20-dione	5β-Pregnan-3α,17α,21-triol-11,20-dione
Tetrahydrodeoxycorticosterone	3α,21-Dihydroxy-5β-pregnan-20-one	5β-Pregnan-3α,21-diol-20-one
Tigogenin	(25R)-5α-Spirostan-3β-ol	(25R)-5α-Spirostan-3β-ol
5α-Tirucallane	5α,13α,14β,17α,20S-Lanostane	5α-Tirucallane
Tircuallol	5α-Tirucalla-8,24-dien-3β-ol	8,24,(5α)-Tirucalladien-3β-ol
Tokorogenin	(25R)-5β-Spirostane-1β,2β,3α-triol	(25R)-5α-Spirostan-1β,2β,3α-triol
Triamcinolone	9α-Fluoro-11β,16α,17α,21-tetrahydroxy-1,4-pregnadiene-3,20-dione	9α-Fluoro-1,4-pregnadien-11β,16α,17α,21-tetrol-3,20-dione
Triamcinolone acetonide	9α-Fluoro-11β,21-dihydroxy-16α,17α-isopropylidenedioxy-1,4-pregnadiene-3,20-dione	9α-Fluoro-1,4-pregnadien-11β,17α,21-triol-3,20-dione 16α,17-acetonide
U		
Uranediol	17α-Methyl-D-homo-5α-androstane-3β,17aβ-diol	17α-Methyl-D-homo-5α-androstan-3β,17aβ-diol
Urocortisol	3α,11β,17,21-Tetrahydroxy-5β-pregnan-20-one	5β-Pregnan-3α,11β,17α,21-tetrol-20-one
Urocortisone	3α,17,21-Trihydroxy-5β-pregnane-11,20-dione	5β-Pregnan-3α,17α,21-triol-11,20-dione
Ursodeoxycholic acid	3α,7β-Dihydroxy-5β-cholan-24-oic acid	24,(5β)-Cholanic acid-3α,7β-diol
Uzarigenin	3β,14-Dihydroxy-5α,14β-card-20(22)-enolide	20(22),(5α,14β)-Cardenolide-3β,14-diol
V		
Vitamin D₁	Ergocalciferol + lumisterol₂	—
Vitamin D₂	*see* Ergocalciferol	9,10-Seco-5,7,10(19),22-ergostatetren-3β-ol

12*

APPENDIX II

SOME RECENT WORK

I. FEEDBACK OF GONADOTROPHINS

The mechanism of the feedback pathways which occur in the human menstrual cycle have been much more difficult to explain. Recently it has been postulated that at the beginning of menstruation, FSH output is low because it has been suppressed by estrogen secreted during the preceding cycle and LH output is low because it has been suppressed by estrogen and progestogen. The cessation of corpus luteum activity enables the release of LH and FSH to escape from this inhibition and FSH output rises leading to the development of a new mature follicle. LH output also rises in a series of diurnal cycles and at first stimulates only estrogen synthesis and output. This blocks any further rise in FSH release but does not affect LH, whose suppression requires the combined action of estrogen and progestogen. It is then postulated that at a critical LH concentration, progestogen appears in significant quantities. This further increases LH output and the positive feedback leads to a surge of LH release and progestogen synthesis. It is believed that this facilitatory surge of LH is only transient and leaves the inhibitory actions of estrogen and progestogen unopposed.

An anovulatory cycle probably proceeds normally up to and including the point where the positive feedback mechanism causes a surge of LH and progestogen output. However, the effect of progestogen on the central nervous system is reversed and the release of LH suppressed before sufficient has been released to ensure ovulation. The fact that anovulatory cycles may be of normal length, or only slightly shorter, suggests that the preovulatory burst of estrogen and progestogen output is sufficient to suppress the output of LH for several days, irrespective of whether or not the steroids continue to be secreted by the corpus luteum.

II. COMPOSITION OF PROTEIN HORMONES

Preparations of FSH from different laboratories tend to have slightly differing compositions. A recent analysis is shown in Table 1.

Table 1. *Composition of human FSH (nmoles/mg)*

Asp	312	Ile	96	D-Galactose	125
Thr	222	Leu	229	D-Mannose	394
Ser	223	Tyr	118	L-Fucose	39
Glu	409	Phe	131	2-Acetamido-2-deoxy-	
Pro	225	Lys	220	D-glucose	824
Ala	218	His	67	2-Acetamido-2-deoxy-	
Val	154	Arg	159	D-galactose	29
Met	46	Gly	199	*N*-Acetyl-neuraminic	
		Cys	244	acid	155
		(half)			

Complete amino acid structures have been published for human growth hormone (Fig. 1) and ovine placental lactogen (prolactin) (Fig. 2). It is now becoming clear that pituitary growth hormone and placental prolactin are very similar in structure. Human placental lactogen has been shown to have an identical sequence of amino acids from at least number 165 to the carboxyl end of the chain at number 188 when compared with human growth hormone. At present the immunoassay and radioimmunoassay methods of protein hormones suffer from cross reactivity problems between different hormones. This is probably due to similar sequences of amino acids in both hormones. In ACTH, it has been shown that amino acids 1-24 are responsible for the biological activity, species variability occurs in numbers 25-33 and immunological activity depends on numbers 25-39. In future it may be possible to differentiate spheres of activity and identify the active sites in the larger protein hormones.

Human growth hormone has a molecular weight of 21,734. Similar, small disulphide loops occur at the carboxyl end of bovine and equine growth hormones.

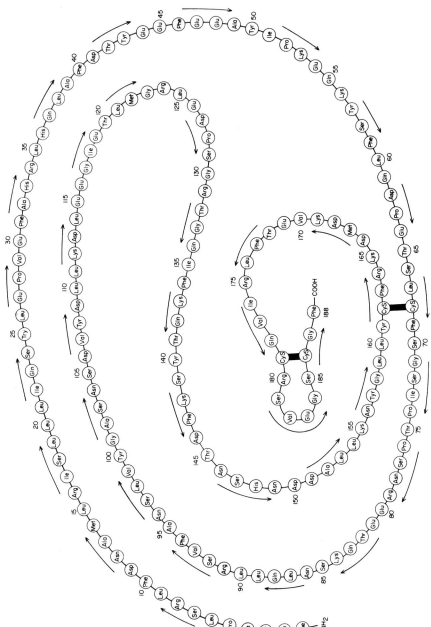

Fig. 1. The complete amino acid sequence of the HGH molecule

NH₂ - Thr - Pro - Val - Cys - Pro - Asn - Gly - Pro - Gly - Asp - Cys - Gln - Val - Ser - Leu - Arg - Asp - Leu - Phe - Asp - Arg - Ala - Val - Met -
1   5   10   15   20

Val - Ser - His - Tyr - Ile - His - Asn - Leu - Ser - Ser - Glu - Met - Phe - Asn - Glu - Phe - Asp - Lys - Arg - Tyr - Ala - Gln - Gly - Lys -
25   30   35   40   45

Gly - Phe - Ile - Thr - Met - Ala - Leu - Asn - Ser - Cys - His - Thr - Ser - Ser - Leu - Pro - Thr - Pro - Glu - Asp - Lys - Glu - Gln - Ala -
50   55   60   65   70

Gln - Gln - Thr - His - His - Glu - Val - Leu - Met - Ser - Leu - Ile - Leu - Gly - Leu - Arg - Ser - Trp - Asn - Asp - Pro - Leu - Tyr - His -
75   80   85   90   95

Leu - Val - Thr - Glu - Val - Arg - Gly - Met - Lys - Gly - Val - Pro - Asp - Ala - Ile - Leu - Ser - Arg - Ala - Ile - Glu - Ile - Glu - Glu -
100   105   110   115   120

Glu - Asn - Lys - Arg - Leu - Leu - Glu - Gly - Met - Glu - Met - Ile - Phe - Gly - Gln - Val - Ile - Pro - Gly - Ala - Lys - Glu - Thr - Glu -
125   130   135   140

Pro - Tyr - Pro - Val - Trp - Ser - Gly - Leu - Pro - Ser - Leu - Gln - Thr - Lys - Asp - Glu - Asp - Ala - Arg - His - Ser - Ala - Phe -
145   150   155   160   165

Tyr - Asn - Leu - Leu - His - Cys - Leu - Arg - Arg - Asp - Ser - Ser - Lys - Ile - Asp - Thr - Tyr - Leu - Lys - Leu - Leu - Asn -
170   175.   180   185

Cys - Arg - Ile - Ile - Tyr - Asn - Asn - Asn - Cys - COOH
190   195   198

Fig. 2. Amino acid sequence of the ovine prolactin molecule.

III. THE HAYNES AND BERTHET HYPOTHESIS OF THE MECHANISM OF ACTION OF ACTH

Reduced nicotinamide adenine dinucleotide phosphate (NADPH, TPNH) is responsible for the oxidations (hydroxylations) of steroid intermediates in the biosynthesis of corticosteroids from cholesterol. An exception is the conversion of pregnenolone to progesterone by 3β-hydroxysteroid dehydrogenase, which requires nicotinamide adenine dinucleotide (NAD, DPN). Large quantities of NADPH are required for steroidogenesis. In 1957, Haynes and Berthet put forward the hypothesis that the action of ACTH, mediated by cyclic-$3',5'$-AMP, brings about an increased activity of phosphorylase and hence increased glycogenolysis to glucose-6-phosphate (Fig. 3). This could then be used as substrate in the reduction of $NADP^+$ to NADPH via the pentose phosphate shunt pathway. In this hypothesis the rate of synthesis of steroids depends largely on the rate of reduction of $NADP^+$ by the pentose phosphate cycle, preformed NADPH being a relatively poor electron donor to the steroid hydroxylating enzymes. The pentose phosphate cycle also seems to be the principle source of ribose sugars for nucleotide synthesis. In all endocrine tissues the activity of the pentose phosphate cycle for the metabolism of glucose-6-phosphate with glucose-6-phosphate dehydrogenase is high. Many endocrine tissues are also rich in $NADP^+$-specific isocitric acid dehydrogenase (in the citric acid cycle) and presumably there is a transfer of the electrons from the NADPH generated, to the electron transport chain. In recent years there has been much dissatisfaction with the Haynes and Berthet hypothesis as G-6-P when used alone *in vitro* does not elicit steroidogenesis, and McKerns has suggested the ACTH exerts a direct stimulation on glucose-6-phosphate dehydrogenase. It is now believed that any substrate which can permeate the adrenal cortical mito-chondrial membrane and which can be oxidized by the proper dehydrogenase in a NADPH-linked reaction will give rise to intramitochondrial NADPH. There will then ensue an electron flow along the cytochrome P-450 chain and steroid hydroxylations will be carried out. In addition, other substrates, e.g. succinate and malate, which are linked in their oxidations to the classical cytochrome chain can also be utilized to bring about steroid hydroxylations in mitochondria and microsomes. One possible route involves reversed electron flow from flavoprotein-linked succinate.

IV. COMPARISON OF THE MENSTRUAL AND ESTROUS CYCLES

Figure 4 shows the plasma progesterone levels throughout the estrous cycle of the pig, cow and ewe compared with the luteal phase of the human menstrual cycle.

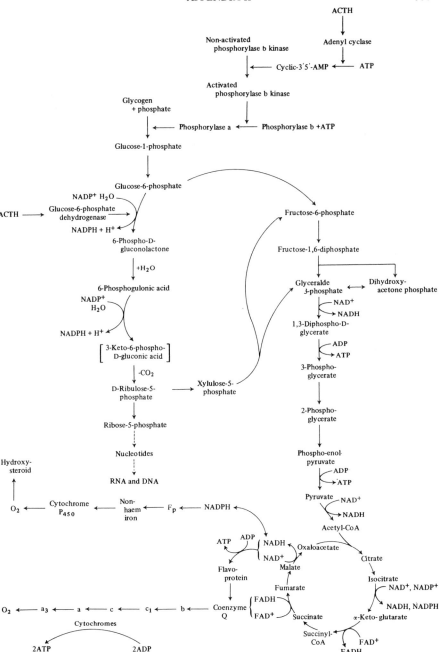

Fig. 3. Metabolic pathways illustrating the hypotheses of *Haynes and Berthet (1957) and of McKerns (1965)* concerning the mechanism of action of ACTH in steroidogenesis.

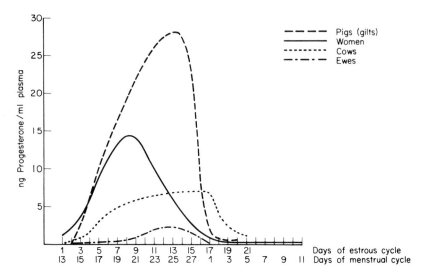

Fig. 4. Plasma progesterone in the human menstrual cycle and in some polyestrous domestic animals.

V. STEROID MUSCLE RELAXANTS

Recently a class of amino-steroids has been developed with potent muscle relaxing powers similar to curare. Curare-like compounds are widely used in surgery so that muscle relaxation can be achieved together with only light anaesthesia. The most commonly used compounds are tubocurarine chloride ("Tubarine"), alcuronium chloride ("Alloferin") and suxamethonium chloride ("Scoline") or bromide ("Brevidil"). The two former compounds are non-polarizing types of muscle relaxant, i.e. neuromuscular transmission is interrupted by competing with acetylcholine for receptor sites on the motor end plate, thus reducing its response to acetylcholine. Their action is rapidly reversed by anticholinesterases. The amino-steroid, pancuronium bromide ("Pavulon") (Fig. 5) has been found to be nearly as powerful as tubocurarine chloride, a 6 mg injection causing complete muscle relaxation in 2-3 min, which lasts for 45 min. Respiration must be assisted. Pancuronium bromide is similar in structure to the naturally occurring steroid alkaloid, malouétine, which also possesses powerful muscle relaxing action but produces hypotension when injected.

It has been postulated that the closeness of the acetyl groups to the amino functions in pancuronium chloride afford some steric compression of rings A and D, so that ring A is held in the intermediate skew position between boat and chair. It is possible that this shape may be optimal for the receptor site in the motor end plate. It seems likely that the steroid part of the molecule allows

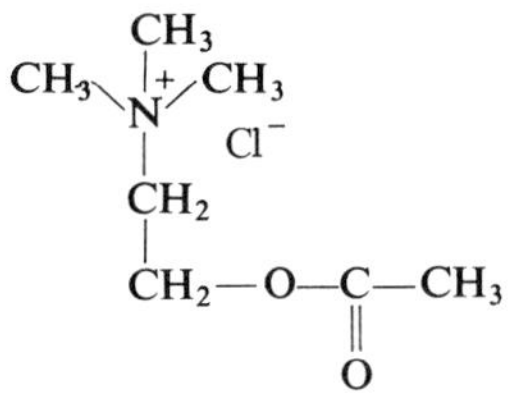

CH$_3$
CH$_3$—N$^+$—CH$_3$
CH$_2$ Cl$^-$
CH$_2$—O—C—CH$_3$
O

Acetylcholine
chloride

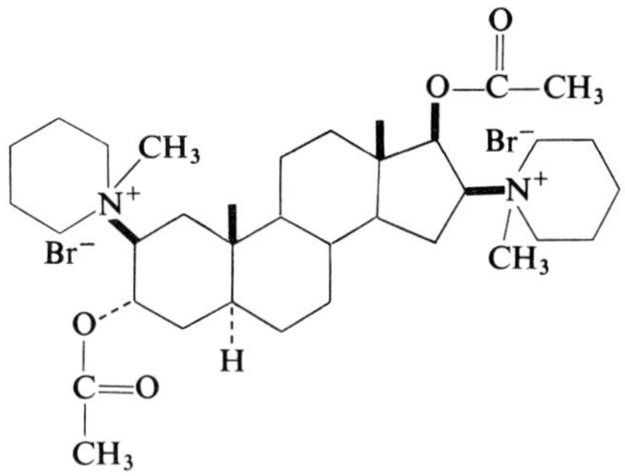

O
‖
O—C—CH$_3$

CH$_3$ Br$^-$

Br$^-$ N$^+$—CH$_3$

N$^+$ H

O
C=O
CH$_3$

Pancuronium bromide
2β, 16β-Dipiperidino-5α-androstane-
3α, 17β-diol diacetate dimethobromide

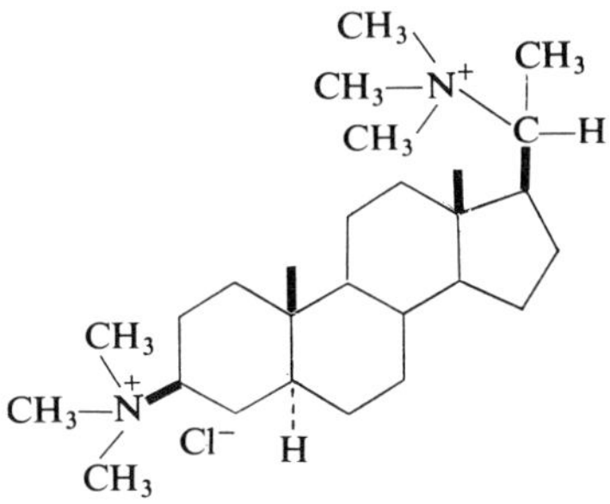

CH$_3$
CH$_3$—N$^+$ CH$_3$
CH$_3$ C—H

CH$_3$
CH$_3$—N$^+$
CH$_3$ Cl$^-$ H

Malouétine
3β,20β-Bisdimethylamino-
5α-pregnane bismethochloride

Fig. 5. Steroid muscle relaxants and acetylcholine.

membrane penetration into the target organ so that the charged amino function can react. Indeed, when an acetylcholine-like structure is incorporated into ring A of 5α-androstane-17-one or 5α-pregnane-20-one weak neuromuscular blocking agents are produced.

VI. PROTEIN BINDING OF STEROIDS

The binding of steroid hormones to blood proteins has been much studied and the effect of molecular modifications on the degree of protein binding has been elucidated. The precise three-dimensional structure of the steroid is very important in relation to its binding properties. Binding to tissue enzymes is believed to depend on the same factors and to be the first step in the enzymatic conversion of the steroids.

A. STEROID STRUCTURE

Figure 6 shows the precise structure of progesterone. It is believed that the two axial methyl groups, C-18 and C-19, shield the front (upper) side of the steroid molecule, from the interaction with approaching molecules. This is evident from the side view which shows the whole steroid molecule as possessing a convex shape, with the upper side forming a curved "surface". The substituents at the rear side appear to be less hindered and therefore more apt to interact. The underside or α-surface of the molecule forms a flat plane which includes the oxygen function at C-3. It is believed that this flat surface permits a close fit between the steroid and the surface of the protein. Protein binding forces are believed to be low energy Van der Waals forces which are highly dependent on distance, Van der Waals forces for spherical atoms being inversely proportioned to the seventh power of the distance between atomic centres. Binding to serum proteins and to certain steroid-metabolizing enzymes has been found to be at the rear or α-surface of the steroids. The relatively high affinity of aromatic steroids (estrogens) for proteins may be explained by the high degree of planarity of their α-surface.

Figure 7 shows the precise structure of cortisone. The molecular modifications which are involved in binding to 11β-hydroxysteroid dehydrogenase have been elucidated. This is illustrated by a projection on a plane normal to a line joining C-8 and C-10. An early hypothesis of association between the enzyme-coenzyme complex and the steroid substrate along the line AA[1] with hydrogen attack on the α-carbonyl bond along the line a has been discarded in favour of association along the line BB[1] with attacks in the direction b. Evidence has been obtained from the effects of substituents, e.g. 9α-chloro and 12α-bromo, on the rate of enzyme action. It is believed that the active site of the enzyme-coenzyme complex requires close contact with the steroid around the upper half of its α-surface and parts of its "top edge"; more specifically, in the region defined by hydrogen atoms 1β, 2α, 12α, (?), 12β and 21 and by carbon atoms 1, 2, 11, 12?, 20 and 21. The dashed line (C) shows the circumference within which a hydrogen atom or hydride ion must approach C-11 before hydrogenation is more likely than recoil.

The configuration of the C-17 side chain is less restricted than the rest of the steroid structure and several arrangements are theoretically possible. Recently the precise conformation of the C-17 side chain of cortisone and a number of similar molecules have been determined from crystallographic data. It has been shown that the carbonyl oxygen atom at C-20 is situated vertically over the D ring but is not equidistant from C-13 and C-16 (when there is not any substituent at C-16). This is illustrated by a projection along the C-17–C-20 bond. There is a torsional angle so that the C-20 carbonyl oxygen is nearer to C-16. For cortisone, this angle is − 27° while eleven other steroids show a range

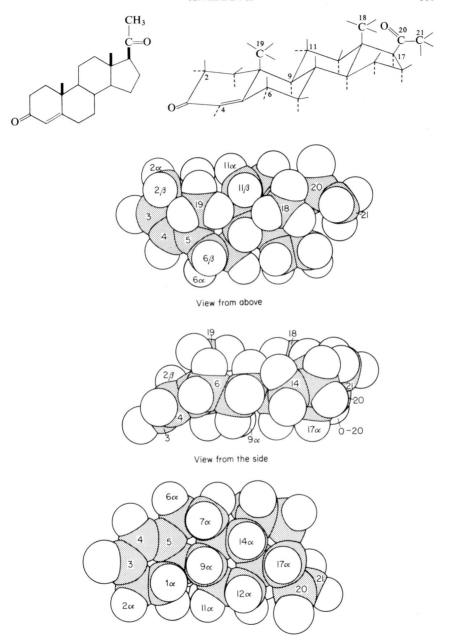

View from above

View from the side

View from below

Fig. 6. Structure of progesterone.

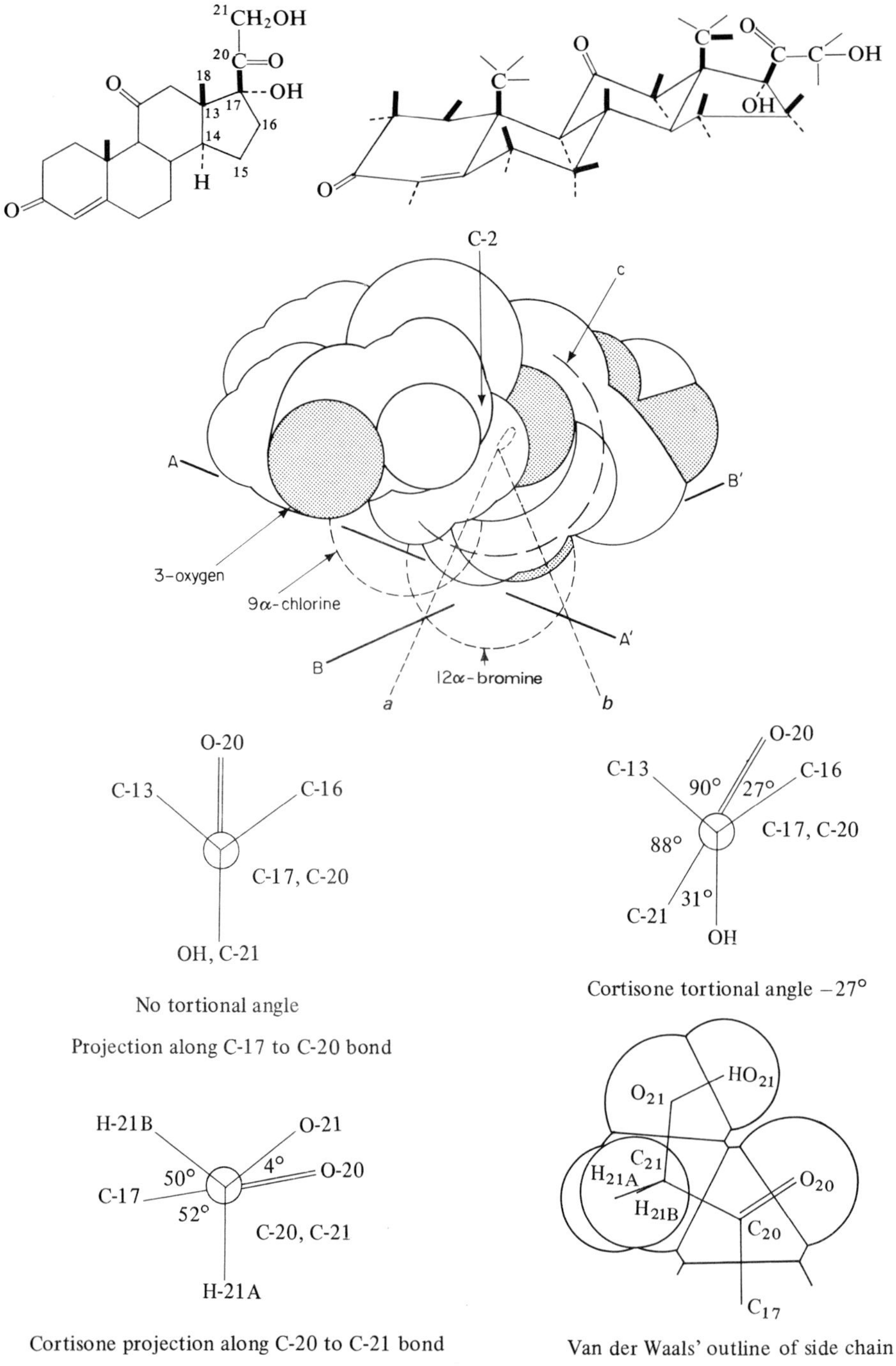

Fig. 7. Structure of cortisone.

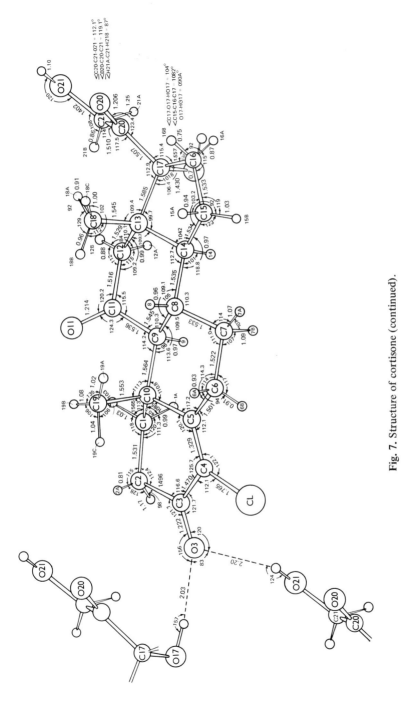

Fig. 7. Structure of cortisone (continued).

of 0-30° with two in the range of -40 to $-45°$. Thus, for cortisone the 17α-hydroxyl group is not coplanar with the rest of the side chain. The side chain atoms C-20, C-21 O-20 and O-21 are all within 0.20 Å of a plane while the 21-hydroxyl group lies 0.16 Å out of this plane with a torsional angle of 7°. The C-21 hydroxyl group is not essential for glurocorticoid activity and does not appear to be protein bound. The complete structure of cortisone also shows that it cannot form an internal hydrogen bond with either the 17α-hydroxyl or the C-20 oxygen. Intermolecular hydrogen bonding occurs in cortisone crystals between the C-3 oxygen and the 17α-hydroxyl group.

B. BINDING IN BLOOD

1. Types of binding

Steroids bind to serum albumin and globulin and also to erythrocytes, e.g. erythrocytes carry about a quarter of the blood estrogen activity. Red cell binding is less strong for cortisol and corticosterone. It is believed that this binding is entirely passive. It is not known whether cortisol binding is to the haemoglobin molecule, the cell membrane being freely permeable to cortisol, or to the cell membrane. Estradiol binding is to haemoglobin.

Binding to serum albumin is weak and non-specific although the binding affinity for most steroids is high. Considerable variation has been observed among the non-aromatic steroids in their binding affinity to serum albumin which is inversely proportional to the number of polar groups in the steroid. A marked stepwise reduction of binding affinity has been observed from "duo-polar" to "tri-polar" to "tetra-polar" bile acids. A similar effect has also been observed for the cardiac glycosides. Proteins for which the "polarity rule" applies appear to be characterized by a preponderance of such side chains, or other structural features which favour the weak Van der Waals forces over hydrogen bonding. These proteins, e.g. serum albumin and β-lactoglobulin, interact more firmly with steroids of low "polarity".

Binding to serum globulin is strong and specific although the binding affinity is low. The introduction of hydroxyl groups enhances the ability of a steroid of the pregnane series to displace cortisol from its protein-bound complex. This binding which is contrary to the "polarity rule" is characterized by proteins with a comparatively high number of hydroxyl groups and serine molecules. It is believed that hydrogen bonds form between the hydroxyl groups of the steroid and those of the protein (or enzyme) which counterbalance and partially replace those between water molecules and the steroid hydroxyl groups. The specific binding globulin for cortisol is known as transcortin. It is believed that the transcortin-bound cortisol is not physiologically active and this may apply to all the globulin-bound steroids in blood. Testosterone and estradiol have been shown to bind to a globulin which is probably the same protein for both hormones. Progesterone binds tightly to an orosomucoid in plasma.

2. Binding constant

The affinity of a steroid for binding to a protein is expressed in terms of the binding constant,

$$K = \frac{[PS]}{[S][P]}$$

where $[PS]$ is the concentration of protein-bound steroid, $[S]$ the concentration of unbound steroid and $[P]$ the concentration of binding protein present in moles/litre. It has the units of litres/mole which is an expression of dilution and is the number of litres to which a gram molecule of protein must be diluted in order that the maximal binding of a tracer be reduced to 50%. The protein concentration remains essentially constant and independent of the extent of binding as long as $[S] \ll [P]$. The protein-bound fraction is usually determined by equilibrium dialysis, e.g. for testosterone to human serum albumin dialysis is performed with 2 ml of 1% albumin in saline against 10 ml of 0.15M phosphate buffer, pH 7.4, containing 110,000 disintegrations/min 1,2[^{3}H] testosterone and 10, 20, 40, 60 and 120 ng non-radioactive testosterone. Dialysis is carried out at a variety of temperatures. The bound fraction (1-α) is calculated as for example

$$1 - \alpha = 1 - \frac{R_o \cdot V_i}{R_i \cdot V_o} = 1 - 0.22 = 0.78 \text{ at } 20°C$$

where α is the unbound fraction, R_o and R_i are the amounts of radioactivity outside and inside the dialysis bag and V_o and V_i are the corresponding volumes. At temperatures over the range 20-37°C the amount of testosterone bound is independent of the concentration of testosterone. The association constant C is expressed as

$$C = \frac{1 - \alpha}{\alpha} \times \frac{1}{P}$$

where P is the binding capacity of albumin $= n/c$, where n is the number of binding sites per mole of albumin, which is assumed to be 1, and c is the albumin concentration in moles/litre $= 10/69,000$, where 69,000 is the molecular weight of human serum albumin. The binding constant K is then expressed as

$$K = C \cdot n = \frac{1 - \alpha}{\alpha} \times \frac{1}{P} = \frac{78}{22} \times \frac{69,000}{10} = 2.45 \times 10^4 \text{ litres/mole at } 20°C$$

At 37°C, $K = 2.02 \pm 0.08$ litres/mole.

Similarly, the binding of cortisol to human albumin has been studied by ultrafiltration through a dialysis bag of a solution of 0.4-400 μg cortisol/100 ml in 3.2% solutions of albumin in buffer at 37°C. The bound fraction was 60% giving $K = 3.25 \times 10^4$ litres/mole.

Table 2 shows some comparative figures for the bound fraction of some steroids with a 4% solution of serum albumin obtained by equilibrium dialysis.

There is evidence that the binding sites of the different steroids are different as there is relatively little interference, i.e. competition, between the steroids. With the adrenal steroids, the Δ^4-3-keto configuration of ring A plays an important part in binding to albumin. Introduction of a hydroxyl group at C-11 interferes with binding whereas hydroxyl groups at C-17 and C-21 do not.

Table 2. *Steroid binding to serum albumin (%)*

Cortisol	72
Cortisone	75
Deoxycorticosterone	83
Corticosterone	85
Testosterone	96
Progesterone	97
Estrone	98
Estradiol	99.5

Similar comparisons can be made for binding to testosterone binding globulin. A 17β-hydroxyl group is essential for binding and the presence of an oxygen function at C-3 is required for high affinity. Hydrogen bonding may take place at these two centres. Dihydrotestosterone and androstanediol have a much higher affinity for this protein than does testosterone (Table 3), although the latter is believed to be the major naturally occurring androgen involved in binding. Estradiol also binds strongly.

Table 3. *Relative binding of androgens to the testosterone binding globulin (relative to testosterone = 100%)*

5α-Androstan-17β-ol-3-one	187
5α-Androstan-3β,17β-diol	121
5α-Androstan-3α,17β-diol	108
5-Androsten-3β,17β-diol	71

3. Proportions of free and bound steroids

If transcortin and albumin each have a single species of binding sites for cortisol with capacities P_t and P_a and equilibrium constants K_t and K_a respectively, then

$$K_t(P_t - B_t) = B_t/F$$

$$P_a K_a = B_a/F$$

$$T = F + B_a + B_t$$

where T is the total cortisol present, F is the free amount, B_a the amount bound to albumin and B_t the amount bound to transcortin. Substitution of the first two equations into the third gives:

$$T - F = P_t + \frac{P_a K_a}{K_t} + \frac{1}{K_t} + \frac{P_a K_a}{F} - \frac{T}{F \cdot K_t}.$$

The total plasma cortisol, T, is usually determined by the fluorometric method of Mattingley and the per cent unbound steroid, F, either by centrifugal ultrafiltration at $37°C$ in the presence of tracer amounts of radioactive steroid or by equilibrium dialysis. By adding cortisol to the plasma in three different amounts, it is possible to obtain three values for T and F, and solve the three simultaneous equations for $P_a K_a$, K_t and P_t. Table 4 shows some typical results.

Table 4. *Binding constants of transcortin and albumin*

$°C$	P_t (moles/litre)	K_t (litres/mole)	$P_a K_a$
10	4.6×10^7	44×10^{-7}	3.7
25	4.9×10^7	26×10^{-7}	3.1
37	5.1×10^7	11×10^{-7}	2.6

In normal plasma, the unbound fraction of cortisol is about 8%, that bound to transcortin is greater than 75% and that bound to albumin is about 15%. Progesterone is distributed as about 37% to transcortin, about 78% to albumin, about 2% unbound and about 36% to an unknown protein(s) which may be an orosomucoid.

Table 5 shows the relative proportions of bound and unbound plasma testosterone. The differences in the amounts bound to both α- and β-globulins is significantly different between males and females. Females have a much lower total plasma testosterone and a higher proportion of it is bound to globulins and therefore probably inert.

Table 5. *Protein binding of plasma testosterone*

	Normal female	Normal male
Albumin	$4.3 \pm 0.40\%$	$6.2 \pm 1.1\%$
β-Globulins	$80.5 \pm 1.9\%$	$69.3 \pm 3.0\%$
α-Globulins	$7.3 \pm 0.80\%$	$14.3 \pm 1.6\%$

4. Alterations in pregnancy

Total plasma testosterone, progesterone and cortisol are much raised in pregnancy but the mother appears to suffer no, or relatively few, ill effects. This is due to simultaneous increase in transcortin and testosterone binding globulin. Recent evidence has tended to suggest that the binding affinity of transcortin is also increased as well as the absolute amount of transcortin. It has now been established that there is a slight rise in the free cortisol during pregnancy and that this probably accounts for the signs of Cushing's syndrome in some pregnant women together with the alteration of carbohydrate metabolism as shown by the glucose tolerance test. Under normal circumstances, the concentration of plasma progesterone is so low as not to play an important role in affecting the binding of cortisol to transcortin. During pregnancy progesterone gradually replaces cortisol from transcortin.

C. COMPETITIVE PROTEIN BINDING ANALYSIS

Competitive protein binding can be used as a sensitive assay of small amounts of steroid hormones in blood, and is a variation of saturation analysis. The principle is shown in Fig. 8. If a protein P is mixed with a steroid substance S for which it has specific binding sites, a complex PS will be formed. Similarly, the

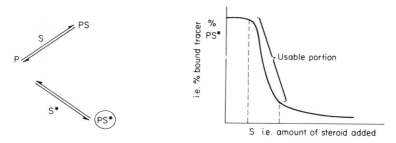

Fig. 8. Principle of competitive protein binding assay.

radioactive form of S, S*, will form a complex PS*. If the concentrations of S and S* exceed the number of binding sites available, they will compete with each other for binding sites in proportion to their concentrations. If the amounts of P and S* are kept constant, then, as non-radioactive S is added, it will displace more and more tracer-S* and the amount of tracer complex will fall. If the amount of bound tracer is plotted against the amount of non-radioactive S added, a curve is obtained as shown in Fig. 8. Maximal binding occurs until the protein-binding sites are saturated. Then as more S is added, the percentage of bound tracer falls rapidly. The same principle applies if a specific antibody is added to estimate an antigenic compound, when the method is called immunoassay or radioimmunoassay; or if a specific enzyme is added as in the assay of vitamin B-12.

It is necessary to remove any specific binding protein present in the plasma sample and this is usually done by extraction of the steroids present with an organic solvent, e.g. methylene chloride, which leaves most of the proteins in the aqueous phase. Radioactive tracer and a preparation of the specific binding protein is then equilibriated with the dried steroid extract at about 10°C to achieve maximum binding, as binding increases with decrease in temperature, probably due to more binding sites becoming available. The specific binding proteins are usually prepared from pregnancy plasma. After equilibriation the bound and unbound fractions are separated, usually by absorption of the unbound substance onto charcoal, fuller's earth, florisil or kieselguhr. The radioactivity in the remaining bound fraction is measured.

Competitive protein binding analysis was first successfully developed for cortisol using transcortin obtained from human pregnancy plasma. The method has now been extended to the estimation of progesterone with transcortin, for whose binding sites it competes with cortisol; testosterone with its specific testosterone binding globulin; and for estradiol using specific proteins isolated from animal tissues. For illustrative purposes a typical method for the assay of testosterone is described.

Carrier [^{3}H] testosterone (1500 disintegrations/min, specific activity 30 Ci/mole) is added to 5 ml heparinized plasma at the beginning of the assay and steroids are extracted with mixed alkali and ether. Testosterone is separated from other steroids in the ether extract by thin layer chromatography and eluted into methanol. A portion of this methanol solution is used to estimate the percentage recovery of the testosterone by liquid scintillation counting.

Radioactive testosterone bound to testosterone binding globulin is prepared from heparinized plasma obtained from subjects in the third trimester of pregnancy. Plasma is diluted 1:100 and 100 ml added to 1.5 ng dried [^{3}H] testosterone (4×10^6 disintegrations/min, specific activity 30 Ci/mole). The binding assay is then carried out by adding one ml of this globulin preparation to a suitable aliquot of the dried methanol extract of testosterone. Binding is allowed to take place at 0°C for 10 min. The testosterone which does not become bound to the added globulin is then removed by adding specially treated charcoal, mixing at 0°C, and centrifuging. The amount of testosterone in the supernatant, which represents that which became protein bound to the added globulin, is then estimated by liquid scintillation counting and related to a standard curve with the range 0.2-2.0 ng. The testosterone present in the original plasma is calculated as

$$\text{Testosterone, ng/100 ml plasma} = \text{ng found} \times \frac{100}{5}$$

$$\times \frac{100}{\% \text{ aliquot of methanol extract analysed}}$$

$$\times \frac{100}{\% \text{ recovery of testosterone from original plasma}}.$$

Results compare very well with double isotope dilution methods and show a mean of 533 ± 259 ng/100 ml for males and 47 ± 19 ng/100 ml for females.

VII. BIOSYNTHESIS OF TRITERPENES

A. BASIC CHEMISTRY

Triterpenes may be defined as C-30 compounds which are built up from six isoprene units. All are believed to be derived from all-*trans* squalene by a series of concerted cyclization and rearrangement reactions. For each cyclization the squalene chain is specifically orientated by being folded into a series of potential chair or boat cyclohexane rings, due to the particular cyclization enzyme. The cyclizations proceed by a sequence of planar *trans* additions to the olefin bonds. Subsequently, Wagner-Meerwein rearrangements and 1,2-eliminations occur. All the transformations between squalene and the final product are envisaged as occurring in a non-stop sequence. Products may be incompletely cyclized, e.g. onocerin, or contain a tetracyclic steroid structure or contain the pentacyclic structure of the true triterpenes. The pentacyclic triterpenes can be divided structurally into the hydropicene type, i.e. all five rings are of six carbon atoms, e.g. β-amyrin, and the cyclopentenobenzophenanthrene type, i.e. the fifth (E) ring has five carbon atoms, e.g. lupane. Triterpenes have been isolated from over 100 families of dicotyledonous plants and also from many of the lower plant orders. About 400 triterpenes have been characterized and the structures of some 300 elucidated.

1. Cyclization

Electrophilic addition to simple olefins (I) proceeds so that the two newly attached groups are in the same plane and *trans* to one another (III). In some cases, e.g. bromination, there is evidence for a symmetrical intermediate (II). This stereoelectronic control is thought to be a consequence of the maximum overlap of π-electrons which is achieved in the intermediate. The *trans* nature of the product is then controlled by the attack of the nucleophile from the opposite side of the molecule to that occupied by the electrophile. Such a *trans* attack results in a minimum of steric interference between the two groups, and the transition state is again one with a maximum overlap of π-electrons.

If the nucleophile is another double bond in the same molecule, there will be a specific stereochemistry for cyclization. Thus, a hexadiene will be folded into a potential chair (IV) or boat (V) conformation to assure the planar *trans* arrangement of the reacting centres and products will be VI and VII respectively.

Chair IV → VI → Trans-trans-trans *(anti)* VI

Boat V → → VII → Trans-cis-trans *(syn)* VII

2. Wagner-Meerwein rearrangements

The essential step is the movement of a carbon-carbon bond from one carbon atom to an adjacent one, via a carbonium ion intermediate.

A carbonium ion may be defined as the product formed by the loss of H^- from methane to give CH_3^+ which is a trivalent ion whose structure cannot be represented by conventional valency diagrams. The formation of the carbonium ion is preceded by either the loss of an anion (e.g. OH^-) from a neutral saturated molecule or addition of a proton (H^+) to a double bond. The discharge of the rearranged ion necessarily involves either the uptake of an anion (OH^-) or loss of a proton (H^+).

Carbonium ions may also be described in non-classical form as bridged ions (VIII) (resonance hybrids) which rearrange so that one of the groups originally attached to the olefin may become the bridge ion.

In the biosynthesis of triterpenes, non-classical bridged carbonium ions are envisaged as occurring between three adjacent methylene groups with a triple overlap of the sp^2 electrons and are prepresented as

$$-CH_2\text{------}CH_2- $$

During rearrangements a group departs with both of the electrons formerly shared with another atom, leaving this atom with only a sextet of electrons. Another group then migrates, with its pair of bonding electrons, onto the electron-deficient atom.

3. 1,2-Shifts

When there is no change in ring size, the substituent which shifts and the group which is displaced from the molecule must be axial and antiparallel (*trans*)

In rearrangements a group departs with both of the electrons formerly shared with another atom, e.g. carbon, leaving this atom with only a sextet of outer electrons. Another group then migrates, with its pair of bonding electrons, onto the electron-deficient atom and so on.

As progressive 1,2-shifts proceed along the triterpene molecule, the orientation of the rings to each other becomes altered. The prefixes *cis* and *trans* denote the stereochemistry of ring fusions. The prefixes *syn* and *anti* denote the terminal orientation of the rings with respect to each other, e.g. if the bond joining rings A and C (C-9 to C-10 in the steroid numbering) has *cis* hydrogens then rings A and C are *syn* with respect to each other and if the hydrogens are *trans*, rings A and C are *anti*. The simplest case where both the *cis-trans* and *syn-anti* nomenclature is required to describe the ring orientations is in the three-ring system of perhydrophenanthrene. Here ten stereoisomers are possible, i.e. four pairs of enantiomorphs (*trans-anti-trans, cis-anti-trans, cis-syn-trans* and *cis-anti-cis*) and two *meso* compounds (*cis-syn-cis* and *trans-syn-trans*). The most stable form is *trans-anti-trans* as all the rings are fused by equatorial bonds. In the triterpenes, the full orientations of the rings have been elucidated in the well-known oleanane and hopane series of 1,2-shifts.

4. Cyclization enzymes

The enzyme(s) involved in the direct production of lanosterol from squalene appear to be the only cyclization enzymes which have been studied so far. It is now believed that two enzymes are involved, first a mixed function oxidase which requires molecular oxygen and $TPNH^+$ for the formation of 2,3-oxido-squalene, and secondly 2,3-oxidosqualene cyclase. Cyclization is initiated by the uptake of a proton at C-3 (steroid numbering) and the four steroid rings are formed as an intermediate cation with a deficiency of two electrons at C-20. The appropriate 1,2-shifts then occur and a proton is eliminated from C-9β to give lanosterol. There is no net loss or gain of elements. The overall reaction of the two enzymes may be denoted by:

$$\text{squalene}\,(C_{30}H_{50}) + O_2 + 2H^+ + 2_e \rightarrow \text{lanosterol}\,(C_{30}H_{50}O) + H_2.$$

All triterpenes are believed to be formed by specific cyclization enzymes, the differences in product being due to some Wagner-Meerwein rearrangements and subsequent 1,2-shifts of the primary cation formed. Some triterpenes do not have an oxygen function at C-3 and it is believed that cyclization is initiated by the attack of a proton onto squalene directly. Most triterpenes with an oxygen function at C-3 have a 3β-hydroxyl group but a few, e.g. cephalosporin P_1 have a 3α-hydroxyl group. This is presumed to be due to the stereospecificity of the first mixed function oxidase.

B. MODES OF CYCLIZATION OF ALL-*TRANS* SQUALENE

1. Chair-chair-unfolded-unfolded-chair (ambrane)

Ambrein (Fig. 9) is apparently produced by cyclization beginning at both ends of the squalene chain, leaving the potential rings in the central part of the molecule unclosed. Cyclization appears to be initiated by a proton attack and is not oxidative. The parent hydrocarbon, ambrane, is usually depicted from above as if the enclosed rings are arranged as chairs.

Chair-chair-unfolded-unfolded-chair

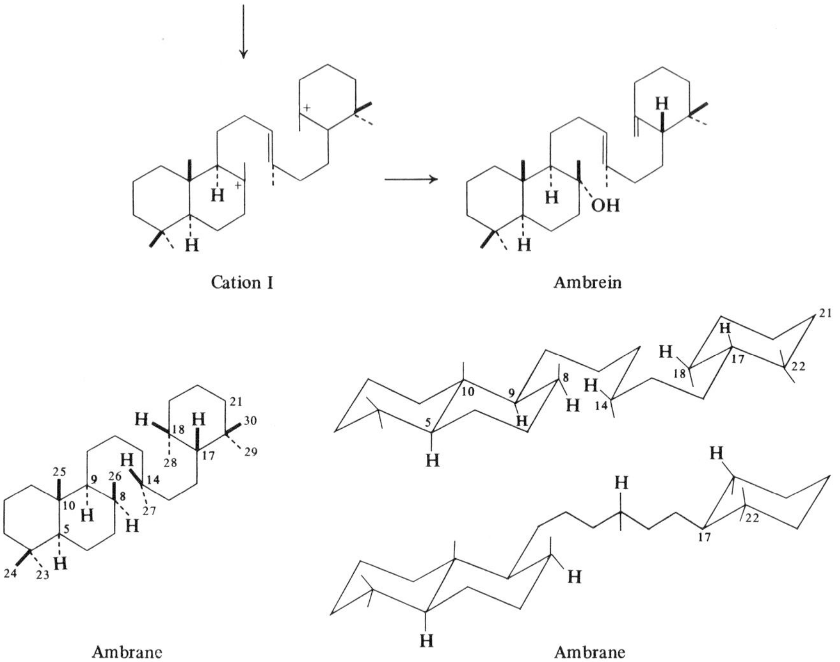

Cation I   Ambrein

Ambrane   Ambrane

Fig. 9. Biosynthesis of ambrane derivatives.

2. Chair-chair-unfolded-chair-chair (onocerane, serratane)

Onocerin (Fig. 10) is produced by the oxidative cyclization of squalene beginning at both ends via cation I. The parent hydrocarbon, onocerane, may be depicted either with carbon atoms 11 and 12 unfolded, or with these atoms folded into the chair conformation, which is more usual. This latter arrangement involves the inversion in space of the D-E ring complex with the result that the methyl group at C-14 is α, the hydrogen atom at C-17 is β and the methyl group at C-18 is α. Onocerane derivatives occur in the fruit peel of *Lausium domesticum* where rings A and E have become broken between C-3 and C-4 and between C-21 and C-22 respectively.

Serratenediol is produced from cation I by a series of 1,2-shifts to cation III which loses two protons. Its parent hydrocarbon, serratane is depicted viewed from the side and from above the molecule. The configurations at C-14, C-17 and C-18 are the same as in onocerane when the latter is depicted with carbon atoms C-11 and C-12 arranged as a chair. A number of serratane derivatives have been isolated from, for example, club moss, *Lycopodium clavatum*, and other lower plants (Table 6).

Table 6. *Some naturally occurring derivatives of serratane*

Serratene	14-Serratene
Serratenediol	14-Serraten-3β,21α-diol
21-Episerratenediol	14-Serraten-3β,21β-diol
Diepiserratenediol	14-Serraten-3α,21β-diol
Sterratenolone	14-Serraten-21-ol-3-one
	14-Serraten-3β,21β-diol-3-methyl ester
	14-Serraten-3β,21α-diol-3-methyl ester
	14-Serraten-3β,21α-diol-3-acetate
16-Oxoserratenediol	14-Serraten-3β,21α-diol-16-one
16-Oxoepiserratenediol	14-Serraten-3β,21β-diol-16-one
16-Oxodiepiserratenediol	14-Serraten-3α,21β-diol-16-one
Serratriol	14-Serraten-3β,21α,24-triol
Lycoclavanol	14-Serraten-3β,21β,24-triol
Lycoclavin	14-Serraten-2α,3α,21β,24-tetrol
16-Oxolycoclavanol	14-Serraten-3β,21β,24-triol-16-one
Tohogenol	Serratan-3β,14β,21α-triol
Tohogeninol	Serratan-3β,14β,21α,24-tetrol

3. Chair-chair-chair-boat-unfolded

This is the most common type of folding encountered and explains the biosynthesis of several major groups of triterpenoids by a series of Wagner-Meerwein rearrangements as shown in Fig. 11. Five different types of triterpene skeleton are produced in turn, from the five primary cations A1 (steroid type), B1 (shionane type), C1 (lupane type), D1 (germanicane or β-amyrin type) and E1 (taraxasterane or α-amyrin type). The two last have firstly two methyl groups in ring E attached to the same carbon atom, and secondly attached to adjacent carbon atoms. It is believed that this sequence of triterpenoid types is also followed after other types of 4-ring folding of squalene and starting at type C cations for 5-ring folding. In Fig. 11 the cations are shown both as the classical carbonium ions and as the bridged ions. In subsequent sequences only the classical form is shown. In the change from cations A1 and B1 to C1, so forming the pentacyclic triterpenoids, the numbering of the carbon skeleton becomes altered. On the steroid system of nomenclature, C-18 becomes inserted between C-16 and C-17 to form the 6-carbon ring E. These atoms are then numbered consecutively as C-16, C17 and C-18 in the pentacyclic triterpenoids.

A number of 3α-hydroxy- and 3-keto-pentacyclic triterpenoids are found in nature. It is believed that these are derived from either the hydrocarbon derivative or 3β-hydroxy derivative which is produced by the cyclization of 3S-2,3-oxido-squalene as a chair in ring A. Cyclization of ring A as a boat from 3R-2,3-oxido-squalene would theoretically produce a 3α-hydroxyl derivative.

Each of the five primary cations shown in Fig. 11 can serve as the terminal

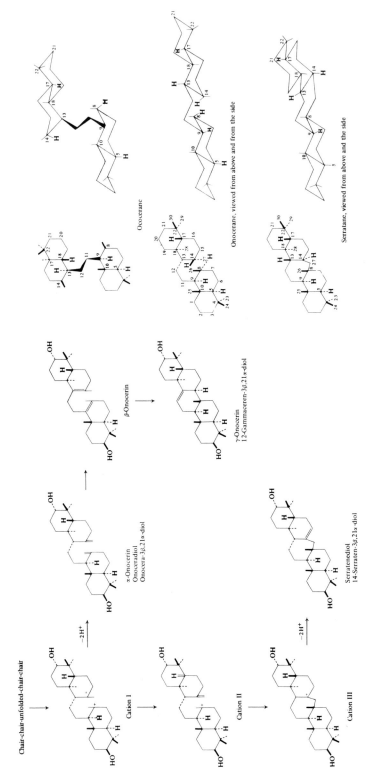

Fig. 10. Biosynthesis of onocerane and serratane derivatives.

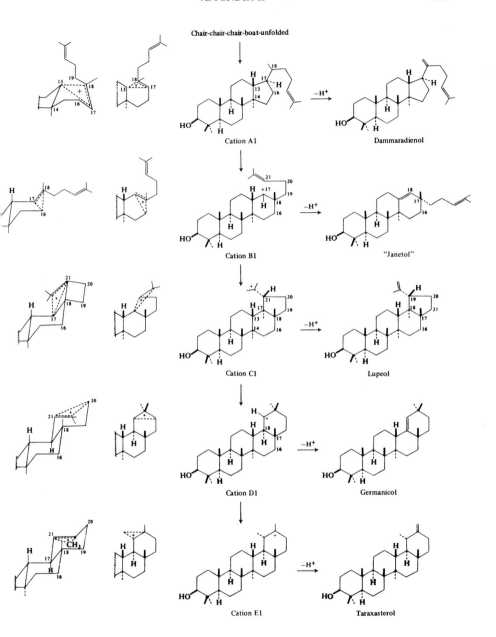

Fig. 11. The five primary types of triterpenes produced by chair-chair-chair-boat-unfolded folding.

13*

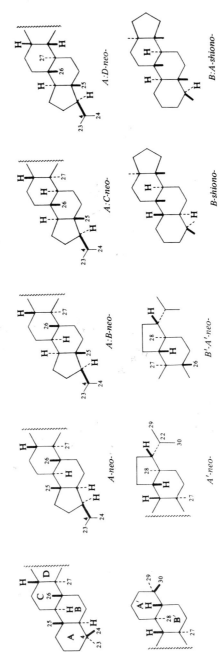

Fig. 12. Ring nomenclature of triterpenoids according to Ourisson and Shioni.

Wagner-Meerwein rearrangement and proceed instead subsequently via a series of 1,2-shifts to produce a series of compounds all with the same basic ring structure. After certain 1,2-shifts a new theoretical parent hydrocarbon is produced. The structure of some of these hydrocarbons have been defined by IUPAC as naturally occurring derivatives of them are well known. Some of the less well-known theoretical hydrocarbons remain nameless. A systematic nomenclature has been developed by Ourisson to describe the hydrocarbons of the pentacyclic triterpenes arising from primary cations of the C, D and E types which use the prefix *friedo* to describe the migration of the angular methyl groups. Thus, when an angular group has moved from C-14 to C-13, at the C/D ring junction, the new compound has the prefix D-*friedo*- followed by the name of the first parent hydrocarbon in the series. Similarly, when a further angular group has moved from C-8 to C-14, the prefix of the new compound is D:C-*friedo*-; when another has moved from C-10 to C-9, the prefix is D:B-*friedo*-; and when another has moved from C-4 to C-5, the prefix is D:A-*friedo*-. The numbering of the angular methyl groups remains the same throughout, as shown in Fig. 12. Contractions of ring A and of ring E are named using the prefix *neo* as shown in Fig. 12. In symmetrical triterpenoids ring E is considered as A' and ring D as B'.

The derivatives of the five primary cations are described separately.

(a) Dammarane, panaxane and euphane derivatives

Figure 13 shows that loss of a proton from cation A1 produces dammaradienol. Two parent hydrocarbons are possible with different configurations at C-20. Dammarane has been defined as having a 20R-configuration like lanostane and is thus 8-methyl-18-nor-lanostane or 14α, 17β, 20R-lanostane. It is proposed that the 20S parent hydrocarbon be called panaxane. Most derivatives of dammarane and panaxane (Table 7) have a hydroxyl group at C-20 which may be formed by the addition of OH⁻ to cation A1. Derivatives of dammarane, which are more numerous than those of panaxane, thus have a 17αH, 20S-ol configuration.

Euphane derivatives (Table 8) arise from cation A5. They have the 20R configuration. (Derivatives of tirucallane have an identical structure to those of euphane except the configuration is 20S. Their biosynthesis from chair-chair-chair-chair-unfolded folding is described later.) IUPAC have defined 5α-euphane and 5α-tirucallane with an 8β H atom, so giving ring C as a boat. The less strained chair form is given if the H atom at C-8 is α.

(b) Shionane derivatives

Shionanone (shionone) (Fig. 14) has been identified as a member of this series. Its parent hydrocarbon may be defined as shionane. The Japanese chemist, Shioni, has also given his name to a system of nomenclature of the

Table 7. *Some naturally occurring derivatives of panaxane and dammarane*

Dammaradienol	20,24(5α)-Dammaradien-3β-ol
Aglaiol	20,(5α)-Dammaren-3β-ol 24,25-epoxide

Panaxane derivatives (14α, 17β, 20S configuration)

Dammarenediol I	24(5α)-Panaxen-3β,20-diol
Protopanaxadiol	14(5α)-Panaxen-3β,12β,20-triol
Panaxadiol	5α-Panaxane-3β-ol 20,25-epoxide

Dammarane derivatives (14α, 17β, 20R configuration)

Dammarenediol II	24(5α)-Dammaren-3β,20-diol
Dipterocarpol	24(5α)-Dammaren-20-ol-3-one
Dryobalanone	24(5α)-Dammaren-20,21-diol-3-one
Betulafolienetriol	24(5α)-Dammaren-3α,12β,20-triol
3-Epibetulafolienetriol 20-Epiprotopanaxadiol }	24(5α)-Dammaren-3β,12β-20-triol

Table 8. *Some naturally occurring derivatives of euphane (13α, 14β, 17α-lanostane)*

Euphol	8,24,(5α)-Euphadien-3β-ol
Basseol Butyrospermeol }	7,24,(5α)-Euphadien-3β-ol
Kulinone 16β-Hydroxybutyrospermone }	7,24,(5α)-Euphadien-16β-ol-3-one
Euphenol	8,(5α)-Euphen-3β-ol

Lanostane has 20R configuration

Table 9. *Some naturally occurring derivatives of the lupane series*

Derivatives of lupane

Lupeol	20(30)-Lupen-3β-ol
	20(30)-Lupen-3-one
Betulin	20(30)-Lupen-3β,28-diol
Betulinic acid	20(30)-Lupen-3β-ol-28-oic acid
Ceanothic acid	20(30)-Lupen-3β-ol-22,28-dioic acid
Glochidione	1,20(30)-Lupadien-3-one
	20(30)-Lupen-3β,16β-diol
	Lupan-3β,20-diol
	Lupan-3β,20,28-triol
Clerodone	Lupan-12-one
Glochidiol	20(30)-Lupen-1β,3α-diol
Clerodolone	20(30)-Lupen-3β-ol-12-one
Lupenone	20(30)-Lupen-3-one

Derivatives of isolupane

	13(18)-Isolupen-3β-ol

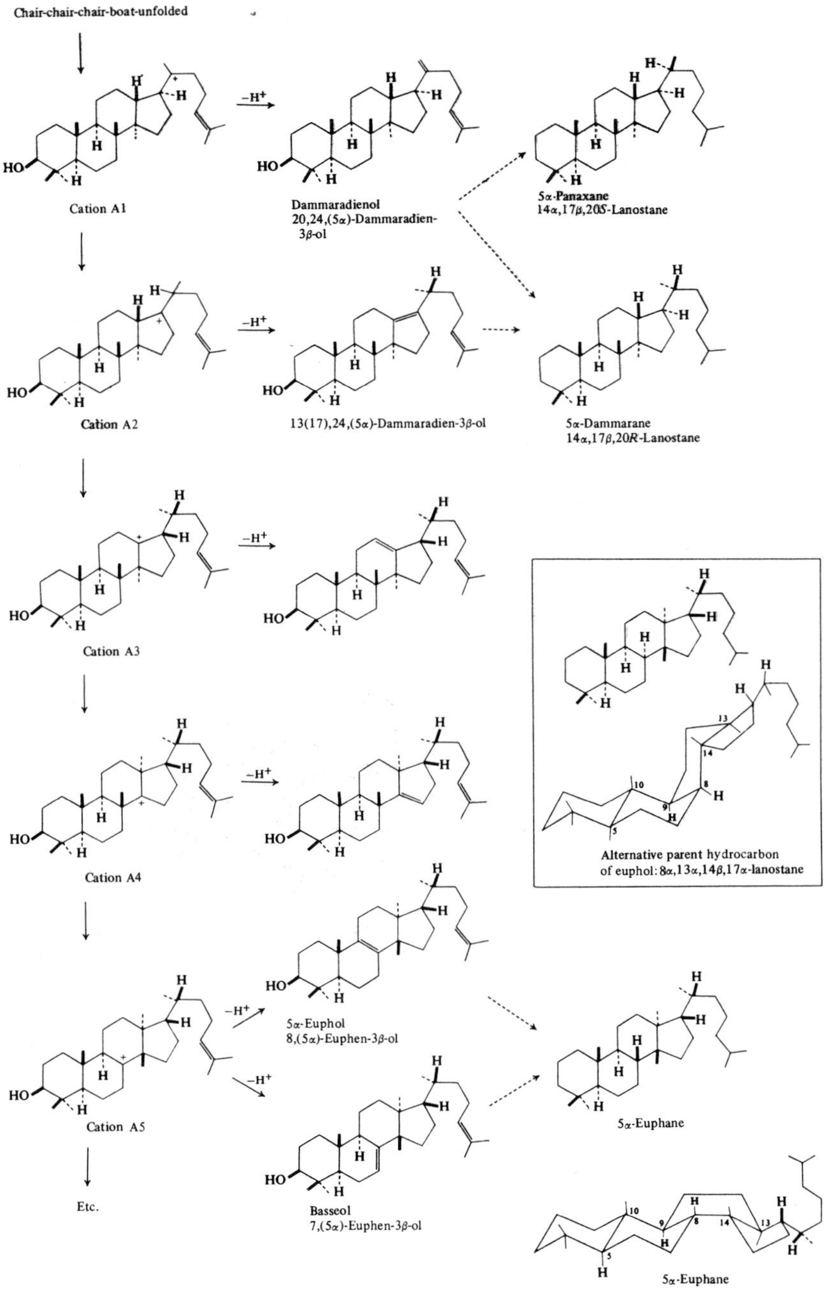

Fig. 13. Biosynthesis of panaxane, dammarane and euphane derivatives.

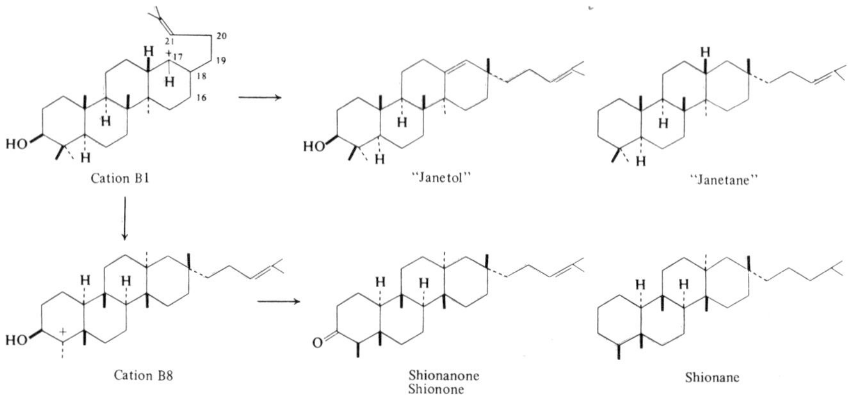

Fig. 14. Shionane derivatives.

products of 1,2-shifts in the steroid (euphane, lanostane and tirucallane series) which uses the prefixes B-*shiono-* and B:A-*shiono-*.

(c) Lupane derivatives

Figure 15 shows the biosynthesis of compounds in this series and Table 9 shows some known derivatives. The first two parent hydrocarbons are lupane and isolupane.

(d) Oleanane (β-amyrane derivatives)

Figure 16 shows the biosynthesis of this series. There are six parent hydrocarbons: 18αH-oleanane, oleanane, taraxerane, multiflorane, glutinane and friedelane. Systematic nomenclature has tended to relate to oleanane which is the most important parent hydrocarbon. Their structure and systematic nomenclature is shown in Table 10. Oleanane derivatives, i.e. related to β-amyrin, are the most abundant plant triterpenoids. Oleanolic acid is the most abundant compound. Some of the known oleanane derivatives are shown in Table 11. A few known derivatives of the other parent hydrocarbons are shown in Table 12. Figure 17 shows some of the several ways of depicting the three-dimensional structure of some of the hydrocarbons.

(e) Ursane (α-amyrane derivatives)

α-Amyrin (Fig. 18) is relatively common in plants but its derivatives are comparatively rare. Some derivatives of taraxasterol and baurenol are known (Table 13).

4. Chair-chair-chair-chair-unfolded (tirucallane)

Derivatives analogous to the dammarane, shionane, lupane and amyrane types of the chair-chair-chair-boat-unfolded type do not appear to be known, with the

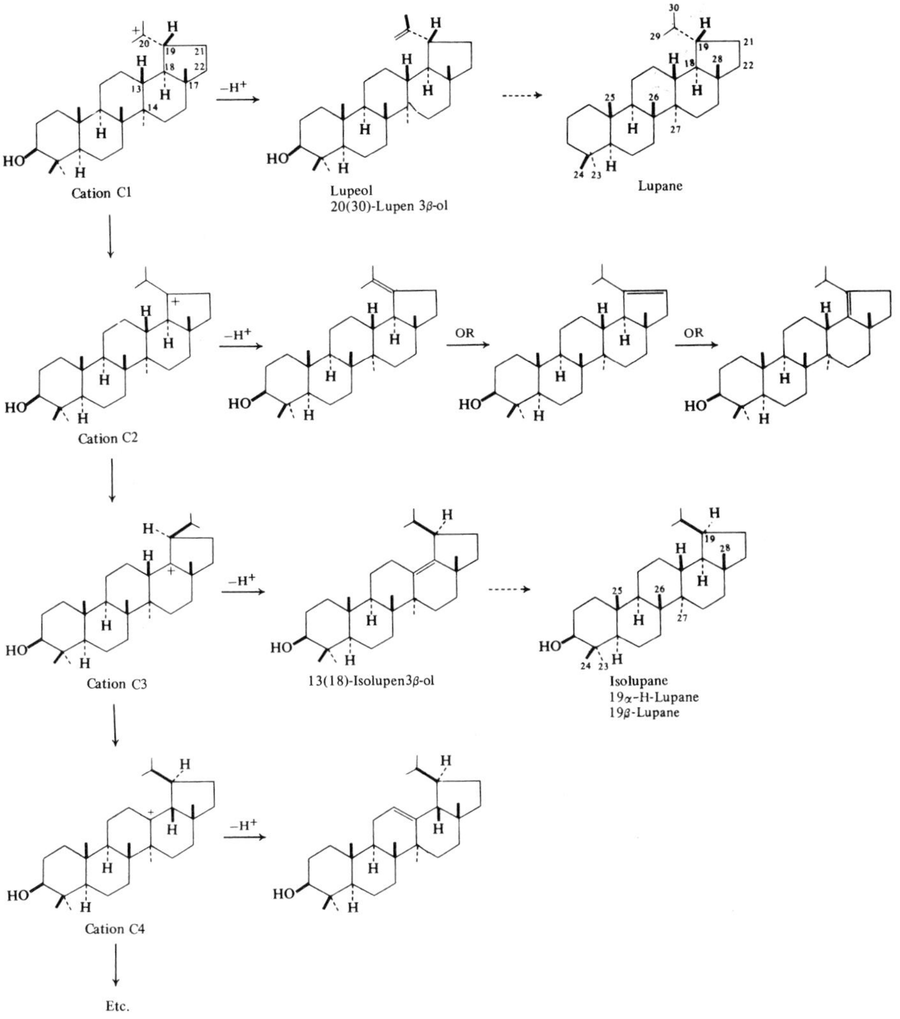

Fig. 15. Biosynthesis of lupane derivatives.

exception of tirucallane derivatives which appear to arise from the fifth cation (A5) of the steroid series (Fig. 19, Table 14). Tirucallane derivatives with an oxygenated ring structure in the side chain are known as melianes and have been found in the seed of *Melia azadirachta* (Nim oil). The biosynthesis of melianone (Fig. 20) may be via flindissol. Cedrelone and its derivatives probably arise from cation A4 in this series, the parent hydrocarbon of which may be designated cedrane.

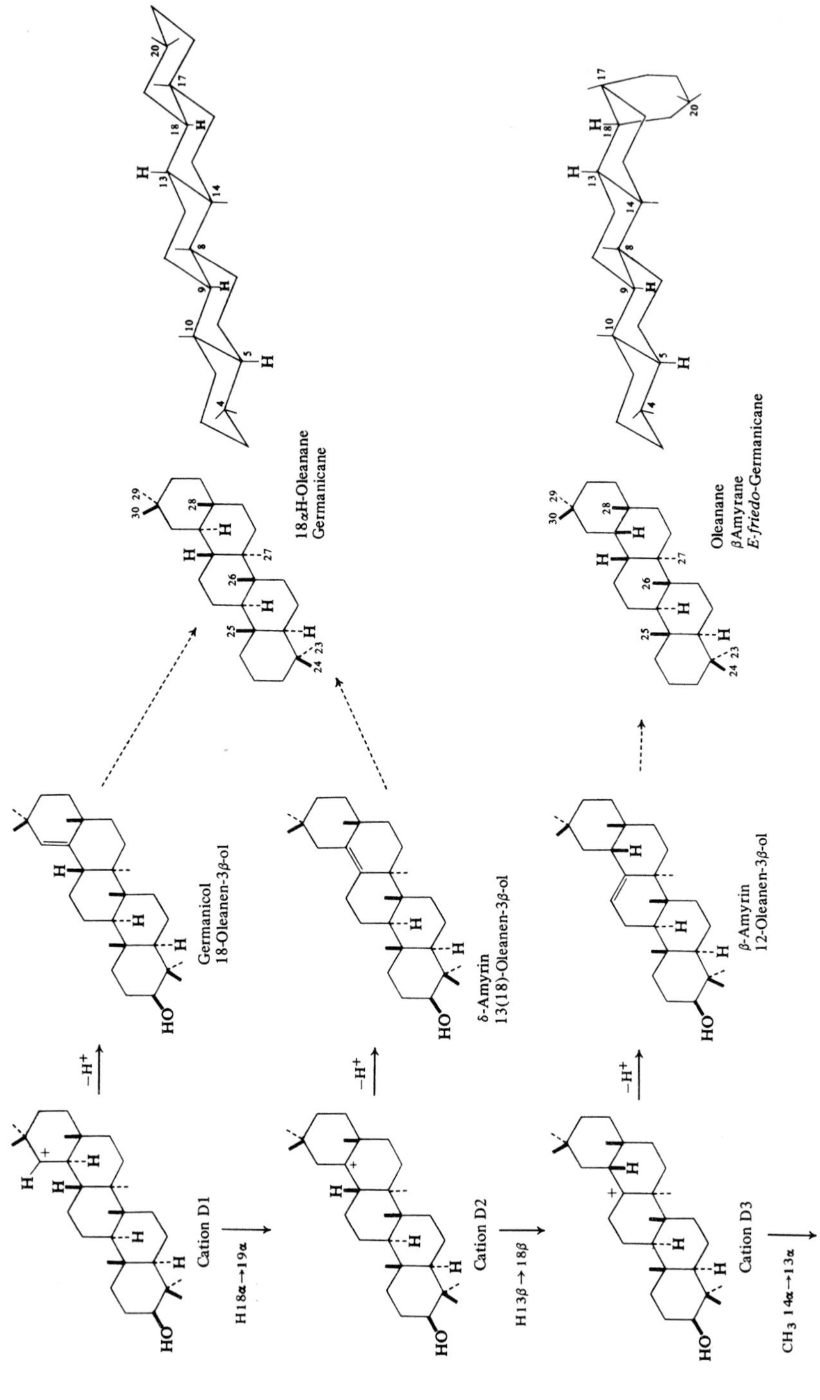

18αH-Oleanane
Germanicane

Germanicol
18-Oleanen-3β-ol

Cation D1

−H+

H18α→19α

δ-Amyrin
13(18)-Oleanen-3β-ol

Cation D2

−H+

H13β→18β

Oleanane
βAmyrane
E-friedo-Germanicane

β-Amyrin
12-Oleanen-3β-ol

Cation D3

−H+

CH₃ 14α→13α

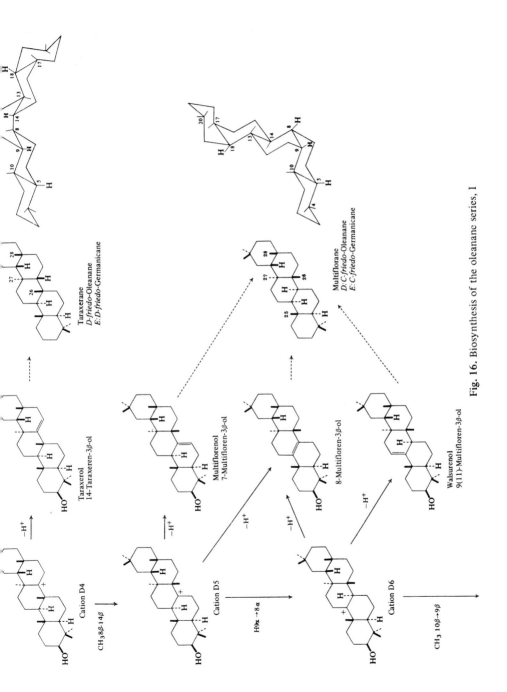

Fig. 16. Biosynthesis of the oleanane series, I

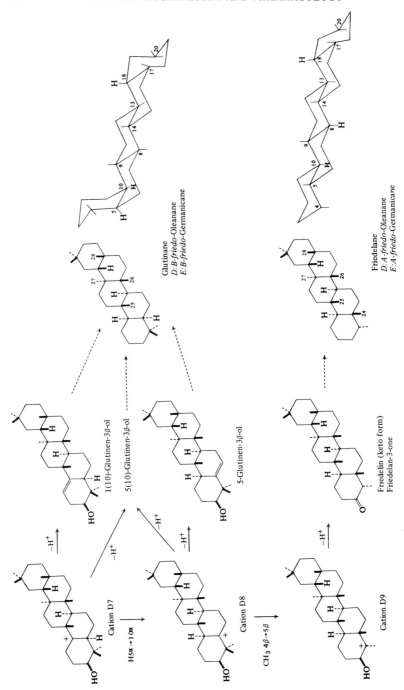

Fig. 16. Biosynthesis of the oleanane series, II.

Table 10. Nomenclature and configuration of pentacyclic triterpenes of the oleanane (β-amyrane) series

	18αH-Oleanane Germanicane†		Oleanane E-friedo-Germanicane	Taraxerane D-friedo-Oleanane E:D-friedo-Germanicane	Multiflorane D:C-friedo-Oleanane E:C-friedo-Germanicane		Glutinane D:B-friedo-Oleanane E:B-friedo-Germanicane		Friedelane D:A-friedo-Oleanane E:H-friedo-Germanicane
Parent Hydrocarbon	D1	D2	D3	D4	D5	D6	D7	D8	D9
From cation number	18		12	14	7	8	1(10)	5(10)	3
Double bond at carbon atom number	13(18)		12	14	9(11)		5		3
Configuration of substituents at carbon atom number									
5	α	α	α	α	α	α	α*	α*	β
10	β	β	β	β	β	β	β	β	α
9	α	α	α	α	α*	α*	α*	α*	α
8	β	β	β	β	α*	α*	α	α	α
14	α	α	α	β*	β	β	β	β	β
13	β	β*	β*	α	β	β	β	β	β
18	α*	α	β	β	β	β	β	β	α
17	β	β	β	β	β	β	β	β	β
Configuration between carbon atoms (ring junctions)									
5/10 A/B	trans	trans	trans	trans	trans	trans	cis	cis	trans
9/10 A/C	anti	anti	anti	anti	anti	anti	anti	anti	anti
8/9 B/C	trans	trans	trans	trans	cis	anti	trans	trans	trans
8/14 B/D	anti	anti	anti	syn	anti	trans	anti	anti	anti
13/14 C/D	trans	trans	trans	trans	trans	anti	trans	trans	trans
13/18 C/E	anti	anti	syn	anti	anti	anti	anti	anti	anti
17/18 D/E	trans	trans	cis	cis	cis	cis	cis	cis	cis
Conformation of ring									
A	chair	chair	chair	chair	chair	chair	chair	chair	chair
B	chair	chair	chair	chair	chair	chair	chair	chair	chair
C	chair	chair	chair	boat	chair	chair	chair	chair	chair
D	chair	chair	chair	chair	chair	chair	chair	chair	chair
E	chair	chair	chair	chair	chair	chair	chair	chair	chair

*H inserted to construct the parent hydrocarbon

† Gammacerane has the same configuration

Table 11. *Some naturally occurring derivatives of oleanane (β-amyrane)*

β-Amyrin	12-Oleanen-3β-ol
Oleanolic acid	12-Oleanen-3β-ol-28-oic acid
Katonic acid	12-Oleanen-3α-ol-28-oic acid
Erythrodiol	12-Oleanen-3β,28-diol
Maniladiol	12-Oleanen-3β,16β-diol
Sophoradiol	12-Oleanen-3β,22β-diol
α-Boswellic acid	12-Oleanen-3α-ol-24-oic acid

Monohydroxyoleanolic acids

Maslinic acid	12-Oleanen-2α,3β-diol-28-oic acid
Sumaresinolic acid	12-Oleanen-3β,6β-diol-28-oic acid
Echinocystic acid	12-Oleanen-3β,16α-diol-28-oic acid
Cochalic acid	12-Oleanen-3β,16β-diol-28-oic acid
Siaresinolic acid	12-Oleanen-3β,19α-diol-28-oic acid
Machaerinic acid	12-Oleanen-3β,21β-diol-28-oic acid
Hederagenin	12-Oleanen-3β,23-diol-28-oic acid
Mesembryanthemoidigenic acid	12-Oleanen-3β,29-diol-28-oic acid
Queretaroic acid	12-Oleanen-3β,30-diol-28-oic acid

Dihydroxyoleanolic acids

Acacic acid	12-Oleanen-3β,16β,21β-triol-28-oic acid
Arjunolic acid	12-Oleanen-2α,3β,23-triol-28-oic acid
Bayogenin	12-Oleanen-2β,3β,23-triol-28-oic acid
Treleasagenic acid	12-Oleanen-3β,21β,30-triol-28-oic acid

Trihydroxyoleanolic acids

Terminolic acid	12-Oleanen-2α,3β,6β,23-tetrol-28-oic acid
Tormentosic acid	12-Oleanen-2α,3β,16α,23-tetrol-28-oic acid
Polygalacic acid	12-Oleanen-2β,3β,16α,23-tetrol-28-oic acid
Caccigenin	12-Oleanen-3β,15α,16β,23-tetrol-28-oic acid

Hydroxyerthyrodiols

Primulagenin A	12-Oleanen-3β,16α,28-triol
Longispinogenin	12-Oleanen-3β,16β,28-triol
Barrigenol	12-Oleanen-3β,15β,16β,27,28-pentol
Barringtogenol	12-Oleanen-2α,3β,23,38-tetrol
Camelliagenin A ⎫ Dihydropriverogenin ⎭	12-Oleanen-3β,16α,22α,28-tetrol
Theasapogenol A	12-Oleanen-3β,21,23,28-tetrol
Chichipegenin	12-Oleanen-3β,16β,22α,28-tetrol
Aescinindine ⎫ Barringtogenol-C ⎭	12-Oleanen-3β,16α,21α,22β,28-pentol
Protoaescigenin	12-Oleanen-3β,16α,21α,22β,24,28-hexol

Dicarboxylic acids

Barringtogenic acid	12-Oleanen-2α,3β-diol-23,28-dioic acid
Cincholic acid	12-Oleanen-3β-ol-27,28-dioic acid
Medicagenic acid	12-Oleanen-2β,3β-diol-23,28-dioic acid
Spergulagenic acid	12-Oleanen-3β-ol-28,29-dioic acid
Phytolaccogenin	12-Oleanen-2β,3β,23-triol-28,30-dioic acid

Table 11.–*continued*

Others

Bassic acid	5,12-Oleanadien-2α,3β,23-triol-28-oic acid
Gypsogenin	12-Oleanen-3β-ol-23-al-28-oic acid
Cyclamiretin	12-Oleanen-3β,16α,28-triol-25-al
Soyasapogenol-A	12-Oleanen-3β,21α,22α,24-tetrol
Soyasapogenol-B	12-Oleanen-3β,21α,24-triol
Soyasapogenol-C	12,21-Oleanadien-3β,24-diol
Soyasapogenol-E	2-Oleanen-3β,24-diol-21-one
Gummosgenin	12-Oleanen-3β,16β-diol-28-al
Machaeric acid	12-Oleanen-3β-ol-21-one-28-oic acid
Quillaic acid	12-Oleanen-3β,16α-diol-23-al-28-one
Bredemolic acid	12-Oleanen-2β,3α-diol-28-oic acid
Liquiritic acid	12-Oleanen-3β-ol-11-one-29-oic acid
Glycyrrhetic acid	12-Oleanen-3β-ol-11-one-30-oic acid
Commic acid C	12-Oleanen-2β,3β-diol-23-oic acid

Table 12. *Some naturally occurring derivatives of 18αH-oleanane, taraxerane, multiflorane, glutinane and friedelane*

Derivatives of 18αH-oleanane (germanicane, δ-amyrane)

Germanicol	18-Oleanen-3β-ol
Miliacin	18-Oleanen-3β-ol methyl ester
Morolic acid	1,18-Oleanadien-3β-ol-28-oic acid
Avenagenin	18-Oleanen-3β,23,28-triol-11-one
Germanidiol	18-Oleanen-2β,3β-diol
Epigermanidiol	18-Oleanen-2α,3β-diol
δ-Amyrin	13(18)-Oleanen-3β-ol
Albigenic acid	13(18)-Oleanen-3β,16α-diol-28-oic acid
δ-Boswellic acid	13(18)-Oleanen-3α-ol-24-oic acid
δ-Amyrenone	13(18)-Oleanen-3-one
Soyasapogenol-D	13(18)-Oleanen-3β,21α,24-triol
Saikogenin-D	11,13(18)-Oleanadien-3β,16α,23,28-tetrol
Saikogenin-A	11,13(18)-Oleanadien-3β,16β,23,28 tetrol
Milacin	13(18)-Oleanen-3β-ol methyl ester

Derivatives of taraxerane (D-friedo-oleanane)

Taraxerol	14-Taraxeren-3β-ol
Taraxerone	14-Taraxeren-3-one
Sawamilletin	14-Taraxen-3β-ol 3-methyl ester
Taraxerene	14-Taraxerene
Myricadiol	14-Taraxeren-3β,28-diol
Myricolal	14-Taraxeren-3β-ol-28-al

Derivatives of multiflorane (D:C-friedo-oleanane)

Multiflorenol	7-Multifloren-3β-ol
Isomultiflorenol	7-Multifloren-3α-ol
Walsurenol	9(11)-Multifloren-3β-ol

Derivatives of glutinane (D:B-friedo-oleanane)

Glutenone	5-Glutinen-3-one
Glutinol	5-Glutinen-3β-ol

Table 12.—*continued*

Derivatives of friedelane (D:A-friedo-oleanane)

Friedelin, friedelan	Friedelan-3-one
Friedelanol	Friedelan-3β-ol
Epifriedelanol	Friedelan-3α-ol
Putranjivadione	Friedelan-3,7-dione
Pachysandiol-A	Friedelan-2α,3β-diol
Cerin	Friedelan-2α-ol-3-one
Roxburgholone	Friedelan-3α-ol-7-one

Table 13. *Some naturally occurring derivatives of the ursane series*

Derivatives of taraxastane (18α,19βH-ursane)

Taraxasterol	20(30)-Taraxasten-3β-ol
ψ-Taraxasterol	20-Taraxasten-3β-ol
Epi-ψ-taraxastanonol	Taraxastan-20-ol-3-one
Epi-ψ-Taraxastanediol	Taraxastan-3β,20-diol
Faradiol	20-Taraxasten-3β,12-diol
Arnidiol	20(30)-Taraxasten-3β,12-diol

Derivatives of ursane

α-Amyrin	12-Ursen-3β-ol
α-Amyrenone	12-Ursen-3-one
Ursolic acid	12-Ursen-3β-ol-28-oic acid
β-Boswellic acid	12-Ursen-3α-ol-24-oic acid
Bryonol acid	12-Ursen-3β-ol-30-oic acid
Ifflaconic acid	12-Ursen-3α-ol-30-oic acid
Quinovic acid	12-Ursen-3β-ol-27,28-dioic acid
Asiatic acid	12-Ursen-2α,3β,23-triol-28-oic acid
Rotundic acid	12-Ursen-3β,19α,23-triol-28-oic acid
Thankunic acid	12-Ursen-3β,5α,6β,24-tetrol-28-oic acid
Madecassic acid	12-Ursen-2α,3β,23-triol-28-oic acid
Tormentic acid	12-Ursen-2α,3β,29α-triol-28-oic acid
Commic acid-D	12-Ursen-2β,3β-diol-23-oic acid
Brein	12-Ursen-3β,16β-diol
Uvaol	12-Ursen-3β,28-diol
Micromeric acid	12,20(30)-Ursadien-3β-ol-28-oic acid
Tomentosolic acid	12,19-Ursadien-3β-ol-28-oic acid
Neoilexonol	12-Ursen-3β-ol-11-one

Derivatives of bauerane (D:C-friedo-ursane)

Bauerenol	7-Baueren-3β-ol
Isobauerenol	8-Baueren-3β-ol
Baueradienol	7,9(11)-Baueradien-3β-ol

Table 14. *Some naturally occurring derivatives of tirucallane*
(13α,14β,17α,20S-lanostane)

Tirucallol	8,24,(5α)-Tirucalladien-3β-ol
Elemolic acid	8,24,(5α)-Tirucalladien-3β-ol-21-oic acid
Masticadienoic acid	8,24,(5α)-Tirucalladien-3-one-26-oic acid
Euphorbol	24-Methylene-8,(5α)-tirucallen-3β-ol
Tirucallenol	8,(5α)-Tirucallen-3β-ol
β-Elemonic acid	8,24,4(5α)-Tirucalladien-3β-one-21-oic acid

Table 15. *Some naturally occurring derivatives of fusidane and protostane*
(4β-methyl-fusidane)

Derivatives of protostane (20R configuration implied in the name)
13(17),24-Protostadien-3β-ol
17(20)[16,21-*cis*],24-Protostadien-3β-ol
17(20)[16,21-*cis*],24-Protostadien-3β,29-diol 29-methyl ester

Derivatives of fusidane (20R configuration implied in the name)

Fusidic acid	17(20)[16,21-*cis*],24-Fusidadien-3α,11α,16β-triol-21-oic acid 16-acetate
Helvolic acid	1,17(20)[16,21-*cis*],24-Fusidatrien-7α,16β-diol-3,6-dione-21-oic acid 7,16-diacetate
Cephalosporin P₁	17(20)[16,21-*cis*],24-Fusidadien-3α,6α,7β,16β-tetrol-21-oic acid 6,16-diacetate
Isocephalosporin P₁	17(20)[16,21-*cis*],24-Fusidadien-3β,6α,7β,16β-tetrol-21-oic acid 7,16-diacetate
Monodesacetyl-cephalosporin P₁	17(20)[16,21-*cis*],24-Fusidadien-3β,6α,7β,16β-tetrol-21-oic acid 16-acetate

Table 16. *Some naturally occurring derivatives of cycloartane*
(9β,19-cyclo-lanostane)

Cycloartenol	24,(5α)-Cycloarten-3β-ol
Mangiferolic acid	24,(5α)-Cycloarten-3β-ol-27-oic acid
Mangiferonic acid	24,(5α)-Cycloarten-3-one-27-oic acid
Isomangiferolic acid	24,(5α)-Cycloarten-3α-ol-27-oic acid
Hydroxymangiferolic acid	24,(5α)-Cycloarten-3β,26-diol-27-oic acid
Hydroxymangiferonic acid	24,(5α)-Cycloarten-26-ol-3-one-27-oic acid
Cycloartanol	5α-Cycloartan-3β-ol-
	23,(5α)-Cycloarten-3β,25-diol

5. Chair-boat-chair-boat-unfolded

This type of folding (Fig. 21) produces the protostane, lanostane, cycloartane and curcurbitane derivatives of the steroid series. Pentacyclic triterpenoids belonging to this series do not appear to be known.

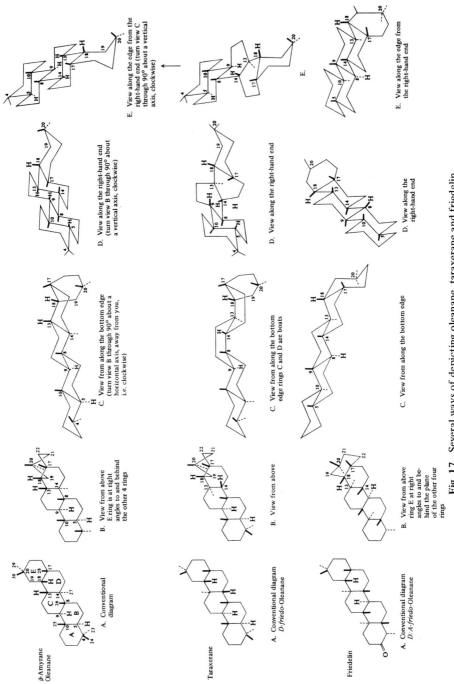

Fig. 17. Several ways of depicting oleanane, taraxerane and friedelin.

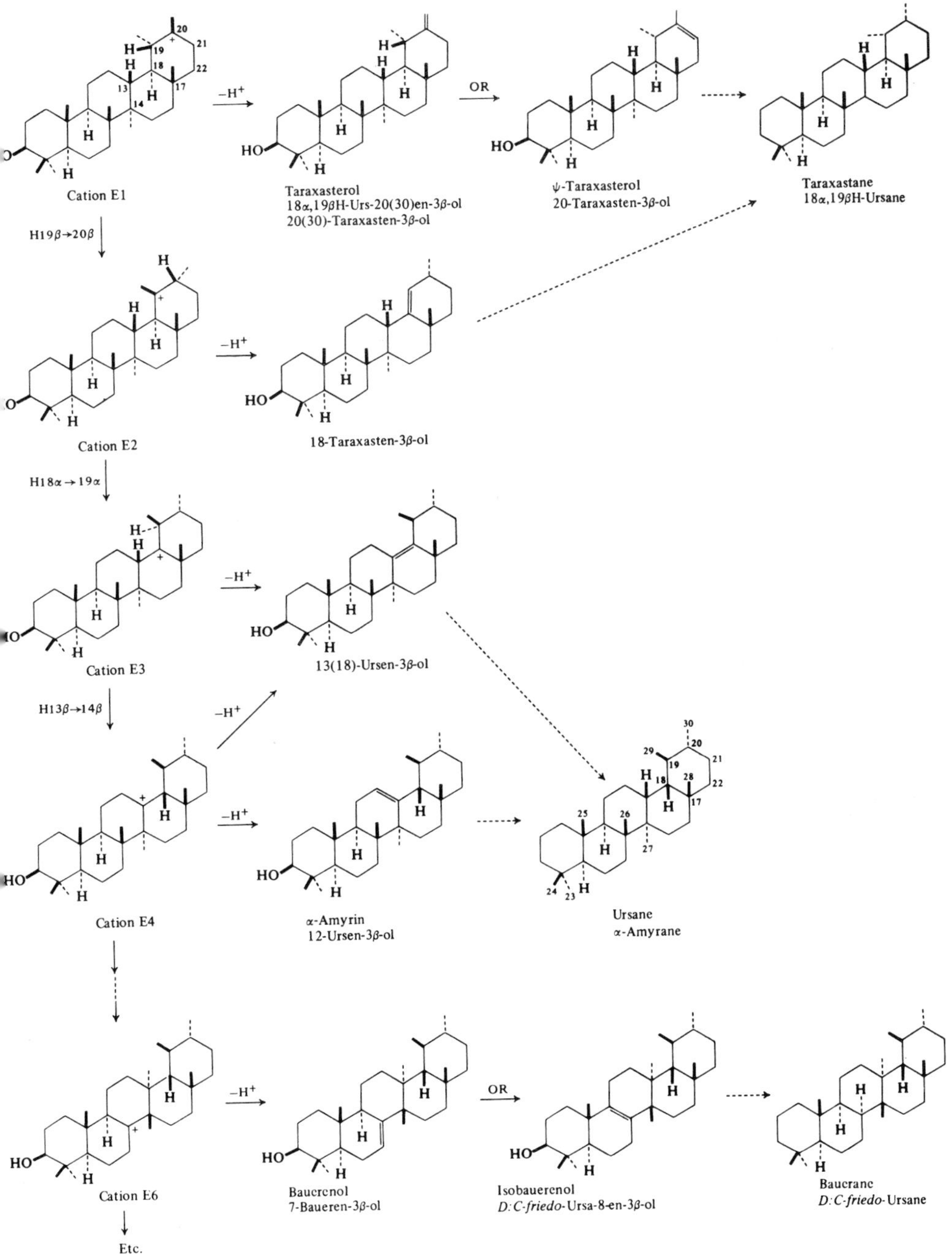

Fig. 18. Biosynthesis of ursane derivatives.

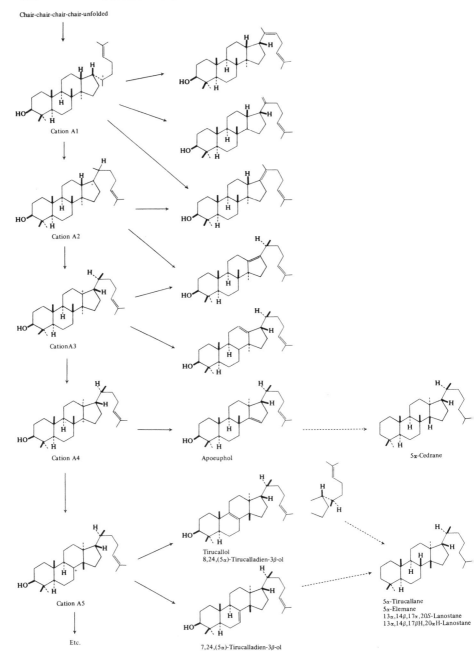

Chair-chair-chair-chair-unfolded

Cation A1

Cation A2

CationA3

Cation A4

Cation A5

Etc.

Apoeuphol

5α-Cedrane

Tirucallol
8,24,(5α)-Tirucalladien-3β-ol

7,24,(5α)-Tirucalladien-3β-ol

5α-Tirucallane
5α-Elemane
13α,14β,17α,20S-Lanostane
13α,14β,17βH,20αH-Lanostane

Fig. 19. Biosynthesis of cedrane and tirucallane derivatives.

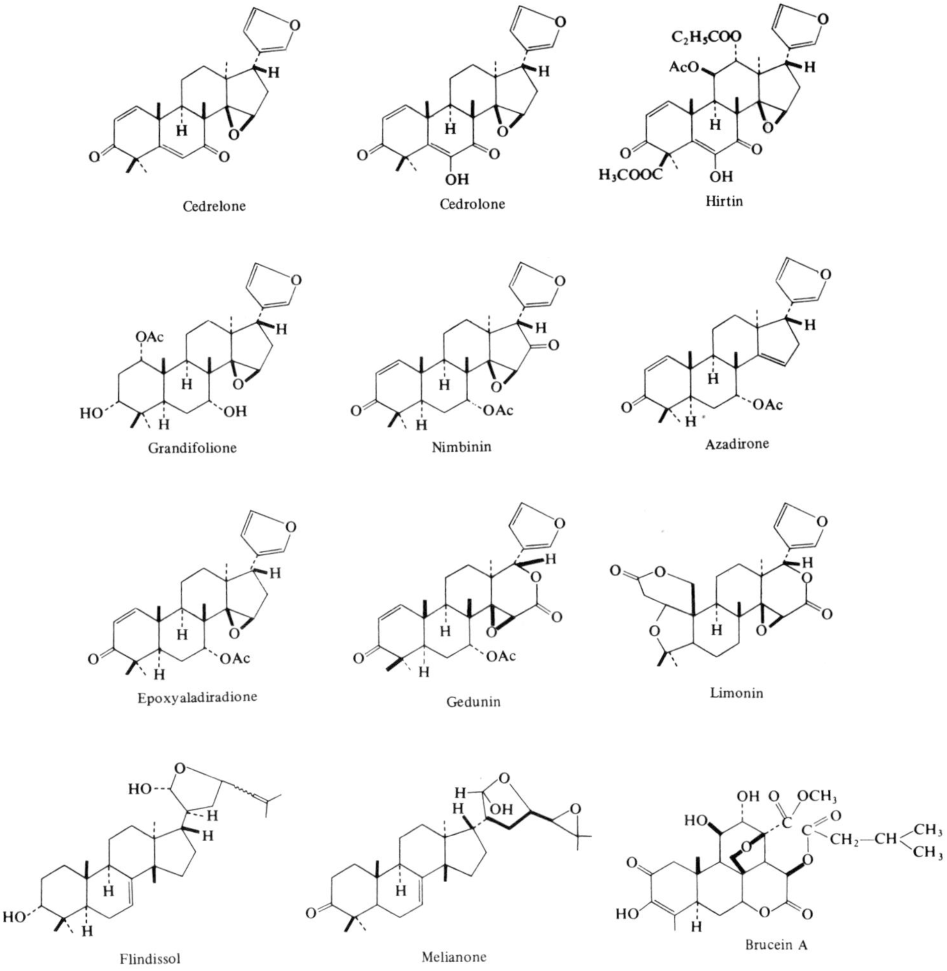

Cedrelone

Cedrolone

Hirtin

Grandifolione

Nimbinin

Azadirone

Epoxyaladiradione

Gedunin

Limonin

Flindissol

Melianone

Brucein A

Fig. 20. Some derivatives of tirucallane and cedrane.

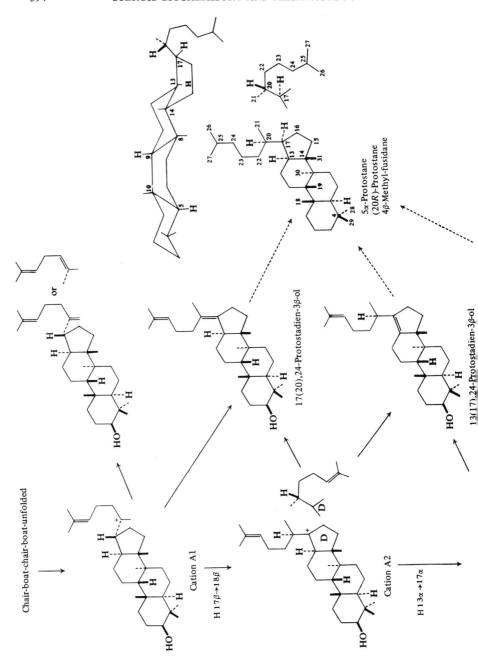

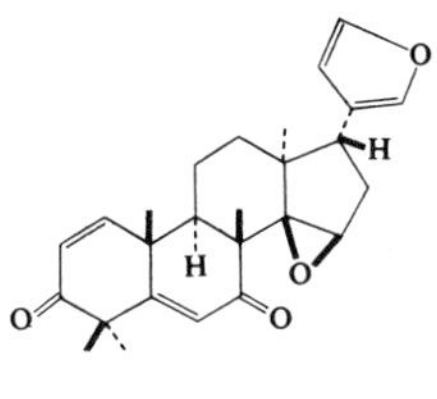

Cedrelone

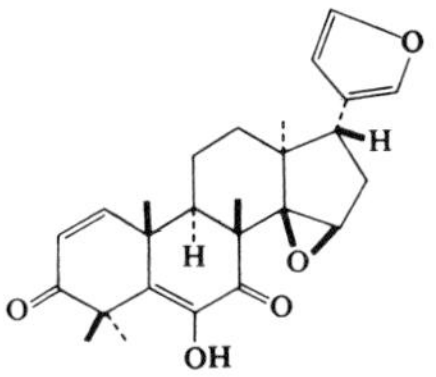

Cedrolone

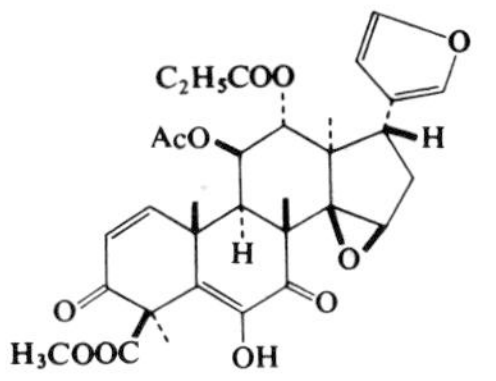

Hirtin

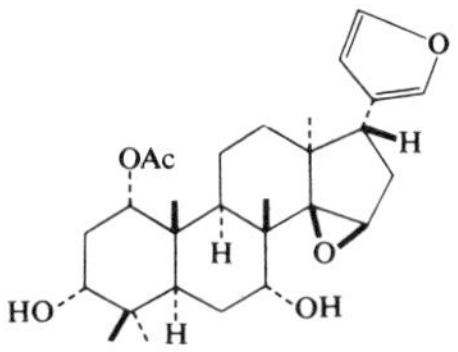

Grandifolione

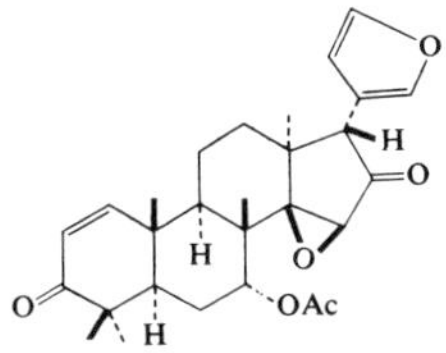

Nimbinin

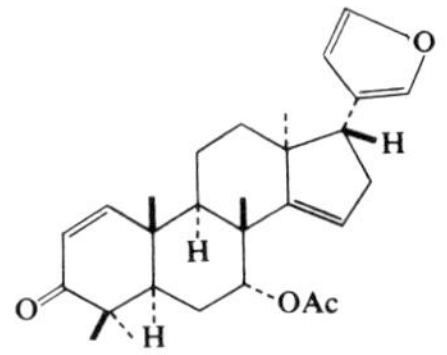

Azadirone

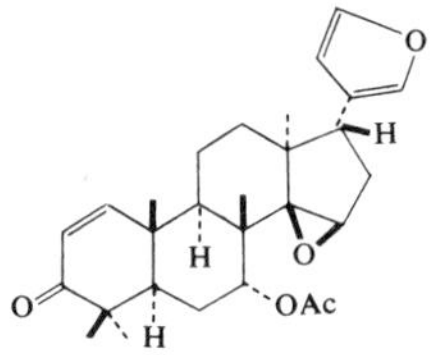

Epoxyaladiradione

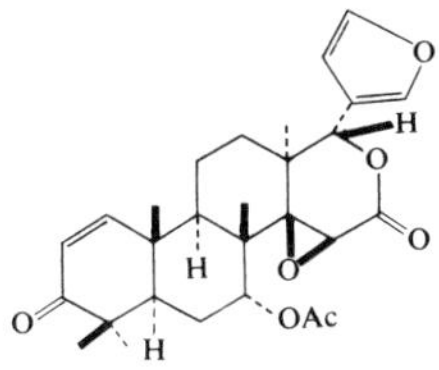

Gedunin

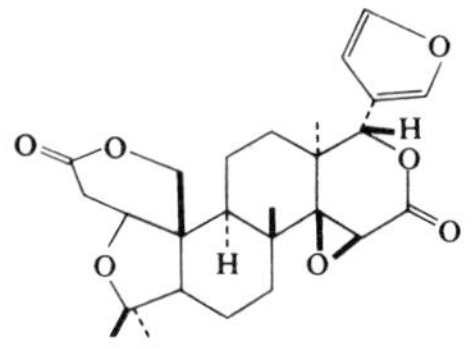

Limonin

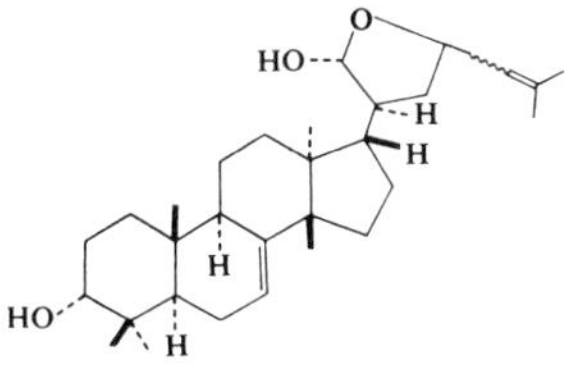

Flindissol

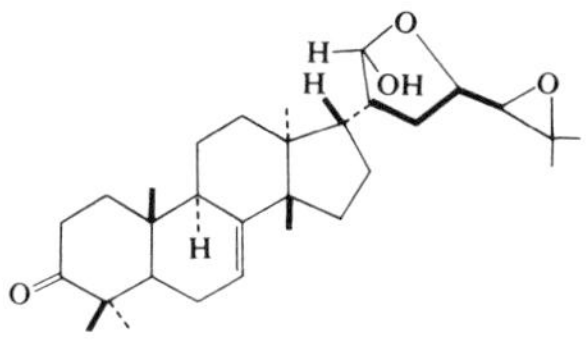

Melianone

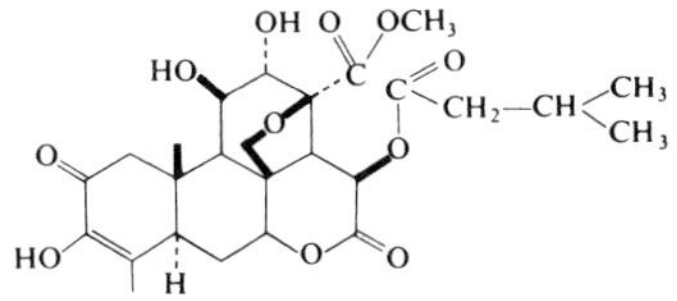

Brucein A

Fig. 20. Some derivatives of tirucallane and cedrane.

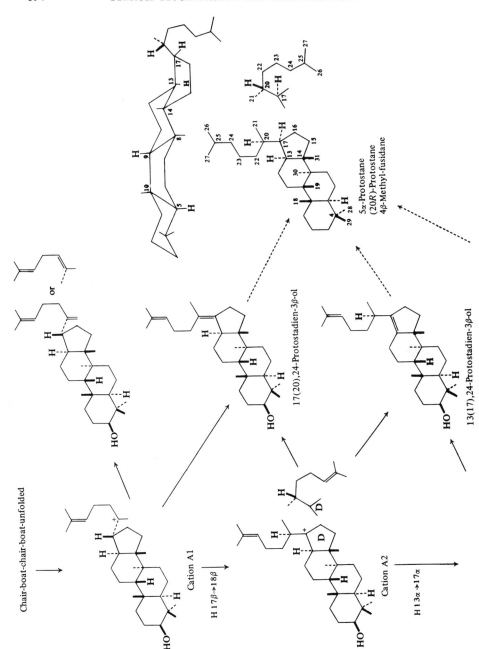

Chair-boat-chair-boat-unfolded

Cation A1

H 17β→18β

Cation A2

H 13α→17α

17(20),24-Protostadien-3β-ol

13(17),24-Protostadien-3β-ol

5α-Protostane
(20R)-Protostane
4β-Methyl-fusidane

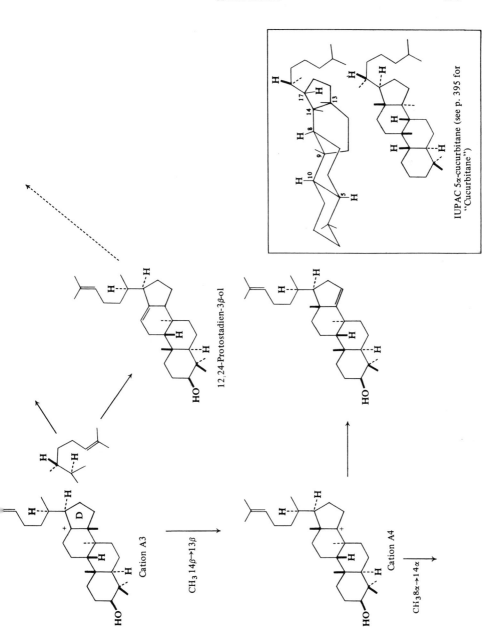

Fig. 21. Biosynthesis of protostane, lanostane, cycloartane and cucurbitane derivatives, I.

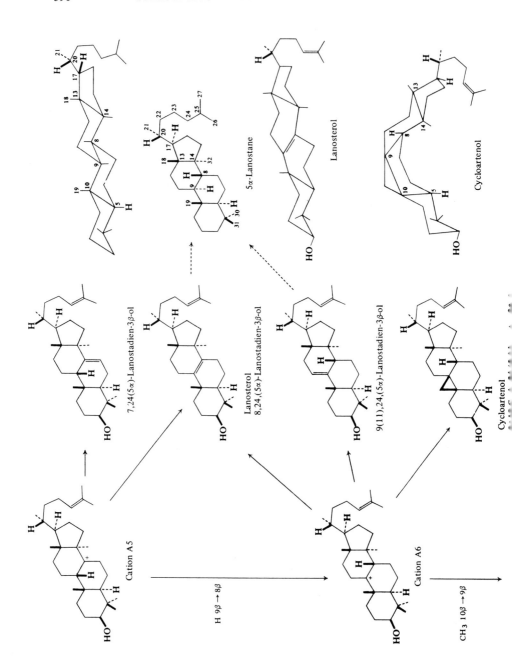

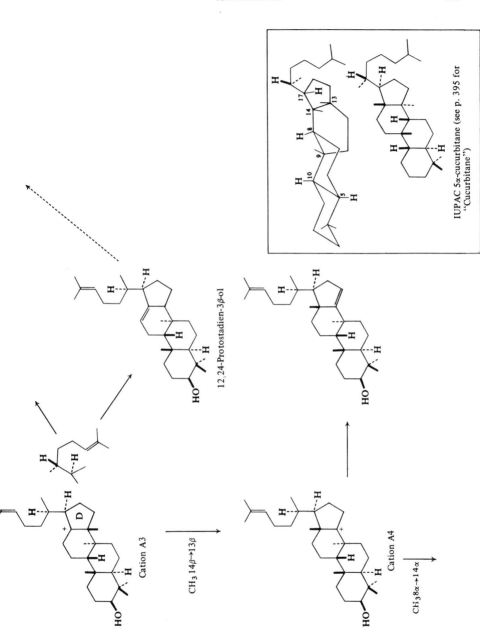

IUPAC 5α-cucurbitane (see p. 395 for "Cucurbitane")

12,24-Protostadien-3β-ol

Cation A3

CH₃ 14β→13β

Cation A4

CH₃ 8α→14α

Fig. 21. Biosynthesis of protostane, lanostane, cycloartane and cucurbitane derivatives, I.

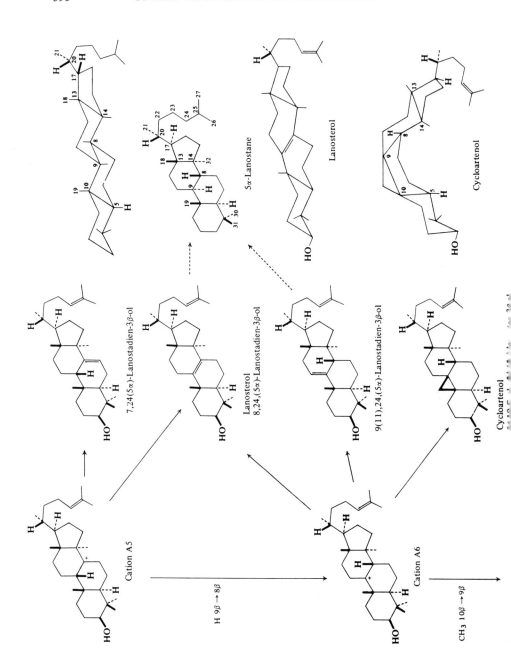

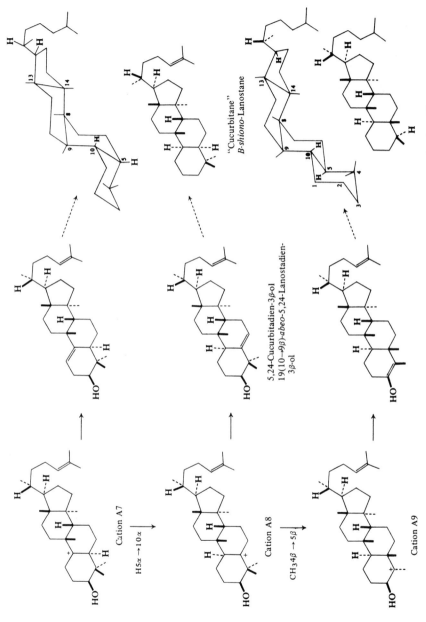

Fig. 21. Biosynthesis of protostane, lanostane, cycloartane and cucurbitane derivatives, II.

(a) Protostane derivatives

These are the fungal antibiotics, i.e. helvolic acid, fusidic acid and cephalo-sporin P1, which have been found in Ascomycetes (Table 15). They are derivatives of the theoretical parent compounds protostane and fusidane (4β-demethyl-protostane) and have a *trans-syn-trans* B-boat configuration.

(b) Lanostane derivatives

All the animal steroids are derived from lanosterol, i.e. corticoids, progesto-gens, androgens, estrogen, bile acids, cholesterol, etc. It is believed that those plant steroids which have a lanosterol type of structure are derived from cycloartenol. The ecdysones are insect moulting hormones which are derived from lanosterol via cholesterol.

(c) Cycloartane derivatives

A wide variety of steroids are found in plants some of which are similar to cycloartenol in structure (Table 16) while others resemble lanosterol. In contrast to the Ascomycetes, Basidomycete fungi produce lanostane rather than proto-stane derivatives. A number of derivatives of 24-methyl-lanostane and 24-methyl-cycloartenol are known. The ring demethylated derivatives have been described previously. The holothurinogenins are a group of compounds found in sea cucumber (family Holothurioideae) which occur as toxic glycosides. They have 7,9-diene structures which are probably the result of the strong acid hydrolysis required to separate them from their glycosides.

(d) Cucurbitane derivatives

The cucurbitacins (Table 17) are a group of bitter compounds occurring in the Cucurbitaceae and are derived from cation A8 which on loss of H^+ gives

Table 17. *Some naturally occurring derivatives of cucurbitane*

Cucurbitacin	A	5,23-Cucurbitadien-2ξ,19,20,25-tetrol-3,11,22-trione 25-acetate
	B	5,23-Cucurbitadien-2ξ,20,25-triol-3,11,22-trione 25-acetate
	D	5,23-Cucurbitadien-2ξ,20,25-triol-3,11,22-trione
	C	5,23-Cucurbitadien-3ξ,19,20,25-tetrol-11,22-dione 25-acetate
	F	5,23-Cucurbitadien-2ξ,3ξ,20,25-tetrol-11,22-dione
	L	1,5-Cucurbitadien-2ξ,20-diol-3,11,22-trione
	E	1,5,23-Cucurbitatrien-2ξ,20,25-triol-3,11,22-trione 25-acetate
	I	1,5,23-Cucurbitatrien-2ξ,20-diol-3,11,22-trione
	J	1,5-Cucubitadien-2ξ,20,24α-triol-3,11,22-trione
	K	1,5-Cucurbitadien-2ξ,20,24-β-triol-3,11,22-trione

5,24-Cucurbitadien-3β-ol. The parent hydrocarbon has 5α- and 10α-hydrogen atoms and may be called cucurbitane. IUPAC has defined 5α-cucurbitane as having a βH atom at C-10, which is different from the cucurbitacins.

6. Chair-chair-chair-chair-(chair or boat)

Figure 22 shows that when ring E cyclizes as a chair, cation C.1b is produced, which yields diplotene, whose parent hydrocarbon is hopane. When ring E cyclizes as a boat, cation C.1a is produced, which yields moretenol, whose parent hydrocarbon is moretane (or 21αH-hopane). As a result of the first proton shift from H at C-21 to H at C-22 both cations produce the same cation C.2. Further shifts produce cations C.3–C.11 and derivatives of fernane, adianane and filicane as shown in Fig. 23. Table 18 shows the precise structure of these hydrocarbons and how they arise from their respective cations. Alternatively, cations C.1a and C.1b can undergo a Wagner-Meerwein rearrangement to give cation D.1 where ring E has six carbon atoms. The parent compound is gammacerane. Cation D.1 can then undergo a series of proton and methyl shifts in the usual way or change to cation E.1 which also does so.

A number of derivatives of the parent hydrocarbons appearing in this series are known, especially from ferns, lichens and other primitive types of plants (Table 19). Optically-active gammacerane has been found in several very ancient shales and its 3β-ol has been found in a primitive ciliated protozoan. This is one of the earliest pieces of evidence for biologically produced compounds on earth.

7. Other

There seems no reason to suppose that other types of folding do not occur, although they are obviously rare. A few compounds are known, whose structure can only be explained on types of squalene folding other than those described above.

Arborane derivatives appear to be derived from chair-boat-chair-chair-boat (or chair) folding (Fig. 24), arborinol being the 3α-hydroxyl derivative of the eighth cation in the C series. Isoarborinol is the 3β-hydroxyl derivative and cyclindrin its methyl ether.

VIII. NOMENCLATURE

The steroid nomenclature used in this book has not been strictly IUPAC. The following systems have been used:

Prefixes are arranged in alphabetical order as in IUPAC, any multiplying parts of simple prefixes being neglected for this purpose, e.g. 6α-Chloro-11β,17α,21-trihydroxy-16β-methyl-1,4-pregnadien-3,20-dione.

According to IUPAC, prefixes are italicized if, and only if, they define either the position of named substituents, e.g. o-, or they define a stereoisomer, e.g. cis

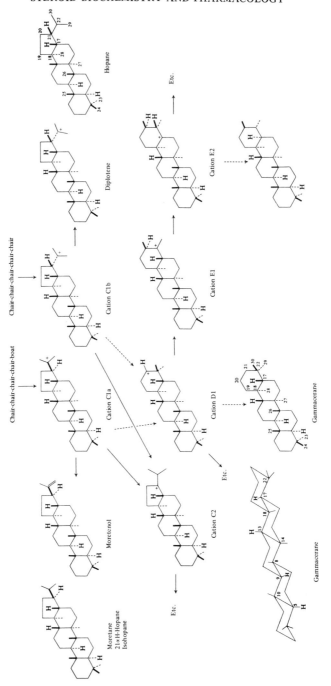

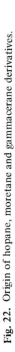

Fig. 22. Origin of hopane, moretane and gammacerane derivatives.

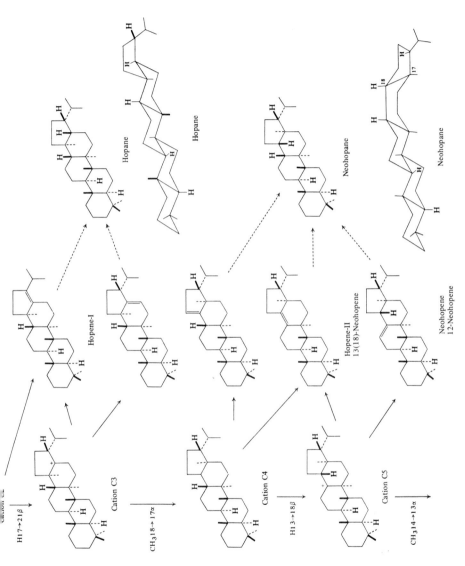

Fig. 23. Biosynthesis of compounds in the hopane series, I.

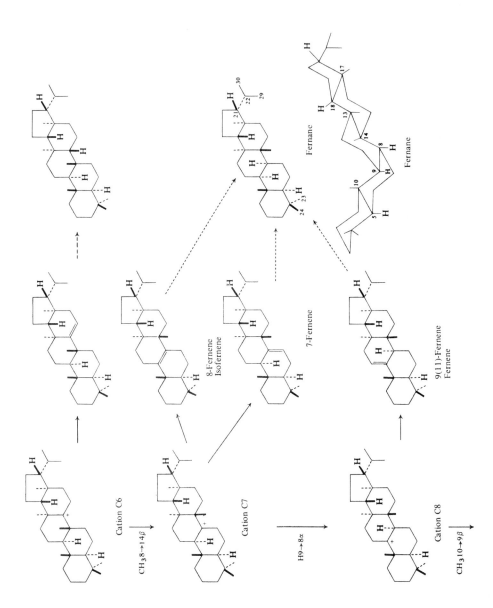

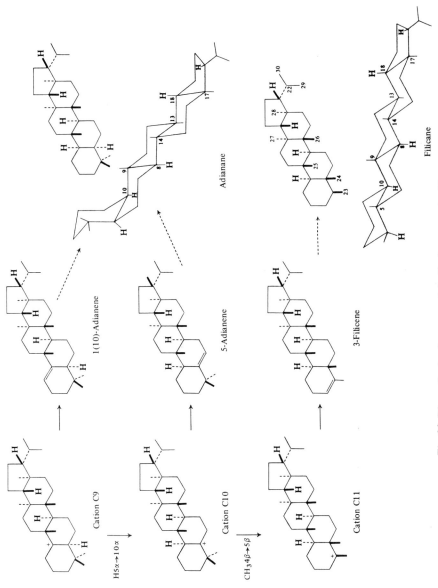

Fig. 23. Biosynthesis of compounds in the hopane series, II.

Table 18. *Nomenclature and configuration of the pentacyclic triterpenes of the hopane series*

Parent hydrocarbon	Hopane†			Neohopane			Fernane		Adianane		Filicane
From cation number	C1a	C2	C3	C4	C5	C6	C7	C8	C9	C10	C11
Double bond at carbon number	22(29)	20	17(21) 16	18	13(18) 12	14	8	7 9(11)	1(10)	5(10) 5	3
Configuration of substituents at carbon atom number											
5	α	α	α	α	α	α	α	α	α	α*	β
10	β	β	β	β	β	β	β	β	α*	α	α
9	α	α	α	α	α	α	α*	β	β	β	β
8	β	β	β	β	β	β*	α*	α*	α	β	α
14 *	α	α	α	β*	β*	α	α	α	α	α	α
13 *	α	α	α	β*	β*	α	α	α	β	β	β
18 *	α	α	α	β*	β*	α	α	α	β	β	β
17 *	β	β	β*	α	α	α	α	α	α	α	α
Configuration between carbon atoms (ring junctions)											
A/B 5/10	trans	trans	trans	trans	trans	trans	trans	trans	cis	cis	trans
A/C 9/10	anti	anti	anti	anti	anti	anti	anti	anti	anti	anti	anti
B/C 8/9	trans	trans	trans	trans	trans	syn	cis	cis	trans	trans	trans
B/D 8/14	anti	anti	anti	anti	anti	trans	anti	anti	anti	anti	anti
C/D 13/14	trans	trans	trans	trans	trans	anti	trans	trans	trans	trans	trans
C/E 13/18	anti	anti	anti	syn	syn	trans	anti	anti	anti	anti	anti
D/E 17/18	trans	trans	trans	trans	trans	trans	trans	trans	trans	trans	trans
Conformation of ring											
A	chair	chair	chair	chair	chair	chair	chair	chair	chair	chair	chair
B	chair	chair	chair	chair	chair	chair	chair	chair	chair	chair	chair
C	chair	chair	chair	chair	chair	boat	chair	chair	chair	chair	chair
D	chair	chair	chair	boat	boat	chair	chair	chair	chair	chair	chair
E	chair	chair	chair	chair	chair	chair	chair	chair	chair	chair	chair

* H Inserted to construct the parent hydrocarbon

† Moretane has the same configuration

Hopane derivatives
Diplotene   22(29)-Hopene
Mollogenol A   Hopan-3β,6α,16β,22-tetrol
Dustanon   Hopan-15α,22-diol
                                       Hopane 17β,21β-epoxide
Leucotylin   Hopan-6α,16β,22-triol
Leucotylic acid   Hopan-6α,16β,22-triol-23-oic acid
Pyxinic acid   Hopan-3β,22-diol-29-oic acid
                                       Hopan-7β,22-diol 7-acetate
Hydroxyhopene-I   17(21)-Hopen-3β-ol
Hydroxyhopene-I acetate   17(21)-Hopen-3β-ol 3-acetate

Neohopane derivatives

                                       13(18)-Neohopene
Neohopene   12-Neohopene
Neomotiol   12-Neohopen-3β-ol

Fernane derivatives

                                       7-Fernene
Fernene   9(11)-Fernene
Isofernene   ⎫
Fernenol   ⎬   9(11)-Fernen-3β-ol
Arundoin   ⎭   9(11)-Fernen-3β-ol methyl ester
                                       7,9(11)-Fernadiene
Fernenediol   9(11)-Fernen-2α,3β-diol
Divallic acid   9(11)-Fernen-24-oic acid
Motiol   7-Fernen-3β-ol
Motidiol   7-Fernen-2ξ,3β-diol

Adianane derivatives

                                       5-Adianene
Simiarenol   5-Adianen-3β-ol
Adianediol   5-Adianen-2ξ,3β-diol
Adiantoxide   Adianan 3α,4α-epoxide

Filicane derivatives
Filicene   3-Filicene
                                       Filicane 3α,4α-epoxide
Filicenal   3-Filicen-23-al
Filicenol A   3-Filicen-6β-ol
Filicenol B   3-Filicen-25-ol

Moretane derivatives
Moretenol   22(29)-Moreten-3β-ol
Moretenone   22(29)-Moreten-3-one
3-Epimoretenol   22(29)-Moreten-3α-ol
Zeorin   Moretan-6α,16β,22-triol

Gammacerane derivatives
Tetrahymenol   Gammaceran-3β-ol
Oxohakonanol   Gammaceran-22β-ol-21-one
γ-Onocerin   12-Gammaceren-3β,21α-diol

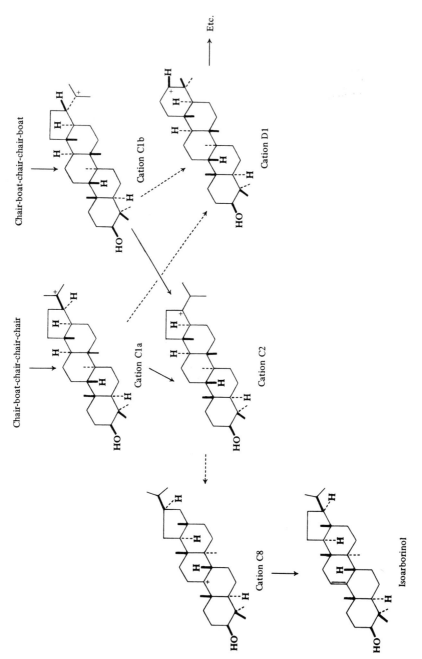

Fig. 24. Arborane derivatives.

but not "iso" in isobutane or "t" in t-butyl. The Biochemical Society prefers *tert.*-butyl. Italicized prefixes are ignored for indexing purposes. For steroids the following systems have been used, and their application explained in the text.

Italics

n-, sec.-, tert.-	e.g. *n*-valerate, *tert.*-Butyl-, *tert.*-butyrate
o-, m-, p-	e.g. *p*-toluene sulphonic acid, *p*-Hydroxyl-
O-, N-, S-	e.g. *O*-Methyl-, *N*-Methyl-, N^4-Acetyl-, *S*-Adenosyl-
R, S	e.g. (24*S*)-24-Methyl-5α-cholestane
E, Z	e.g. *Z*-24(28)-Stigmastene
A, B, C, D, E, A', B'	e.g. *A*-Homo-5α-androstane
friedo-	e.g. *E* : *C-friedo*-Oleanane
neo-	e.g. *A-neo*-Oleanane, *B'* : *A'-neo*-Gammacerane
abeo-	e.g. 19(10-9β) *abeo*-5α-Lanostane
cis, trans, syn, anti	e.g. *cis-trans-anti*-Phenanthrene
ent- = *enantio-*	e.g. *ent*-Testosterone
d- = *dextro-* = (+)-	= dextrorotatory
l- = *laevo-* = (−)-	= laevorotatory
meso = (±)-	= optically inactive
(+)-*rel*- or (−)-*rel*-	= dextrorotatory (or laevorotatory) form of two enantiomers of known relative, but unknown absolute, configuration
rac- = *racemo-* = *dl* = DL	= racemate, i.e. a mixture of the dextrorotatory and laevorotatory forms of two enantiomers, and being optically inactive

Non-italics

cyclo	e.g. 9β,19-Cyclo-24-lanosten-3β-ol
nor, dinor	e.g. 24-Nor-5β-cholane, *A*-Nor-5β-pregnane
homo, dihomo	e.g. *A*-Homo-5α-androstane
seco	e.g. 9,10-Seco-5,7,10(19)-cholestatrien-3β-ol
bisnor	e.g. 22,23-Bisnorcholanic acid
allo	e.g. Allopregnane
epi	e.g. Epiandrosterone
iso	e.g. an isosapogenin, Isoandrosterone
neo	e.g. a neosapogenin
D-, L-	= absolute configuration relative to D-glyceraldehyde

Confusion has arisen over the use of D, L, *d* and *l* for steroids as no official ruling has been made concerning the use of D and L to indicate absolute configuration as has been done by biochemists for amino acids and sugars. In 1955 Reichstein recommended that the absolute configuration related to D-glyceraldehyde of steroids should be related to the configuration at C-10. If C-10 is not asymmetric, as in estrone, the C-13 centre is the point of reference. If neither C-10 nor C-13 is asymmetric, the compound should be named as the phenanthrene derivative. Reichstein used *d* and *l* and many chemists retain these to indicate absolute configuration. Biochemists prefer to use D and L and retain *d* and *l* to indicate the optical rotation. Cholesterol has the D configuration and is laevorotatory.

When suffixes follow a parent hydrocarbon, according to IUPAC the terminal "e" of the hydrocarbon is elided if the first suffix begins with a vowel but not if it begins with a consonant. This is done independently of interruption by a number, e.g.

5α-Cholestane-3β,6α-diol   5α-Cholestan-3β-ol
5α-Androstane-3β,6α-diol   5α-Androstan-3β-ol
5,7,22-Ergostatriene-3β,6β-diol   5,7,22-Ergostatrien-3β-ol
4-Pregnene-3,11,20-trione   4-Pregnen-3-one

This system has not been followed, the terminal "e" being elided in all cases.

BIBLIOGRAPHY

Allard, S. and Ourisson, G. (1957). Remarques sur la nomenclature des triterpènes. *Tetrahedron* **1**, 177-83.

Basu, N. and Rastogi, R. P. (1967). Triterpenoid saponins and sapogenins. *Phytochemistry* **6**, 1249-70.

Berti, G. and Bottari, F. (1968). Constituents of ferns. *In* "Progress in Phytochemistry", Vol. 1, pp. 589-685 (edited by L. Reinold and Y. Liwschitz). John Wiley, New York.

Bethell, D. and Gold, V. (1967). "Carbonium Ions: An Introduction". Academic Press, London and New York.

Borteau, P., Pasich, B. and Ratsimamanga, R. (1964). "Les Triterpenoids en Physiologie Vegetale et Animale". Gauthier-Villars, Paris.

Buckett, W. R., Marjoribanks, C. E. B., Manvick, F. A. and Morton, M. B. (1968). The pharmacology of pancuronium bromide, a new, potent steroidal neuromuscular blocking agent. *Br. J. Pharmac.* **32**, 671.

Chon, T. S., Eisenbraun, E. J. and Rapala, R. T. (1969). The chemistry of steroid acids from *Cephalosporium acremonium*. *Tetrahedron* **25**, 3341-57.

Coffey, S. (ed.) (1969). "Rodds Chemistry of Carbon Compounds", 2nd Edn., Vol. IIc. Elsevier, Amsterdam.

Cooper, A. and Duax, W. L. (1969). Structure and conformation of the cortisone side chain. *J. Pharm. Sci.* **58**, 1159-61.

Dean, P. D. G., Ortiz de Montellano, P. R., Bloch, K. and Corey, E. J. (1967). A soluble 2,3-oxidosqualene sterol cyclase, *J. biol. Chem.* **242**, 3014-15.

Friesen, H. C., Suwa, S. and Pare, P. (1969). Synthesis and secretion of placental lactogen and other proteins by the placenta. *Recent Prog. Horm. Res.* **25**, 161-205.

Goad, L. J. and Goodwin, T. W. (1966). The biosynthesis of sterols in higher plants. *Biochem. J.* **99**, 735-46.

Goldie, D. J., Hasham, N., Keane, P. M. and Walker, W. H. C. (1968). Temperature dependence of cortisol binding to plasma proteins. *Nature, Lond.* **217**, 852-53.

Hattori, T., Igarashi, H., Iwasaki, S. and Okuda, S. (1969). Isolation of 3β-hydroxy-4β-methylfusida-17 (20) [16, 21-*cis*], 24-diene and a related triterpene alcohol. *Tetrahedron Lett.* **13**, 1023-6.

Hills, I. R., Smith, G. W. and Whitehead, E. V. (1968). Optically active spirotriterpane in petroleum distillates. *Nature, Lond.* **219**, 243-46.

Horrobin, D. F. (1969). The female sex cycle. *J. Theoret. Biol.* **22**, 80-88.

IUPAC (1968). Revised tentative rules for nomenclature of steroids. *Biochim. biophys. Acta* **164**, 453-86.

Keane, P. M., Pearson, J. and Walker, W. H. C. (1969). Binding characteristics of transcortin in human plasma in normal individuals, pregnancy and liver disease. *Endocrinology* **43**, 517-79.

Kennedy. J. F. and Butt, W. R. (1969). Periodate oxidation studies of human pituitary-stimulating hormone. *Biochem. J.* **115**, 225-229.

Kitagawa, I. (1967). Chemistry of triterpenoids. *Jap. J. Pharm. Chem.* **38**, 343-80.

Klyne, W. (1965). "The Chemistry of the Steroids". Methuen, London.

Lavie, D. and Levy, E. C. (1969). A compound linking melianes with meliacins. *Tetrahedron Lett.* **40**, 3525-28.

Li, C. H., Dixon, J. S., Lui, W. K. (1969). Human pituitary growth hormone. *Archs Biochem. Biophys.* **133**, 70-91.

Li, C. H., Dixon, J. S., Lo, T. B., Pankov, Y. A. and Schmidt, K. D. (1969). Amino acid sequence of ovine lactogenic hormone. *Nature, Lond.* **224**, 695-96.

McKerns, K. W. (ed.) (1968). "Functions of the Adrenal Cortex". North Holland Publishing Co., Amsterdam.

Moss, G. P. and Nicolaidis, S. A. (1969). Terpenoid biosynthesis: the stereochemistry of squalene cyclization. *J. chem. Soc.* **18**, 1072-73.

Murphy, B. E. P. (1969). Protein binding and the assay of non-antigenic hormones. *Recent Prog. Horm. Res.* **25**, 563-610.

Ourisson, G., Crabbé, P. and Rodig, D. R. (1964). "Tetracyclic Triterpenes". Herman, Paris.

Ponsinet, G., Ourisson, G. and Oehlschlager, A. C. (1968). Systematic aspects of the distribution of di- and triterpenes. *In* "Recent Advances in Phytochemistry", Vol. 1, pp. 271-302. North Holland Publishing Co., Amsterdam.

Richards, J. H. and Hendrickson, J. B. (1964). "The Biosynthesis of Steroids, Terpenes and Acetogenins". W. A. Benjamin Inc., New York.

Roller, P., Djerassi, C., Cloetens, R. and Tursch, B. (1969). The isolation of three new holothurinogenins and their chemical correlation with lanosterol. *J. Am. chem. Soc.* **91**, 4918-20.

Rosenfield, R. L., Eberlein, W. R. and Bongiovanni, A. M. (1969). Measurement of plasma testosterone by means of competitive protein binding analysis. *J. clin. Endocr. Metab.* **29**, 854-59.

Rosenthal, H. E., Slaunwhite, W. R. and Sandberg, A. A. (1969). Transcortin: a corticosteroid-binding protein of plasma X. Cortisol and progesterone interplay and unbound levels of these steroids in pregnancy. *J. clin. Endocr. Metab.* **29**, 352-67.

Rosner, W. and Deakins, M. (1968). Testosterone binding globulins in human plasma: studies on sex distribution and specificity. *J. clin. Invest.* **47**, 2109-16.

Ruzicka, L. (1959). A history of the isoprene rule. *Proc. chem. Soc.* 341-60.

Sengupta, K. and Mukhopadhyay, J. (1966). Terpenoids and related compounds, VII, Triterpenoids of *Phyllanthus acidus* skeels. *Phytochemistry* **5**, 531-34.

Shahenfeldt, G. H., Holt, J. A. and Ewing, L. L. (1969). Peripheral plasma levels during the ovine estrous cycle. *Endocrinology* **85**, 11-15.

Tsuda, Y., Hatanaka, M. and Fujimoto, T. (1969). Triterpenoids of *Lycopodium clavatum*: the structure of 21-episerratriol. *J. chem. Soc.* **18**, 1040-43.

Vermeulen, A. and Verdonck, L. (1968). Studies on the binding of testosterone to human plasma. *Steroids* **11**, 609-35.

Westphal, U. (1961). Interactions between steroids and proteins. *In* "Mechanisms of Action of Steroid Hormones", pp. 33-89 (edited by C. A. Villee and L. L. Engel). Pergamon Press, Oxford.

INDEX

411

Etianic acids, 10
Euphane derivatives, 273, 276, 377
Expectorants, steroidal, 274, 286
Exudate, inflammatory, 147

F

Faeces,
    bile acids in, 83
    progestogens in, 231
Fallopian tubes, 96
Feedback mechanisms, 24, 25, 203-6, 350
Fertile Eunuch syndrome, 254
Fever, steroidal, 262
Fernane derivatives, 399
Fibrin, 147, 214
Fibroblasts, 50, 159
Fibroids, 258
Filicane derivatives, 399
Finkelstein-Forschielli-Dorfman method, 244
Fluocinolone, 164
Fluorescence, of steroids, 199, 225, 230
Fluorinated steroids, 165, 326
Foetal-placental unit, 236
Follicle stimulating hormone (FSH) (*see also* Gonadotrophins)
    activity of HCG, 47
    biological assay of, 219
    effects of oral contraceptives on, 114
    effects on ovaries, 45
    effects on testes, 124
    for induction of ovulation, 224
    immunoassay of, 220
    in blood and urine, 220
    in control of estrous cycle, 99
    in Klinefelter's syndrome, 251
    secretion of 30, 33, 44
    structure of, 33, 351
Friedelane derivatives, 380
Friedman test, 222
Frohlich's syndrome, 252
Fungi, steroids of, 266
Furostane derivatives, 288-9
Fusidane derivatives, 294, 398

G

Galactorrhea, 254
Gall stones, 187

Gammacerane derivatives, 399
Gas-liquid-chromatography (GLC),
    of androgens in blood, 245
    of estrogens in urine, 226
    of progestogens in blood and urine, 234
Genes, 87, 247
Genins, steroidal, 276-94
Germanicane derivatives, 380
Giant cells, 150
Giantism, 253
Girard reagent, 226, 302
Glinski's syndrome, 253
Globulin permeability factor, 156
Globulins, 35, 151, 197, 362
Glucocorticoids (*see also* Corticoids)
    biological assay, 145, 157
    effects on inflammatory and immune responses, 135
    effects on lysosomal and mitochondrial membranes, 176
    effects on target organs, 139, 144
    effects on wound healing, 161
    secretion, 37
Glucuronic acid, 75
Glucuronides, 75, 80-1, 176
Glutinane derivatives, 380
Glycine, conjugates with bile acids, 83
Glycogen deposition, 122, 145
Glycyrrhetic acid, 247
Goldzieher-Nakamura method, 233
Gonads (*see also* Testis, Ovary)
    abnormal functioning of, 247
    agenesis (dysgenesis) of, 248
    structure of, 40-6
    tests of function, 260
Gonadotrophins [*see also* Follicle Stimulating Hormone (FSH), Luteinising Hormone (LH), Interstitial Cell Stimulating Hormone (ICSH)]
    effects on growth, 122
    feedback mechanisms of, 350
    for induction of ovulation, 224
    human chorionic (HCG), 47, 219, 236
    human menopausal (HMG), 219
    human pituitary (HPG), 219
    pregnant mare's serum (PMSG), 219
    secretion of, 30, 31